'Professor Vivian Nutton's *Renaissance Medicine* is an astonishing achievement. Deeply and widely read in primary sources as well as in the wealth of secondary literature that has been generated in the field of medical history over the years, Nutton surveys the entire world of sixteenth-century European medicine. His book is also a global history, tracking the impact of new drugs and diseases on European medicine and populations, stemming from both East and West – the Indies and the Americas – in the late renaissance.'

—Jonathan Sawday, *Saint Louis University*, USA

'Vivian Nutton has written a magisterial survey of the lively world of Renaissance medicine. Drawing on sources from all over Europe (and with a particular focus on the large German-speaking territories), he looks at the major debates and developments – among them the crucial role of Galenism as well as the new horizons and challenges, from the recovery of ancient medical theories and the rise of neoplatonic ideas to the encounter with new diseases and exotic drugs and the laborious work at the dissection table. A must-read for anyone interested in this formative period in the history of Western medicine.'

—Michael Stolberg, *University of Würzburg*, Germany

Renaissance Medicine

This volume offers a comprehensive historical survey of medicine in sixteenth-century Europe and examines both medical theories and practices within their intellectual and social context.

Nutton investigates the changes brought about in medicine by the opening-up of the European world to new drugs and new diseases, such as syphilis and the Sweat, and by the development of printing and more efficient means of communication. Chapters examine how civic institutions such as Health Boards, hospitals, town doctors and healers became more significant in the fight against epidemic disease, and special attention is given to the role of women and domestic medicine. The final section, on beliefs, explores the revised Galenism of academic medicine, including a new emphasis on anatomy and its most vocal antagonists, Paracelsians. The volume concludes by considering the effect of religious changes on medicine, including the marginalisation, and often expulsion, of non-Christian practitioners.

Based on a wide reading of primary sources from literature and art across Europe, *Renaissance Medicine* is an invaluable resource for students and scholars of the history of medicine and disease in the sixteenth century.

Vivian Nutton FBA is emeritus professor of the History of Medicine at UCL. He has written widely on pre-modern medicine. His many books include *Galen, a Thinking Doctor in Imperial Rome*, Routledge, 2020. He is at present revising his *Ancient Medicine* (2nd edition, Routledge, 2013).

Renaissance Medicine

A Short History of European Medicine
in the Sixteenth Century

Vivian Nutton

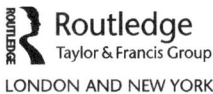

Routledge
Taylor & Francis Group

LONDON AND NEW YORK

Cover image: Triumph of Jacobus Castricus, woodcut by Hans Holbein the Younger, circa 1530 © INTERFOTO/Alamy Stock Photo

First published 2022
by Routledge
4 Park Square, Milton Park, Abingdon, Oxon OX14 4RN

and by Routledge
605 Third Avenue, New York, NY 10158

Routledge is an imprint of the Taylor & Francis Group, an informa business

British Library Cataloguing-in-Publication Data
A catalogue record for this book is available from the British Library

Library of Congress Cataloging-in-Publication Data
Names: Nutton, Vivian, author.
Title: Renaissance medicine : a short history of European medicine in the sixteenth century / Vivian Nutton.
Description: Milton Park, Abingdon, Oxon ; New York, NY : Routledge, 2022. | Includes bibliographical references and index.
Identifiers: LCCN 2021048118 (print) | LCCN 2021048119 (ebook)
Subjects: LCSH: Medicine—History—16th century. | Renaissance.
Classification: LCC R128.6 .N88 2022 (print) | LCC R128.6 (ebook)
    DDC 610.94—dc23/eng/20211124
LC record available at https://lccn.loc.gov/2021048118
LC ebook record available at https://lccn.loc.gov/2021048119

ISBN: 978-1-032-12124-6 (hbk)
ISBN: 978-1-032-12123-9 (pbk)
ISBN: 978-1-003-22318-4 (ebk)

DOI: 10.4324/9781003223184

Typeset in Sabon
by Apex CoVantage, LLC

Contents

Figures

Unless otherwise stated, all images are taken from Wellcome Collections, under the rubric of CC-BY=40 or Public Domain Mark.

Maps

Acknowledgements

This book is the fruit of many years of travel and research in libraries and archives across Europe, aided by the labours of all those who have catalogued and published the sources on which historians rely. Modern methods of communication have allowed Renaissance books and manuscripts to be available at one's desk at the touch of a button, an amazing privilege with only one drawback – the reduction in opportunities to meet the librarians themselves and learn from them of treasures still uncatalogued or accessible only to those who have made the journey to their institutions. The list of those I have visited is far too long to name individually, and my thanks to them and their staffs must be generic. Special mention, however, must be made of institutions which have played a role in my development as a scholar or with which I have been associated for many years. The Archivio di Stato at Mantua provided me with the documentation for one of my first papers on the Renaissance, and its staff guided my faltering decipherment of Italian handwriting. In the Universitätsbibliothek in Basle Prof. Martin Steinmann introduced me to the riches of its Renaissance letter collections, as well as to some manuscript mysteries. I was a guest on several occasions of the Herzog August Bibliothek at Wolfenbüttel with its unrivalled collection of Renaissance books on medicine and science, many of them from the long-departed university of Helmstedt. I retain fond memories also of the Ratschulbibliothek in Zwickau and the Stiftsbibliothek in Zerbst, which gave me a lasting insight into the spread and usage of less familiar medical publications in sixteenth-century Germany. For many years the libraries of the Warburg Institute, The Classical Institute, London, the British Library and the Cambridge University Library have been, and continue to be, remarkable resources for any researcher in the medical history of Europe, whether at a global, European or local level. The Wellcome Library, to which I owe so much, would have been on that list, were it not for the decision of its management to change its focus and concentrate on the public understanding of medicine. Its priorities appear now to be confined largely to the local and the anglophone. In a pleasing contrast, I have for many years been involved with the Biblioteca Communale at Fermo in Italy, which houses a major collection of works on ancient medicine and science from before

1720, many associated with Queen Christina of Sweden and her personal physician, Romolo Spezioli. I have been welcomed there by Maria Carla Leonori, its librarian, and by the officials of the Studio Fermano per la storia della medicina, especially Alfredo Serrani and Fabiola Zurlini. The meetings of the Studio gave me the opportunity not only to revisit the library, now open again after suffering earthquake damage, but also through discussions with other members of the Studio to learn about Renaissance Italy from an unfamiliar perspective, a distant province of the Papal States that maintained close links with the intellectual and medical life of Rome.

The writing of this book began shortly before the Covid virus disrupted academic life, not least by preventing access to major libraries and forcing me to rely on my own personal library and 50 years of notes and xeroxes, as well as on the material accessible online. This has had both positive and negative consequences. Online access to the most recent articles in even the most familiar journals has been scanty, that to those less familiar and non-anglophone often impossible, while coverage of secondary printed books has been a matter of chance, and I have often been forced to cite some of my own publications of decades ago. This may explain some of the obvious gaps in my citation of relatively recent literature; others are the result of my own ignorance, for which I apologise. But against these lacunae must be balanced the opportunity to read (or reread) large numbers of original documents from the sixteenth century, many of them unfamiliar to specialists even when available online. My earlier work in Germany also imparted a bias towards the German-speaking areas of the sixteenth century that, together with Michael Stolberg's recent book, will, I hope, direct readers' attention away from a traditional concentration on what was taking place in Northern Italy. Medicine in the sixteenth century was, as now, an international enterprise, and one of the aims of this survey has been to include examples from across the European republic of letters, a term that came into use in this period. I am aware that many gaps still remain, particularly in French material, not all of them the result of a deliberate policy of selection or of a wish to avoid duplicating unduly some of the excellent work on the social history of medicine over the last 20 years. I am especially grateful to Hannah Marcus, Bruce Moran, Caroline Petit and Michael Stolberg for generously sending me copies of their recent books, as well as to many other friends who have sent me offprints and articles. Dr Antoine Haaker of the Wrocław University Library very kindly sent me digitised images of the Crato correspondence there, and Frau Manuela Rösch supplied me with a splendid photograph of the plague memorial at Großrückerswalde in Saxony.

I have been fortunate over the years to have been able to teach or to attend meetings around Europe and beyond, enlarging my understanding of even familiar figures through conversations with specialists in their local histories and traditions. I have spent time in such major centres of Renaissance medicine as Bologna, Florence, Leipzig, Padua, Pisa, Siena and Wittenberg as well as Paris and Rome, and I have been invited to Alkmaar, Forlì, Strasbourg, Vagli Superiore and Verona to celebrate natives of the town who became famous around Europe in the Renaissance. My work on Vesalius has allowed me to address conferences in many places in Europe, America and, thanks to the Belgian government, Denmark and Kazakhstan, and, not least, to develop many friendships with Belgian Vesalians, especially Maurits Biesbrouck, Theo Godderis, Omar Steeno, Francis Van Glabbeek and Bob Van Hee.

I owe a great deal over the years to discussions with Alessandro Arcangeli, Jon Arrizabalaga, Elena Berger, Fabrizio Bigotti, Ron Blumenfeld, Ann Carmichael, Giancarlo Cerasoli, Sam Cohn, Andrew Cunningham, Theo Dirix, Paula Findlen, Marie-Madeleine Fontaine, Stefania Fortuna, Anthony Grafton, Clare Griffin, Hiro Hirai, Teresa Huguet-Termes, Annemarie Kinzelbach, Tom Kaufmann, Lauren Kassell, Cynthia Klestinec, Monique Kornell, Sachiko Kusukawa, Chris Lawrence, David Lines, Ian Maclean, Hannah Marcus, Dan Margócsy, Outi Merisalo, Bruce Moran, Marjorie O'Rourke Boyle, Alessandro Pastore, Richard Palmer, Antoine Pietrobelli, Caroline Petit, Stuart Rose, David Soulier, Roger Smith, Nancy Siraisi, Claudia Stein, Jane Stevens Crawshaw, Michael Stolberg, Laurence Totelin, Alain Touwaide, Maria Tutorskaya, Alice Tyrell, Soren Urbansky, Ilona Ventura, Gerry Vogringic, Jacqueline Vons, Tilmann Walter, Andrew Wear, Charles Webster, Barbara Zipser and Fabiola Zurlini. My editor at Routledge, Laura Pilsworth, has been consistently helpful as always. Among those no longer with us, I owe a great debt to 30 years of friendship with the late Luis García Ballester, whose work on the Moriscos, discussed in Chapter 11, first opened my eyes to the significance of religion in the medicine of this period. Several of these friends read individual chapters, and some the whole book, and offered me a range of criticism and suggestions. They are not to be held responsible for any of the mistakes and omissions to be found here.

My wife, as always, read through various drafts with a critical eye. It was she who accidentally occasioned my first paper on the medical Renaissance, the result of comments made during a conference on Montaigne that I attended as her guest, and she has continued to improve my knowledge of matters French ever since.

For five years I had the privilege of teaching students at the I. M. Sechenov First Moscow State Medical University. I am grateful to them for their insights into the history of medicine, as well as their eagerness to debate wider medical themes with me. My work there was made possible first by Dmitri Balalykin and Natalya Shok, and then by Evgeniya Panova and Borislav Lichterman. I also discussed many aspects of this book there with Elena Berger, Yulia Kuzmina, Tatiana Sorokina and Maria Tutorskaya, and presented some of its ideas in lectures at the New Economic Research University, Moscow; the Russian Peoples Friendship University, Moscow; the University of Kazan and, during the lockdown of 2020, at a Zoom seminar organised by staff of the Moscow Museum of the History of Medicine.

My experiences there strengthened my belief in the universality of scholarly endeavour, even if critical thought is not always encouraged by those in power, as well as opening my eyes to a Russian perspective on their European Renaissance heritage. This book is dedicated to my Russian colleagues with thanks for their manifold assistance to an ever-inquisitive friend.

Introduction

The main square of the North Italian town of Forlì is dominated by the mighty bell tower of the abbey of San Mercuriale, built in 1180 after a disastrous fire had destroyed a much earlier building. Like many other Italian churches, it houses some fine works of art, especially in a chapel at the east end that was completed in 1606. Save for one epitaph (of a son of the donor who died young in 1597 while a student in Spain), there is nothing to tell today's visitor who had paid for this chapel, erected "with wonderful sumptuousness", and the paintings and frescos within it.[1] But for Italians at the time there was no need to spell this out, for the magnificent painting above the altar shows the Madonna between the two saints to whom the chapel was dedicated, on the left S. Girolamo, the scholar saint of the fourth century, and on the right, S. Mercuriale, a bishop and patron of Forlì. Together they reveal the name of the wealthy benefactor, Girolamo Mercuriale (1530–1606), physician, scholar and native of the town. Contemporaries could also recognise him in one of the large paintings that flank the altar in the guise of the elder of the two deacons assisting S. Mercuriale on his return from Jerusalem: his surviving son, Massimiliano, is also likely to have been the model for the other.[2] During his long career, Girolamo Mercuriale acted as doctor and confidant to the influential Cardinal Alessandro Farnese, and was called in to help treat a Pope, Gregory XIV, as well as holding prestigious chairs in Padua, Bologna and Pisa at a time when these universities had an international reputation for medicine. He wrote many large tomes on subjects as varied as poisons, cosmetics, paediatrics and plague, and he was in overall charge of major editions of the works of the two most influential doctors of Antiquity, Hippocrates and Galen. His most famous work, *De arte gymnastica*, *On the Art of Physical Exercise*, was for centuries the standard account of the importance of physical exercise in medicine and was lavishly illustrated with drawings by Pirro Ligorio, a leading artist of the day.[3] Mercuriale was a friend of leading antiquarians, and corresponded with distinguished medical colleagues around Europe, regardless of their religious affiliations. His *palazzo* at Forlì, furnished on a royal scale, housed an extensive library as well as a collection of paintings second to none in the Romagna, evidence of the great wealth that he had

DOI: 10.4324/9781003223184-1

amassed from his medical practice and of the respect in which he was held by scholars across Europe.[4]

While many aspects of his career can be paralleled from those of doctors of 200 years earlier, others mark a major difference from what had gone before and justify talking of him as a typical example of a Renaissance physician of the sixteenth century. In its appeals to the Greek and Roman Classics his medicine can be rightly termed 'Renaissance', as he shared with almost all of the leading practitioners the belief that by turning directly to their ancient past they were removing erroneous and potentially dangerous medieval interpretations of the medical doctrines that had originated then.[5] But there is a major difference in the recovery of ancient medicine from that of literature or art, where the initial impetus came from Latin in the fourteenth century and the contribution of the Greeks became significant from the 1440s. As we shall see, it was only from the 1490s, and arguably not until the late 1520s, that the two major ancient authors on medicine, Galen and Hippocrates, became available in the Greek original and in a form that could be widely accessed.[6] Recourse to the original Greek not only revealed errors and confusions in the standard medieval Latin translations but also provided remarkable 'new' information on medical botany and anatomy. Until at least the 1560s, learned physicians like Mercuriale could easily assimilate any novelties as supplements to what had earlier been written by the Greeks, which in turn served only to confirm the validity of their presuppositions. Something that had survived for so long and had centuries of apparently successful cures to its credit could not be dismissed as worthless. Similarly, contemporary literary authors who described disease, sickness and death frequently relied on ancient precedents: Thucydides the Greek historian, the Latin poets Lucretius and Vergil, and the Bible, as well as medical texts, to organise or adorn their narratives.[7] Knowledge of Greek, which until the 1530s had been confined to a tiny number of elite physicians, also became more widespread as more schools and colleges taught it to an increasing number of students, and the availability of new and more accurate Latin translations, as well as modern treatises written in elegant humanist Latin, helped to distinguish further the learned Renaissance physician from his humbler and often non-Latinate rivals in the healing arts. In a period when style mattered as an index of one's social worth, the physician could easily demonstrate his qualifications to be regarded as a member of the cultural elite.

This emphasis on the recovery of a classical heritage provides one justification for using the term 'Renaissance medicine', and for seeing it as a part of a movement that in art, literature and architecture can be traced back to Italy, and to Northern and Central Italy in particular, in the middle and late fourteenth century. Nancy Siraisi also drew attention to the impact on medicine of the contemporary development of new civic institutions in the same region.[8] Elsewhere in Europe the transition from the medieval was much slower, sometimes scarcely begun even a century and a half later. Major urban centres, particularly commercial cities or those closely linked with royal courts, were relatively quick to adopt many of the institutions of the Italian city states and embrace the cultural priorities of rulers such as the Medici. Regions on the fringes of Western Europe, however, or whose contacts with the Mediterranean world had been disrupted by conflicts such as the Hundred Years War between England and France lagged considerably behind. Thomas DaCosta Kaufmann in his wide-ranging study of art and culture in Central Europe has extended this argument yet further, stressing the different speed and reactions to Italian art in the late fifteenth and sixteenth centuries in different localities from the Rhine and even as far as Russia.[9] A similar pattern can be discerned in medicine where, until the 1550s and arguably until the end of the century, it was Italy that led the way, even if developments in France and Germany often modified, and sometimes challenged, ideas emanating from there.

As Nancy Siraisi explained in ending her excellent survey of medieval and Early Renaissance medicine around 1500, medicine, and science in general, remained medieval in outlook well down into the fifteenth century, if not the sixteenth.[10] Indeed, a student who had learned his medicine at Bologna, Paris, Oxford or Prague in 1350 would still have followed the same curriculum and attended similar lectures 150 years later, confident that he was being instructed in an ancient medical tradition that had stood the test of time. As late as 1524, Wolfgang Reichart, a graduate of Padua, was advising his student son that all he needed for his studies there was a copy of the so-called *Articella*, a short collection of Latin translations of Byzantine and Classical Greek texts, including Galen's *Art of Medicine*, that had been first assembled in Salerno at least three centuries earlier.[11] Modern medicine, he argued, was merely an extension of these fundamental (and largely Galenic) principles.

His successor 100 years later would still have acknowledged the strength of that classical tradition, but it was now both defined and interpreted differently. Not only was there an abundance of new material available directly from the Greek, but the drugs that had been described originally in Arabic pharmacopoeias were now challenged by alternative therapies and supplemented by new data gained from voyages across the Atlantic and, via Africa, to the Far East. Medical institutions had also developed considerably in size, influence and number during the sixteenth century. By 1600 universities, medical colleges and public health regulations were common across Western Europe, even in its furthest regions such as Scotland or Poland, although England, typically, followed a more idiosyncratic course. Anatomy, medical botany and, in the last decades of the century, chemical medicine occupied a larger place within medicine than ever before. Medical ideas were also spread more quickly thanks to a more efficient postal service, and among newly literate groups through the medium of print and, increasingly, in their own vernacular languages that were beginning to supplement, although not yet replace, Latin as a scientific language. Whether collections of prayers for use against pestilence or massive tomes of academic learning, their appearance in print allowed the wider and more rapid circulation of new ideas as well as initially granting even greater authority to the works of earlier writers.

But all was not well in society. True, warfare, except on the fringes of Europe, was not as ubiquitous as it had been, or as devastating as it was to become in the first half of the next century, but the steady population rise across Europe that characterised the late fifteenth century began to slow from the middle of the sixteenth, when the advent of the Little Ice Age from around 1540 reduced harvests and exposed many to a greater threat of famine and disease as more mouths were now required to be fed. France was "crammed as full as an egg", wrote one Frenchman around 1572.[12] New diseases, most notably syphilis and the English Sweat, manifested themselves, rivalling bubonic plague and smallpox as diseases that not even the newly arrived drugs from the Americas and the Indies could cure. In return, although less remarked upon at the time in medical writings, European diseases ravaged the Americas even more ferociously. Although there were strong continuities with the past, there quickly developed a general sense among both sixteenth-century doctors and their patients that their new medicine was a considerable improvement over what had gone before, and that those who failed to adopt it were thereby inferior. It faced challenges, not least from the Paracelsian alternative from 1560 onwards, but it was also flexible enough to adopt many of its therapies and even some of its ideas, while leaving aside many of its more revolutionary notions. Precise observation and, at the end of the century, experiment became more valued than the simple repetition or logical analysis of academic doctrine. But the practices of physicians and surgeons were only one component in the world of healing. They existed alongside domestic medicine, as well as a near-universal belief in spirits, demons and magic that could be blamed for illness, and, it was alleged, could also be invoked to help in curing.[13] If medicine was thought to be insufficient against such adversaries, one could have recourse to the medicine of the church, the miraculous healing powers offered by Christ and his saints. To describe this new medical world of the late Renaissance is the theme of this book.

I have chosen to begin this survey in 1490, the year that saw the first printing of the collected works of the Roman doctor Galen in Latin. According to its editor, Diomedes Bonardus, a physician from Brescia, it included everything that he could find of Galen's writings conserved in the educational establishments, *gymnasia*, of Italy, most of them translated from Arabic intermediaries and often subsequently found to be spurious. These two massive volumes provide one benchmark against which to measure the change from medieval to Renaissance medicine, for a similar Latin Galen published a century later had been largely purified of Arabic influence and was a far more extensive and more accurate representation of what Galen had written. Finding a suitable end point was more difficult. The second half of the next century certainly has a very different feel from what was happening around 1610. The Thirty Years War and civil wars in France and Britain had disrupted the European world of learning, while the shift in economic power away from the Mediterranean to Northern Europe and the Atlantic led to a diminution in the role of Italy as the dominant medical centre. The growth of academies also subtly altered the position of medical colleges and universities as the predominant sites of intellectual endeavour. But there is no easy marker in the first 30 years, and the decision to confine the book to the sixteenth century rather than continue until, for example, the publication in 1628 of William Harvey's *Anatomical Exercises on the Movement of the Heart and Blood in Animals*, the treatise that ultimately, although not immediately, led to the abandonment of Galenist physiology, requires some justification beyond that of my own ignorance.

The seventeenth century is a period of both feast and famine. There has been a great deal of excellent modern work on the development of chemistry and alchemy in this period, Paracelsianism transformed, as it were, and the Harvey industry has done much to illuminate his intellectual origins, but, save for France, the history of learned medicine in Europe in the years before 1628 still remains to be studied in the detail already available for the medicine of the sixteenth century. The evidence for the social history of medicine in this period, particularly in England, France and to a certain extent Italy, has also burgeoned in the last 30 years, but anglophone historians have rarely ventured across the Channel. I have the impression, and I use that word advisedly, that our knowledge of the seventeenth century, and particularly of the first two decades, resembles that of the sixteenth 50 years ago – an aerial view of a series of mountain peaks rising out of a nigh-impenetrable jungle. Merely to summarise the findings of historians or to conduct a series of sondages into the unfamiliar, as I have tried to do over many years for the sixteenth century, would have added considerably to the time required for the book's completion. A third reason for the decision to end in 1600 is that many of the major themes that would need to be covered, had I decided to continue onwards, arise out of debates, discoveries and developments of the previous 30 years. To build on what I have discussed here and to write a wide-ranging history of medicine in the seventeenth century, or even in its first 30 years, is a challenge I happily leave to others.

Such a periodisation of the medical Renaissance of the sixteenth century is not new, and the names of a few individuals within it, such as Vesalius and Paracelsus, are familiar today. But the traditional account leaves out much, and has, until recently, been dominated by two interrelated preconceptions. The first is that the story of the medical Renaissance is the recovery, triumph and then relatively quick decline of Galenism. The Galenic medicine of the late sixteenth century, despite its ubiquity, is thus dismissed as a tragic mistake or an irrelevance in the march of medical progress. The second is that the torch of modernity, which burned brightly in Italy, was passed on to France and then, with varying degrees of effectiveness, elsewhere. The result of this unhappy conjunction has been a lack of attention given to developments in the late sixteenth century, and a concentration on a small number of progressive individuals and an even smaller number of medical specialties. If many of Galen's ideas on anatomy were generally regarded as outdated by the end of the century, Galenist therapeutics long remained the dominant force in medicine and there were vigorous debates among Galenists around Europe on a whole range of topics. Late sixteenth-century Italy, let alone the German-speaking world, was far from being the intellectual backwater that has often been assumed from the general absence of modern studies. Religious differences may have at times prevented Northern European Protestants from travelling to Bologna, Padua or Rome, but they did not inhibit Catholics from doing so or impede research and critical argument internationally. I make no apology for choosing to draw attention to, some might say concentrate upon, practitioners like Crato and Van Foreest who enjoyed a Europe-wide reputation then but who have subsequently been forgotten because they contributed relatively little to the development of modern medical science, or upon others like Fracastoro and Fernel who have been praised for modernising achievements that are not properly theirs.

More serious has been the consequent lack of interest, apart from purely local or national historians, in medical developments outside Italy and France.[14] Spain is often dismissed as an unfortunate backwater (although that condemnation could more easily apply to England for much of the century), while medicine in the Low Countries is viewed largely in the light of the triumphs of the century that followed.[15] The situation in the German-speaking lands, which stretched from the Rhine to Transylvania and contained far more universities than anywhere else in Europe at the time, has been largely forgotten until very recently, in part because few Anglophone historians now read German. How rich this material is can be glimpsed from the pages of Mary Lindemann's *Medicine and Society in Early Modern Europe*, in many ways a pioneering book, but she chose to focus on the seventeenth and early eighteenth centuries rather than on the sixteenth and in emphasising the social history of medicine she said little about those who participated in medical debates.[16] Most recently, Michael Stolberg's remarkable survey of Renaissance medicine as viewed through the notebooks of Georg Handsch, a German doctor from Bohemia who worked in Prague and later at the court of the Tyrol, offers a wonderful insight into the daily life of one practitioner, as well as a valuable short introductory survey. The forthcoming English translation will emphasise to those without German the importance of German evidence for the social history of medicine in the sixteenth century.[17] The fact that, although agreeing with him in so much of his exposition, I have selected almost entirely different examples of German medical life, shows the richness of the material that has previously been neglected.

To cover the history of medicine in Europe in the sixteenth century requires a considerable amount of selection and simplification, particularly as I have tried to give an idea of what was typical rather than focus simply on a few high points. For that reason, I have chosen at times to discuss some unfamiliar writers such as Thomas Jordanus who, although serving the elite, are more typical in their intellectual interests than Vesalius or Paracelsus. I have also selected examples from across Europe, where there was a general similarity of institutions, organisations and expectations, including hospitals and plague regulations, with Britain as a notable exception. If the result appears piecemeal and the journey often convoluted, this should be seen as conveying something of the kaleidoscope of healing in this period. Likewise, exceptions can be found to almost all generalisations. A concentration on physicians and surgeons risks undervaluing the role of those they considered their inferiors, and it goes without saying that the environment of health (in all its aspects) differed from place to place depending on wealth and access to wider communications.

This survey has also tried to steer a path between those who have looked for the wellsprings of medical modernity and those who have concentrated upon the social institutions and assumptions that constrained the practice of medicine. Hence the plan of the book, which falls in three sections: contexts, people and beliefs. It begins by looking at some of the consequences of the widening horizons in this period, including the new botany and the spread of 'new' diseases. The second chapter discusses the deadliest of these diseases, plague, and the institutions that were developing to safeguard public health. An increasingly literate society more and more obtained its medical information from printed books, and not only from the small number of major academic works singled out by historians of printing to exemplify the transformative power of print. Better communications also allowed information and even objects to be passed on through networks of correspondents across Europe in what became known as the republic of letters. Most doctors, and many of their patients, placed great emphasis on the humanist rediscovery of long forgotten or misinterpreted classical texts, notably but not exclusively Galen, as marking a major improvement over what they termed the errors of their medieval predecessors. The three middle chapters describe the kaleidoscope of healing, from physicians, surgeons and apothecaries to so-called charlatans and domestic or women's medicine. It also considers some of the perceptions of patients and the reasons behind their choice of healers. The last section examines different aspects of the medical debates of the time, including anatomy, both in the university and in art, contagious disease and, from the 1560s, Paracelsianism. The final chapter considers the consequences for medicine of the religious divisions of the period, including their impact on non-Christians. In short, I want to give a broad view of the variegated medical life of the entire sixteenth century for those who may be familiar with some of the great names in literature or art but know almost nothing about the medicine. This has demanded a considerable selectivity, even when dealing with major figures and crucial developments in medicine or surgery, in order to present what was more typical of medical theory and practice. After all, not every professor was a Mercuriale, not every artist a Leonardo, not every book a European best-seller. To forget that is to misunderstand the medical world of the sixteenth century.

Notes

1 Marchesi 1678: 737–8, 751–2, who, p. 693, lists other benefactions to the city in 1559; Colombi Ferretti *et al.* 2000.
2 Bonoli 1826: II, 426–8, a description of this "star of stars", his chapel and his palazzo; Colombi Ferretti *et al.* 2000: 20–1, 33–3, and pl. II, viii–ix.
3 Mercuriale 2008. For a discussion of his writings, see below, pp. 79. 84. 116. 234–5.
4 Cerasoli 2004. He enjoyed an enormous salary, increased further to 200 gold scudi at Pisa.
5 For alternative views on the meaning of 'Renaissance' in different contexts, see Woolfson 2005.
6 Wilson 1992.
7 For France, see Hobart 2020.
8 Siraisi 1990.
9 DaCosta Kaufmann 1995.
10 Siraisi 1990: xii, 190–3.
11 Ludwig 1999: 265–9. The title *Articella*, 'Little Art', is not attested before the age of printing, and may have been student slang. Cf. Manardi, *Ep.* I, 1: 1556: 1: "Who of us over 40 has not worshipped his *Articella* like Mosaic law?", a letter of 1518.
12 Sieur de Brantôme, quoted by Braudel 1986: I, 172; and, in general 170–3.
13 Waddell 2021.
14 Webster 1979, an excellent survey, concentrates mainly on England; the similarly valuable Brockliss and Jones (1997) on France.
15 Cf. now López Terrada 2007; Huguet-Termes *et al.* 2009; Slater *et al.* 2014 for a revision of the place of Spain.
16 Lindemann 2010; the first edition appeared in 1999.
17 Stolberg 2021a, 2022.

Contexts

1 New Lands, New Drugs and New Diseases

New Lands

In 1508/9 a doctoral candidate at the North Italian university of Ferrara challenged his audience by declaring that the traditional ideas on geography and climate had been utterly overthrown by the recent discoveries of voyagers across the Atlantic and to the Far East. Giovanni Manardi (1461–1536), who later became professor of medicine there, had learned from Portuguese sailors that the torrid zone, far from being uninhabitable as Aristotle had supposed, was teeming with people. A doctor friend from Florence who had a relative now living in India had also told him that the seasonal pattern there differed from that of Europe in having two winters and two summers, none excessively hot or cold.[1] This did not mean that the new lands were paradises of health, like the fabled Kingdom of Prester John, for, as was already becoming clear, they had their own diseases appropriate to their own climates. The regions around the Senegal and Gambia rivers might host an abundance of plants and animals, but there were also deadly fevers, allegedly arising from the impure air issuing from the mouths of mines on the Gold Coast.[2] This link between climate and health, established two millennia earlier by the great Greek physician Hippocrates, explained why, after all, it was far better to live in the middle of Avicenna's sixth, temperate zone, particularly in a city like Ferrara under the benevolent rule of Alfonso d'Este.[3]

By the end of the century opinions like Manardi's had become commonplace as Europeans ventured further and further afield in larger numbers. Eager naturalists reported on the birds and fishes that could be found on the stormy shores of the North Atlantic.[4] Russian fur traders penetrated into the distant wastes of Siberia, while missionaries followed conquistadors across the seas to the Americas and the East.[5] The Jesuit historian of the New World, José d'Acosta (1540–1600), recalled how on his first voyage to the Indies in 1570 he had been brought to realise the flaws in the classical tradition in which he had been brought up when, on nearing the equator, the hottest region on earth according to Aristotle, he shivered in the cool wind.[6] Writing around 1580, Francisco Sanches, a Portuguese

DOI: 10.4324/9781003223184-3

physician and sceptical philosopher at the University of Toulouse, declared that a new world had been discovered in New Spain and the West and East Indies whose new realities rendered many previous assumptions out of date. Experience had demonstrated the falsity of the notion of a world surrounded by the Ocean and revealed that the southern zone below the equator and the North closer to the poles were far from being uninhabited, as the ancients had believed. There were animals and plants there that could no longer be fitted into traditional categories, and who knew what remained to be discovered? (See Figure 1.1 for the use of new information.)[7]

But to focus solely on trans-oceanic voyages and conquests as a catalyst for change is to misunderstand their place within a greater expansion of knowledge about people, places and their environment within Europe itself. Printing made maps more accessible, and the stories of travellers, especially those collected by Giambattista Ramusio (1485–1557) and published between 1550 and 1559, supplemented the only slightly more sober accounts of those who preferred to describe the history and geography of their own European region or town.[8] Doctors now travelled great distances to serve on official business in such commercial outposts as the Venetian colonies in the Eastern Mediterranean or the Portuguese and later Dutch

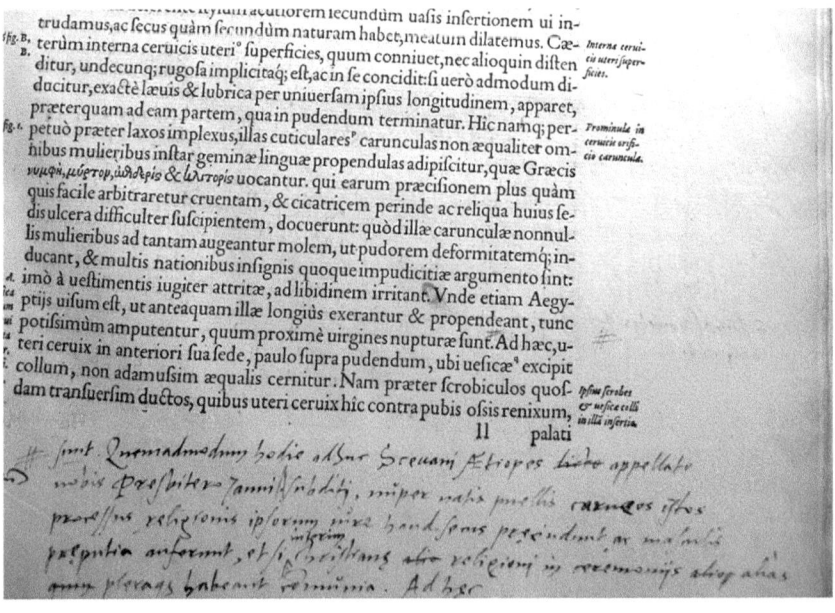

Figure 1.1 Female genital mutilation in Ethiopia. This annotation, based probably on an account of 1550, was made by the anatomist Andreas Vesalius at the foot of his discussion of female anatomy in the 1555 edition of his *De humani corporis fabrica*. Basle: J. Oporinus: 653. The Thomas Fisher Rare Books Room, Toronto University Library. Copyright G. Vogringic.

settlements in Goa and further east in Indonesia.[9] Three English members
of the London College of Physicians, a licentiate Ralph Standish, and two
Fellows, Robert Jacob and Mark Ridley, even made their way to Moscow
where they furthered the interests of Edward VI and, later in the century,
Elizabeth I at the court of the Tsar.[10] Other doctors extolled the history and
antiquities of their own country for the benefit of a European learned readership. In Vienna, Johannes Cuspinianus (1473–1529), doctor, humanist, poet
and diplomat, composed a lengthy description of the territory of Austria,
with its Marches, Duchies and Archduchies, to show that Austria had no
equal among nations.[11] The Englishman John Caius (1510–73) devoted the
second book of his *History of Cambridge University* to a detailed account of
the city of Cambridge, describing its streets, churches, institutions and cus-
toms in the same precise way as he listed elsewhere rare animals and birds
of the British Isles. In his topographical and local historical pursuits he was
part of a wider trend in England that culminated in John Stow's *Survey of
London* and William Camden's *Britannia*.[12] He also exchanged specimens,
drawings and detailed descriptions of the natural world of the British Isles
with the Swiss Conrad Gessner (1516–65), whose correspondence with fellow naturalists stretched around Europe and across religious divides. Gessner was a polymath and a prolific editor and translator of classical medical
texts, but he was also keen to inform others of new discoveries.[13] One such
publication was his short study of some German healing waters, along with
an even longer list of names of spas, which he compiled and published in
1553, and then transmitted to another English friend, William Turner.[14]
Turner (d. 1568) a physician and later a very Protestant Dean of Wells,
included some of Gessner's information in his account of the waters of Bath
and of other places in Germany and Italy.[15] It was through contacts and
publications like this that medical men learned about the many medicinal
substances that had been discovered (or at least made widely known) for the
first time in Europe and beyond, and developed strategies for including them
in a new intellectual landscape. Some, however, still preferred to treat local
diseases with local remedies.[16] Timothie Bright (1551?–1615), a Cambridge
and later London practitioner, aimed to show "the suffiiciencie of English
Medicines, for cure of all diseases, cured with medicine". Whatever would
not grow in English gardens indicated its hostility to English bodies. Instead
of remedies from the hippopotamus or ibis he recommended others made
from earthworms or woodlice to cure tertian fevers, pains in the ears, jaundice and quinsy.[17]

New Drugs and Old Texts

This expansion to both East and West was driven in part by a desire to
gain access to the riches of India and the areas further east, and particularly to the trade in spices that had for centuries been transported overland
to Venice through what had become a hostile Turkish Empire. The rulers

of Portugal were quick to appreciate the economic potential of their new trade routes, especially for pepper and spices like cinnamon which had been known and used for centuries.[18] The drugs of the New World were much slower to enter use, for trade was much smaller at first, serious study took time and Spanish monopoly practices were a further hindrance to their easy distribution. Spanish apothecaries in sixteenth-century Mexico were few, and the herbs they used were overwhelmingly those with which they were already familiar in Spain, whence they needed to be imported.[19] By contrast, before 1540 only one indigenous American remedy was in widespread use in Europe. Guaiac wood was being imported as early as 1508 from the Caribbean, where it had been observed in use by the natives against a treponemal disease, yaws, and it was soon in common use in Spain against a new and reportedly similar disease, syphilis.[20] Nicolaus Pol and Leonard Schmaus, a protégé of the Fuggers of Augsburg, had publicised its benefits even before the appearance in 1519 of the treatise on guaiac by the humanist Ulrich von Hutten, who believed that he (and many others) had been cured by drinking a decoction of it.[21] It was his book, swiftly translated into German, French and English, that established guaiac as a prime therapy for the disease, and that some years later led to the accusation that it had provided the Fugger family with an opportunity for profiteering.[22] Not everyone adopted this wonder drug immediately. Antonio Musa Brasavola (1500–55) reported from Ferrara that he first saw it in 1529 but did not himself begin to employ it against syphilis until 1534.[23] But by the middle of the century, it was so common that it could be mentioned almost incidentally in literature alongside the disease, a "a tree of salvation for those who have thought themselves lost to the disease of youth", as a Spanish poet called it in an attack on court culture.[24]

A second non-European remedy against the same disease came to prominence in the 1530s, the so-called China root, *smilax china*, imported from the East Indies as early as 1525, and widely used by 1535 because it was thought to expel the noxious humours of the disease by stimulating perspiration. It was also recommended against gout and was believed by the wealthy to be a panacea. When, however, his employer, the Emperor Charles V, demanded to use it, Vesalius demurred, and wrote a tract ostensibly about its misuse, but mostly devoted to defending his own controversial ideas about human anatomy against attacks by Jacobus Sylvius.[25]

Similarly, vigorous arguments over the identity and properties even of well-known medicinal herbs had taken place earlier following a debate provoked in 1491–2 by Manardi's teacher, Niccolò Leoniceno (1428–1524).[26] In a learned discussion at the court of Ferrara he had first challenged the traditional identifications of many plants used in medicine on philological grounds, but it soon became obvious that the problem was more complicated than that. Even if one could agree that the Greek accounts were the sources for much of later pharmacology, the properties of the herbs with which Italian botanists and apothecaries were familiar did not always correspond to what had been said about them by the writers of Ancient Greece and Rome. Besides, the herbal of the Greek author on whom most depended, Dioscorides (c. 70 CE) was overwhelmingly focussed on the world of the Eastern Mediterranean and on exotic substances from India. The plants added in medieval Arabic pharmacological writings available in Latin translation only intensified this Eastern bias. As knowledge of the natural world in Italy and particularly beyond the Alps increased, the deficiencies in Dioscorides's coverage became ever clearer, although he still retained his pre-eminence until the 1560s, if not beyond.

One early example will suffice to show how doctors went about trying to check the information they derived from Dioscorides. He had given a detailed description of rhubarb in Book III of his *Materia medica*, and subsequent writers on pharmacology had added yet more information and advice on its use. But although it had been known for centuries that it had been brought from somewhere east of the Black Sea (hence its Latin name *rha ponticum*, Pontic rhubarb), and was widely used, not everything in his description appeared to fit what was on sale in Italy. Dioscorides had said that it was odourless, but what was available in an Italian market had a distinctive smell. Besides, it was claimed to be both a laxative and an astringent, to appear in several different forms and to come from various parts of the East. Marcello Adriani Virgilio in his commentary on Dioscorides contented himself with a warning about careless identification and against assuming that the plant called *rhacoma* by the Elder Pliny was the same as Dioscorides's rhubarb. The two accounts were similar, but Pliny ascribed a much greater range of medicinal properties to his plant.[27]

Other scholars had been similarly puzzled. Manardi and Leoniceno had already discussed this at a meeting in Ferrara around 1512 in the house of Professor Opizzoni. When soon afterwards Manardi accompanied his new employer, the King of Hungary, to a conference at Bratislava, he learned from the doctors of the King of Poland that during the recent war with Moscow a plant corresponding to that of Dioscorides had been found growing in Muscovy and was indeed totally odourless. Manardi had been given a powder made from it, and, after several fruitless enquiries, he finally managed to track down this fabulous plant that was growing at the eastern end of the Black Sea. To avoid confusion, he then cut a slice from the stem and sent it to Leoniceno. One can only imagine what condition it was in after over three months in transit since it was picked.[28]

This Ferrara tradition of medical botany was continued by Manardi's student and successor as professor, Antonio Musa Brasavola, who took his copy of Dioscorides on herborising expeditions with his students, often mislaying his glasses in the process. He compared what Dioscorides had written about rhubarb with what he could buy in Venetian shops and also with the properties of another common herb, the greater centaury.[29] William Turner, who had spent some time in Ferrara in the early 1540s and who knew Brasavola well, thought that *rha ponticum* was in fact the Arabic pharmacologist Mesue's *raued turcicum*, although not all of it came from Turkey, and that it could be compared for its efficacy with the British dock, called by the ignorant 'Monk's rhubarb'. By the end of the century, several other identifications had been proposed for Dioscorides's plant, sometimes rightly associated with China but also including the 'true rhubarb of the Arabians', which grew on Mount Lebanon.[30]

If learned Europeans had difficulty in identifying a medicinal plant whose uses had been recorded for centuries, the first European traders and settlers in India and Ceylon found it even more difficult. That was why King Manuel in 1512 sent an apothecary, Tomé Pires, to India and further east with a list of some 25 plants, including rhubarb, that he and his court thought might have originated there and which, presumably, had commercial value. Pires, who spent three years in the East using Malacca as his base, replied with a carefully detailed report that distinguished between those substances that were valuable and others that might just as well be tossed into the sea. He had observed far more things than Manuel had asked for, but, at this stage, there was no official eagerness to introduce any more exotic plants to Europe.[31] Besides, European botanists were revealing the existence of more species of useful plants closer to home. A young Parisian graduate of 1523, Robert Delevesmont, for example, was praised for always carrying his Dioscorides with him as he investigated the herbs around his native town of Lisieux in Normandy.[32] About 1550 the humanist circle in Rome associated with the Spanish diplomat Diego Hurtado de Mendoza eagerly traversed the countryside to investigate local plants and herbs. A little later, a local apothecary from Verona, Francesco Calzolari (1521–1600), organised learned botanising expeditions to the nearby Monte Baldo, listing some 350 plants in that area.[33] What was found was then described in detail in printed herbals like those of Otto Brunfels (1488–1534) in Strasbourg, Euricius Cordus (1486–1535) in Marburg and, above all, Leonhard Fuchs (1501–66) in Tübingen. Fuchs's *Historia Stirpium, Enquiry into Plants*, published at Basle in 1542 (Figure 1.2), set new standards of accuracy as well as being illustrated with more numerous and more beautiful woodcuts than ever before.[34] The artist and the engraver were deservedly depicted at the close of the large volume, which, should a purchaser require it, could be painted in the exact colours specified by the author. This was a luxury item, but also a practical one. One owner had extra pages bound into his copy onto which he stuck the leaves of various plants and shrubs: the leaves themselves have disappeared but their outlines can still be viewed today.[35]

Equally as significant as Fuchs's herbal in the development of medical botany were the commentaries on Dioscorides by Pietro Andrea Mattioli (1501–78). A graduate of Padua, he worked in his home town of Siena as well as in Rome before moving to Northern Italy around 1529, soon becoming doctor to the powerful Cardinal Clesio, archbishop of Trento. He published his first book, a tract on syphilis in 1533, as well as gaining a reputation for his poetry and his elegant Italian translations of the Classics.

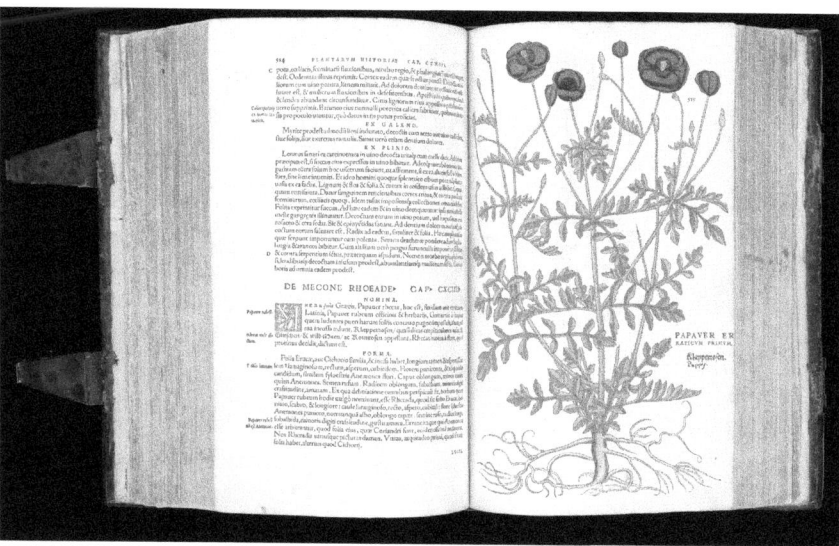

Figure 1.2 The poppy. Leonhard Fuchs, *De historia stirpium commentarii*. Basle:
     M. Isingrin, 1542, pp. 514–5.

Dismissed by Clesio's successor, he moved to Gorizia on the frontier of
the Hapsburg Tyrol in 1535, remaining there for 20 years until he was
appointed doctor to Archduke Ferdinand of the Tyrol. This brought him
into close contact with the Hapsburg Emperor Ferdinand, and he continued
to serve both him and his successor Maximilian II almost until the end of his
life. Although he did not find Gorizia entirely to his liking, he was able while
there to carry on his investigations into plants in the Alpine regions of Italy
and to publish in 1544 the first version of his commentary on Dioscorides.[36]

Written in Italian, it was aimed at an Italian readership, and it contained
no illustrations of plants. In his commentary Mattioli clearly and succinctly
explained Dioscorides's meaning, summarising the various debates about
plant identification and adding many observations of his own. But it was
only when he found a new publisher, Vincenzo Valgrisi in Venice, and
published a revised and enlarged edition with illustrations in 1550 and a
Latin version in 1554 that he moved to the centre of the world of medical
botany and natural history (for Dioscorides had also included animal and
mineral substances).[37] His court connections gave him access to contacts
across Europe and to wealthy patrons who encouraged him to produce ever
more lavishly illustrated and coloured editions in Latin, German, French
and Czech that are works of art in themselves and were correspondingly
expensive.[38] He preferred to sit at the centre of a huge network, expecting
others to do the investigative work for him since, so he claimed, increasing

age and his imperial duties no longer allowed him to carry out field work. When he heard that an Italian gentleman, Gherardo Cibo (1512–1600) had made some wonderful reproductions of plants, now among the treasures of the British Library, he immediately wrote to see if he could obtain a copy.[39] His own well-known refusal to acknowledge all of his debts in his pages amounted to a sentence of academic death for aspiring members of the botanical republic of letters whom he failed to mention.[40] His disagreements with other botanists such as Gessner or Luigi Anguillara, "Luigi the Eel-Skinner" (1512–70), the first Director of the Padua Botanic Garden, sometimes go on for many pages, as Mattioli discusses the possible modern identifications of these classical herbs, noting the names for the plants in a variety of regions and dialects.[41] The later revised and extended editions, many hundreds of folio pages long, are prefaced by massive indexes of plants, their applications and the ailments for which they might be used.

Mattioli's commentaries mark the culmination of the first stage of Renaissance botany. Although Dioscorides continued to be the subject of academic lectures for well over a century longer, no subsequent commentator approached Mattioli in such abundance of detail. However, his expensive volumes were beyond the pocket of many practitioners, who preferred short guides to medical botany that were more relevant to their daily needs and to the substances on sale in local shops. In any case, the ancient text was becoming outdated as more and more individuals were finding plants, animals, birds and fishes that had not been recorded even without leaving their own country.[42] Travellers also explored countries that were unfamiliar to them. William Turner wandered in fields of flowers along the Rhine near Siegburg, and another Englishman, Thomas Penny (d. 1589), was said to have made a hazardous expedition to Majorca while he was studying in Montpellier in 1566, before going on to Germany and possibly the Baltic.[43] Prospero Borgarucci (1540–78) took advantage of his brother's employment at the court of Queen Elizabeth I to botanise in the Welsh mountains in 1564, talking to the native Welsh in what he thought was their native tongue – a dialect of modern Greek.[44] The incomprehensibility seems to have been mutual. Others ventured still further afield. Luigi Anguillara, before he began teaching at Padua, explored Crete around 1540 in the company of a druggist, Constantino Rodioto, and described 32 new species of plants they found there. Prospero Alpini (1553–1616) investigated the medicinal plants of Egypt in 1580–81, arranging for specimens to be sent back to Italy where they were eagerly adopted by owners of botanical gardens, both private and official.[45] At the same time the Augsburg physician Leonhard Rauwolf (1535?–96) travelled around the Middle East, taking notes on plants for inclusion in his book of 1582 and bringing back samples for his own herbarium, which, after a brief stay in the Prague library of the Emperor Rudolf II, became part of the collection of another celebrated botanical garden, that of Leiden.[46]

Meanwhile medical botany was becoming institutionalised. Chairs in simples were founded, at Rome in 1514 (although it was soon to be suspended in the chaos that followed the Sack of Rome in 1527) and then at Padua in 1533, Bologna in 1534 and Perugia in 1537.[47] Oecolampadius's 1533 plan for the medical Faculty at Basle stipulated that students should be shown plants in summer, and any deficiencies in the herbs in the pharmacists' shops should be pointed out to them, and to the Basle Senate as well.[48] It was not long before these lectureships were followed by the creation of dedicated gardens. The first may have been at Ferrara as early as 1540, but little is known about it.[49] More famous is the botanical garden at Pisa, established in 1543, with a former lecturer in simples at Bologna, Luca Ghini (1490–1556) as its first prefect. Others quickly followed Pisa's example – Padua in 1545, Florence in 1550, Rome in 1563 and Bologna in 1568.[50] The importance of having such a garden was also recognised north of the Alps. When the university of Helmstedt was founded in 1576, its first professor of medicine, Johann Bökel (1535–1605), immediately arranged for the planting of a garden, thus anticipating by 14 years the much more famous botanical garden at Leiden.[51] In the last decade of the century Basle gained a great reputation as a place where one might study medical botany, with vigorous discussions taking place both within and without the university.[52] Otto Brunfels's vigorous denunciation in 1530 of the book-bound learning of physicians and of their unwillingness to learn the basics of pharmacology that even a barber could pick up in six weeks might have been true at the beginning of the century, but this was no longer so 100 years later.[53]

New Drugs and an Old Paradigm

From the middle of the sixteenth century onwards, the abundance of new substances, and still more of detailed information about them and their uses, altered perspectives on the classical heritage as mediated through Arabic and later humanist pharmacologists.[54] It also allowed for the wider introduction of substances from the Americas and the East that had been examined and tested by men who had spent a considerable time in the Tropics, even if they were regarded at first mainly as substitutes for other better-known drugs.[55] Two books, published almost simultaneously, provided the first substantial accounts of the medical botany of the increasingly familiar lands in the East and the Americas. Nicolas Monardes (1493–1588), who in 1536 had written that American medicinal drugs were inferior to those of Spain itself, gradually changed his mind, and in 1565 published the first of three parts of a large book dealing with all the things that were brought from the Americas. Parts 2 and 3 appeared later in 1571 and 1574, a Latin abridgement followed in 1575, an Italian version in 1576 and an English one by John Frampton in 1577, titled *Joyfull Newes out of the New Founde World*. Although some of his family travelled to New Spain, Monardes remained throughout his life in Seville, gaining his knowledge of plants from what he could find imported and from his interviews with administrators, sailors, priests and travellers of all kinds about their medicinal usages. The first part of his book dealt with resins, purgatives, remedies for syphilis (including guaiac and sarsaparilla) and Peruvian balsam; the second covered a variety of substances from animals, including the armadillo and cayman, and began with a long section on tobacco (which he regarded as a panacea), as well as on sassafras. In the third part, Monardes discussed Tolu balsam, the granadillo and coca. He described at length how the native Indians prepared and chewed coca as a way of warding off hunger and giving them stamina, but warned also that they deliberately used it neat or mixed with tobacco whenever they wished to rob themselves of their wits and simply have a pleasurable experience.[56] In using the language and standard categories of Galenic medical botany, he, like others reporting on distant exotica, was assimilating these new plants and drugs into a European medical and intellectual environment as well as providing his readers and other travellers with a template for understanding other new things they might encounter.

It is not clear whether Monardes knew of and used the codex of Nahuatl medicine in the Spanish Royal Library that had been prepared by a native convert, Martin De la Cruz, in 1552 and translated into Latin the following year.[57] Equally unclear is his role in the appointment of Francisco Hernandez as chief physician of New Spain by King Philip II in 1570 with instructions to gather as much information as possible about the properties of all the medicinal plants of New Spain.[58] But it was certainly Monardes's work that allowed Europeans in general to make fuller use of substances from the New World that had earlier circulated largely in Spain: their properties and their medicinal uses were now explained in terms that all doctors, surgeons and apothecaries could understand.[59] But progress was still slow. Although botanists like Aldrovandi eagerly took note of these new discoveries, the herbs themselves do not appear to have been widely exported from Spain to elsewhere in Europe or distributed through Spanish apothecaries' shops, with a few exceptions, until the end of the century. Two major Florentine pharmacies in the 1560s sold a variety of guaiac and one sold sarsaparilla, but do not appear to have offered other New World drugs. Similarly in London in 1567, guaiac was the only new drug being imported, perhaps because, as Thomas Paynell put it, "no man wolde lightly go unto a medicine that came from so strange a place". Twenty years later, it had been joined by china root and sarsaparilla, but the large-scale importation of exotics from the New World occurs only in the last decade of the century.[60] Whether, as Teresa Huguet-Termes suggests, these drugs were somehow passed on in private, or even in an underground way, remains to be decided.[61]

Two years before Monardes, a similar exposition of medicinal substances from the East Indies was published in Goa by Garcia D'Orta (1501/2–68). His *Dialogues on Simples and Drugs and Medicinal Matters from India* appeared first of all in Portuguese in Goa, and then in a shorter illustrated Latin translation by Carolus Clusius (1526–1609) at Antwerp in 1567.[62] Unlike the stay-at-home Monardes, Garcia D'Orta had spent 29 years of his life in 'Golden Goa', the centre of Portuguese trade in India, first as doctor to the governor but later as an independent physician. In his earliest years in the East he had travelled on official business around India and Ceylon, but later he was largely confined to Goa.[63] This was no great handicap, for medicinal substances came there to be traded, and the city itself was crowded with merchants and travellers from all over the East. There were also Portuguese apothecaries there, like Tomé Pires and Simao Alvarez, who were interested in local drugs and who reported back with details of substances that might be traded profitably.[64] Their reports provided the mental and geographical framework for D'Orta's activities, but he went far beyond them in many ways. He too had been educated in the humanist tradition of Leoniceno, Manardi and Brasavola, and followed the Dioscoridean method of description. But whereas Pires and Alvarez were mainly concerned with discovery and identification of new drugs, he was heavily involved in practical medicine, not only in treating foreign diseases but also in observing the work of native healers in their communities, meeting and discussing their therapies with them.[65] At first sceptical of their claims, he later came to appreciate what they were trying to do and to understand why many members of the Western community in Goa came to rely on them. He was also conscious of the suspicions of the Goan authorities, especially Jesuit missionaries, about his links with Hindus, and he was careful in his mediation of native remedies to warn of possible subversive uses. Chewing betel leaves was disgusting, opium was morally and physically harmful, and hashish, "which is not one of our remedies, . . . made a fool of those who took it".[66]

D'Orta's books, like those of Monardes and the slightly later *Tractado de las Drogas y las Medicinas de las Indias Orientales*, *Tract on Drugs and Medicines from the East Indies*, 1578, by Christovao da Costa (1515–80), who had travelled as far as Malacca and China, brought new plants and therapies to the notice of Europeans.[67] Indeed, a writer in 1603 complained that [doctors and apothecaries] "wish to put Africa, Asia, Europe and the New World together into their recipes, continuously concocting new things for their sick patients [that are] both dangerous and untested".[68] But at least, unlike their predecessors in the first quarter of the century, they could now read descriptions of many exotic plants that used familiar categories and explained their value for a wide range of European diseases.

New Epidemic Diseases[69]

It was no coincidence that two of the earliest drugs to be widely adopted from the Americas, guaiac and sarsaparilla, were employed in the treatment of a new disease, the French disease, later called syphilis, that was often associated with that region, where a treponemal disease, yaws, with similar symptoms was endemic.[70] Whether syphilis itself was a mutation of that disease in the Americas or of a form of non-venereal syphilis already known in Europe or North Africa is still a matter of scientific controversy, but there can be little doubt that the opening up of Europe at the very least allowed formerly local diseases to spread further and faster or to be better reported as something 'new' or 'unknown before'.[71] The most famous European scholar of the day, Erasmus of Rotterdam (1466–1536), devoted much of the preface to his *Lingua* (*The Tongue*) in 1525 to a comparison between the ways in which words and diseases could cause harm. Some like the English Sweat suddenly appeared but remained relatively localised (an opinion he was to revise substantially only a few years later in 1529). Others, like plague, never entirely died away, but suddenly erupted to threaten the whole of humanity. Still others, like typhus or smallpox, remained a steady threat. In Erasmus's view, the most serious of all epidemics was a disease of uncertain origin and with a variety of names, the French pox, the Spanish pox, or the Neapolitan disease (different regions blamed it on outsiders near and far). It broke out quickly, and swiftly covered the known world. It was easily transmitted, and defied medical aid. It was painful, disfiguring the face and then other parts of the body, and even if it seemed to have been checked, it would suddenly return, like gout.[72] Forty-five years later, the French novelist Pierre Boaistuau (1500–60) came to a similar conclusion. He began the third book of his musings on human life with a discussion of the miseries caused to mankind as a result of God's punishment for sin. He singled out pestilences, from ancient Athens and Rome to the French disease, whether caused by poison or bad air, as well as the plague that affected Germany and England (what we know today as the English Sweat) and the localised epidemic that followed the siege of Boulogne in 1545.[73] He recalled how at Aix en Provence in 1546 a new disease broke out, killing people within two days, even as they ate or drank, with the result that some preferred suicide by leaping from windows to suffering its torments. Neither Boaistuau nor Erasmus was a medical man, although they had many medical friends, but they had themselves experienced various epidemics and their observations of them are typical of those in the community at large.[74]

Both men insisted on the severity and speed with which the French disease affected the whole of Europe. (It was no surprise that the Turks should have called it the Christian disease, as it appears to have moved East somewhat later.) It was first reported in Naples in 1495 among the French troops then occupying the city and spread rapidly northwards as the army retraced its steps. It had reached Germany by 1496 at the latest and Scotland in 1497 and was recorded in Eastern Europe by 1499. Its ubiquity resembled that of plague itself, although its symptoms were noticeably different.[75] Its most obvious manifestations were pains, sometimes so severe that the patient cried out and even contemplated suicide, and sores all over the body that sometimes penetrated deeply under the skin. One early sufferer, a canon of Orvieto, first felt severe pains in 1496 in his knees, back and buttocks. The pain returned in 1498, this time in his arms and in his bones so that he could hardly sleep. His body was covered in boils, and his mouth became so sore that he could eat only soft bread for over a month. Others reported that as the disease progressed it gnawed away parts of the body, such as the nose.[76] Erasmus thought that it combined the worst features of every disease because of its range, speed and ease of transmission, its painfulness and near-incurability, as well as the extremely loathsome aspect of those it affected.[77]

That this was an epidemic disease was abundantly clear almost from the outset, but both doctors and patients regarded this categorisation as only the first stage in identifying it and proceeding to a cure. The earliest recorded debate about it took place not in a university but at the court of Ferrara in spring 1497, when it was rampant in the city and was shortly to affect several members of the ducal family, and possibly the Duke himself. The participants discussed whether or not this was a new disease.[78] Leoniceno, a familiar figure in such courtly disputes, argued that it had been known to the ancient Greeks and, like all epidemics, was the result of changes in the atmosphere that produced the warm, wet climate in 1495–6 that had been ideal for the putrefaction that produced the genital sores. It was a generic disease, whose exact manifestations differed according to an individual's humoral constitution.[79] The second speaker, Sebastiano dall'Aquila (c. 1440–1510), agreed that this was no new disease, but one described by Galen as 'elephantiasis', a form of leprous skin disease, spread partly by air and partly by contagion or propinquity. There were three main sources of direct infection, sexual intercourse or sharing a bed with an infected person and being suckled by an infected woman. Their appeal to the Greeks alone was rejected by Coradino Gilino (fl. 1468–99), a local man who also lectured at the university.[80] He accepted that this disease was in some way a divine judgement and brought about by a planetary alignment, but it had been identified long ago by Celsus and by Avicenna as *ignis sacer* or *ignis persicus*, the result of an excess of black bile. He spent longer than the others in explaining why it attacked the genitals, and recommended avoiding intercourse, for those who caught the disease in this way he had found to suffer greater torments. But those who had a good constitution, were young and used to it might still indulge in sex in moderation. All the participants agreed that it was possible to find evidence for earlier outbreaks of this 'new' disease in the older literature, and that, once found, these precedents provided a means towards a cure. But they differed substantially in the authorities that they preferred, and consequently in the treatment they proposed. Gilino, for example, favoured cauterising the sores, while Leoniceno emphasised an individual dietetic approach.

Similar debates, whether in a formal university setting, among intellectual courtiers, or in a series of pamphlet wars, took place in Bologna, Rome, Leipzig and probably elsewhere.[81] They raised many similar questions. Was this disease the result of an astrological conjunction, and hence could be predicted in the future, or of unpredictable climatic changes? Was it curable or not? (Doctors' experiences varied, not least because of the disease's pattern of remission, but later in the century Italian hospitals for syphilitics were labelled 'for the incurable'.) Which of the ancient skin diseases did it most resemble? Was it, indeed, a single disease or the conjunction of several? The evidence of autopsies was used almost from the beginning, but what they revealed was far from clear. Some believed they had found a phlegmy matter collecting in the joints, like gout, others that it gathered in the nerves and muscles. Was the phlegm to be found in the bones, or in the pustules visible all over the body? On the other hand, Giorgio Vella reported in 1515, probably at second hand, that the *gumma* on the bones was in fact dry, thus excluding putrefaction as a cause.[82]

Other writers, and particularly non-medics, wondered about the relationship between this new disease and that described in the Old Testament in the Book of Job as a loathsome skin disease sent by God.[83] Preachers, almost from the beginning, had proclaimed that this was a divine call to repentance, and Emperor Maximilian I had issued a series of rulings against blasphemers who had brought this disease down upon his Empire.[84] It was no coincidence that Ercole d'Este in Ferrara embarked on a moral crusade at this time, under the influence of the austere Girolamo Savonarola, who is more famous for his activities in Florence. Although none of the early debaters associated the disease with sexual intercourse exclusively, for its symptoms were not confined to the genitals and both Maximilian and Ercole focussed on the sinful nature of all their citizens, there was a growing appreciation that this was the major means of transmission. Most people were familiar with the medieval story of the girl so filled with poison that she killed all her lovers, and it was only too easy to single out marauding soldiers from elsewhere or filthy prostitutes as the main source of infection.[85] In 1526, the Lutheran town council of the German town of Zwickau in Saxony justified their decision to close the town brothel primarily on moral grounds but also because "so many young journeymen had been poisoned there with the French disease".[86] Shakespeare was merely referring to what was common knowledge when he had Lucio in *Measure for Measure*, Act I, Scene 2, chaff with fellow gentlemen about how easy it was to catch the disease, and many others as well, in Madame Overdone's brothel, now about to be closed down by an overzealous and moralising Angelo.

The tragicomic failure of Angelo's schemes also reveals how by the end of the sixteenth century syphilis had lost the dire reputation that it had when it first appeared. Writing as early as 1530 Erasmus lamented that such a dreadful disease had now become a joke. A gentleman was now considered a worthless clod if he had not caught the disease and waved two fingers at God the chastiser.[87] His observation can be confirmed from Royan in South-West France, where one of the titles borne by the heads of the associations of young men was 'Grand Patriarch of Syphilitics'.[88] Doctors also noticed a change in the behaviour of the disease. In the final section of his book on linctuses and syrups of 1553, Brasavola reported that the symptoms of the disease had altered since Leoniceno's day and that new ones had appeared even in the 1530s. He believed that it now showed a large number of variations, sometimes following each other in a well-defined sequence, including loss of hair, teeth and hair to blindness and 'gonorrhoea'.[89] Whether this was due to the disease itself becoming old, as he argued, more effective treatment or better standards of personal hygiene were questions for academic discussion, but there was general agreement that it was much less serious and had, like plague, become in its gravest and nigh incurable manifestations a disease primarily of the poor.[90]

In part, this was because many of the remedies on offer were beyond the reach of the poorest in society. Brasavola in passing noted the high cost of treatment by guaiac or other exotic woods, suggesting that a few shavings might be enough at least to mitigate its pains.[91] The china root was also an expensive import, while the recommended treatments to drive out the poison by sweating required a large amount of free time to be effective. One of the few named individuals not from the upper classes in Brasavola's account, the head bellringer at the cathedral, Doro Batano, was praised for curing himself of very severe pains in the joints by extremely vigorous and prolonged sessions of pulling on the ropes of the great bell.[92] Brasavola, however, cautioned that this hard physical exercise, although helping the joints to move, might not always work and might even lead to greater pains in those who were unused to it, not a strong recommendation for those accustomed to a wealthy lifestyle. Intensive sweating treatment with mercury, which was also frequently prescribed, had dangerous side effects, and by the middle of the century was being considered suitable only for those of a strong constitution, and far inferior to guaiac. The poor, transported to a hospital for the incurable, were subjected to even harsher regimes that might include beating and flogging.[93]

The best evidence for the normalisation of the pox among the upper classes from the 1520s onwards is provided by the Latin poem that, many years later, gave the disease its familiar name, syphilis. Projected in the early 1510s, but not published until 1530, *Syphilis sive morbus Gallicus, Syphilis or the French Disease*, is a poem in three books by the Veronese physician, Girolamo Fracastoro (1478–1553) (Figure 1.3).[94] Although he acknowledged the horrible nature of the disease, the fact that he could make an extremely elegant (and well received) poem out of it shows that it no longer held the same terrors it once had. In the first book, he explains the astral causes of the pox and its symptoms, expounding, in very preliminary way, the ideas on contagion that he was to develop further over the following decades and that will be discussed later in more detail, later (pp. 225–8). His model was the Roman poet Lucretius, whose exposition of Epicurean philosophy combined factual detail with literary digressions. So, in Book Two Fracastoro not only described the various ways in which the disease was treated but also ended it with the story of the discovery of the healing properties of mercury by a hunter and keeper of a sacred garden, Ilceus, aided by the nymph Callirhoe.[95] The third book is concerned with another discovery, that of guaiac, by the sailors of Columbus on their first voyage to Hispaniola. They first encountered sufferers from the disease when they were attending a feast with the natives, who told them how they had learned to cure it by drinking decoctions of guaiac. The second part of the book contains the story of the shepherd Syphilus, who having prayed in vain to the Sun and the other gods for relief for his flocks from the heat of summer, turned in prayer to the king. King Alcithous, highly pleased with the sacrifices made to himself, then forbade the worship of other deities. The Sun in anger sent the new disease on the kingdom and on its first victim, Syphilus. Only when everyone had repented and set up a festival in honour of the gods did Juno send from heaven the seeds of a tree that would end their suffering. While in this part of the poem, Fracastoro imagines an American origin for the disease, a claim that first appeared in print only a matter of months before the poem was published, he then goes on to describe the amazement of the sailors on their return to Europe that the same disease was already rampant there. The poem ends with further praise of guaiac as a powerful remedy.

Although *Syphilis* adumbrates much of what Fracastoro was to conclude in his later notes and writings on this disease, including his conviction that

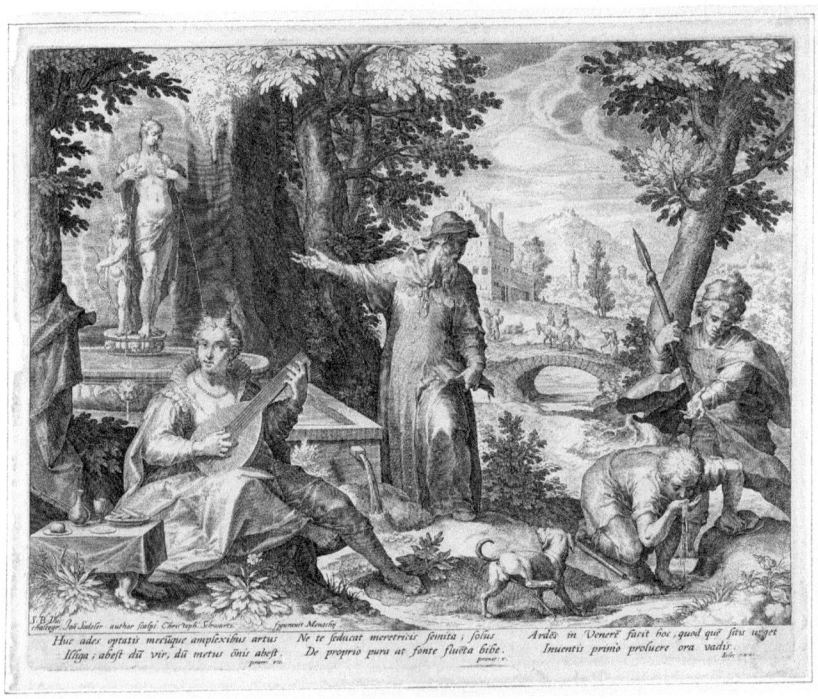

Figure 1.3 Girolamo Fracastoro shows the shepherd Syphilus and the hunter Ilceus a statue of Venus to warn them against the danger of infection with the pox. The warnings below are versifications of biblical injunctions against immorality. Engraving by Jan Sadeler I, around 1588/1595, after Christoph Schwartz.

the European outbreak was not, as some suggested, the result of contact with the Americas, it should be considered above all as a poem.[96] It shows his mastery of a variety of genres within the poem – the two small epics, the lament for lost youths, praise of his native land, as well as anguish over recent political and military catastrophes – that would have been instantly recognised by his learned contemporaries.[97] It turns what had been, and still often was, a painful tragedy for those who suffered from the disease into literary entertainment to be appreciated by those for whom the worst was in the past. It was now a disease that one could live with.

The English Sweat

If doctors in the sixteenth century were reasonably confident themselves about the origins, transmission and treatment of the French pox among the new diseases singled out by Erasmus, this could not be said of another one, the English Sweat, whose identification remains almost as problematic today as it did then. DNA analysis has so far failed to resolve the debate about whether it was some kind of viral disease, and about its relationship with other equally problematic diseases from Britain and Northern France such as the (later) Picardy Sweat.[98] The first detailed description of the English Sweat, by the Rouen physician Thomas Le Forestier, described it as a "pestilential rabid fever" that arrived in London in 1485 among the troops that had landed from France with Henry Tudor on his way to defeat Richard III at the battle of Bosworth Field.[99] He had observed it in London, and wrote a short tract first in English soon after, and then repeated his observations in a Latin version in 1490/1 and in French in 1495.[100] His explanation was the standard one for any plague: divine punishment and a planetary conjunction, and he followed Avicenna and the Arabs in describing the humoral imbalances that were thus produced. His English version also emphasised the filthy condition of London's streets and the speed with which "false lechys" took advantage of a frightened population to sell their services, even advertising their remedies on church doors.[101] Three things distinguished this plague from others. It was characterised by a fever and a continuous sweat, with pains in the back, limbs and liver. It came on very suddenly, and death occurred often within 12 hours: people dropped dead in the street before they could even make their confession. Not surprisingly, some compared it with poison, and, like John Caius later, recommended further sweating to follow nature's way of driving out the venom. The third unusual feature of the Sweat was that it frequently attacked boys and young men in the prime of life.[102]

Le Forestier may have been wrong in his supposition that the disease originated in France, for there is evidence of an outbreak of a pestilential fever in the north of England before Henry's landing in summer 1485, but the army, like the French army after their capture of Naples, may have been the major vector. This would account for deaths in rural England and in towns such as St Albans along their route south.[103] It then seems to have disappeared until 1508, but there were subsequent outbreaks in 1517, 1528 and 1551, after which nothing further is recorded. Despite Le Forestier's fears, only the outbreak of 1528 seems to have spread to the continent, where it ravaged the Netherlands, Germany and Switzerland in 1529–30, unless the infection had an independent origin somewhere in the Baltic region.[104] It was probably the expectation of another major continental outbreak that impelled John Caius to publish at Louvain in 1556 a Latin version of his 1552 English treatise for the benefit of his European colleagues who could not read English.[105]

All writers stress the speed with which the initial symptoms were often followed by death within a matter of hours. Those who joked at lunchtime might be dead before dinner. No one was safe, whether they fled to the countryside or shut themselves up at home. Anyone might be attacked, but it was often those in the prime of life and the wealthy who were most affected (or whose demise was most noticeable). Two Lord Mayors of London died in 1495, and many members of the court and judiciary died in 1517.[106] Caius, who gives a very detailed account of the outbreak of 1551, says that most who died were "either men of welthe, ease and welfare, or of the poorer sorte such as wer idle persones, good ale drinkers, and Tauerne haunters," hence the common term for the disease 'Stopgallant'.[107] Ever the curmudgeonly conservative looking back to the good old days of merry England, he put the blame less on the poison in the air than on modern lifestyle. He recommended a fish diet above all, but

> we are nowe a daies so vnwisely fine and womanly delicate, that we may in no wise touch a fisshe. The olde manly hardnes, stoute courage and peinfulnes of Englande is vtterly driuen awaye, in the stede whereof, men now a daies receive womanliness and become nice, not able to withstande a blaste of wynde or resiste a poor fisshe. And children be so brought vp, that, if they be not all daie by the fire with a toste and butire, and in their furres, they be streight sicke.[108]

Parish records have extended Caius's remarkable account, although they say nothing about hot buttered toast. They show a pattern of spread from the Welsh border in both north-westerly and south-easterly directions, and from London westwards along the Thames valley. Deaths occurred in small clusters, often with many fatalities within the same household, and usually over a short period. The Sweat lingered on beyond September 1551, Caius's terminal date, and there may have been other isolated outbreaks between 1528 and 1551. There is a preponderance of males in the London records; although, apart from the deaths of two young relatives of Henry VIII, there was no aristocratic massacre to compare with 1517. Overall mortality appears to have been relatively low, around 2%, and many places were not touched, but the epidemic of 1551 was long remembered and used as a measure in later outbreaks of epidemic disease.[109]

Neither Le Forestier nor Caius says much about any public action on the part of the authorities, except to bemoan its absence. The response in the Netherlands and Germany was very different, in part, as we shall see (p. 47), because of their more sophisticated administrative structure and higher literacy.[110] Doctors throughout the region swiftly produced short plague regimens against the Sweat, sometimes at the behest of local rulers or simply providing local versions of the writings of others. John Flood counts at least 89 such productions, often from areas remote from the immediate path of the disease, evidence of the higher literate culture and market for self-help literature there compared with England as well as the fear that this disease instilled in those already familiar with plague. In 1529 Northern Europe could also draw on the experiences of England the previous year, and the authorities in Lubeck may have been assisted in their response by an English ex-friar, Robert Barnes, an Evangelical exile from Henry VIII.[111]

The Sweat arrived first in the Netherlands at Antwerp, and it was to Antwerp that the doctors further west in Ghent wrote to see what advice its physicians could offer. Their answer was discouraging. Most doctors had already fled from Antwerp with their families, some had died, and the rest were occupied day and night with treating the sick. Jacobus Castricus, the town physician, however, did send his own short response to Ghent, recommending similar treatment to that for plague. He was joined in the fight against the disease in Antwerp by two other local doctors, Jean Thibault and the much more famous Heinrich Cornelius Agrippa von Nettesheim (1486–1535). Agrippa had the sad experience of having his wife die of the disease, which he described in a letter to one of her relatives, Guillaume Furbity, in Paris. Both this letter and that of Castricus to Ghent were quickly printed in Paris in case the Sweat should break out there. Both pamphlets emphasised the experiences of their authors, that of Agrippa also having been shown to and improved by other doctors both in Antwerp and at the Burgundian court in nearby Mechlen. The ending of the Sweat was marked in Antwerp by a woodcut produced by an Antwerp designer, Dirk Vellert. It shows Castricus, flanked by Theory and Practice, sitting in a chariot under a triumphal arch, while Melissa (a honey balm), Mint and Artemisia lead their beasts over the prostrate and chained emblematic bodies of Plague, Fever and Dropsy. This unusual woodcut, even if somewhat fanciful in its detail, attests the relief felt at the departure of the Sweat and the gratitude felt to the town physician. Agrippa gained a more lucrative reward, posts as physician to Margaret of Burgundy (who, alas, died the next year) and then as physician to the Archbishop of Cologne. Thibault fared less well, being involved in disputes in both Flanders and Paris over his astrological prognostications before his death in 1544 or shortly afterwards.[112]

New and Old Diseases

Both syphilis and the Sweat caused confusion and fear when they first appeared as both the general public and their doctors tried to make sense of them against the background of earlier diseases, particularly plague. Some emphasised the role of divine punishment, while others looked for precedents in the medical classics, whether those deriving from Antiquity or from more recent attempts to deal with plague.[113] By the middle of the century, however, doctors and officials had become more sophisticated in their understanding of widespread diseases, beginning with Fracastoro's *De contagione et morbis contagiosis*, *Contagion and Contagious Diseases*, of 1546, and were applying new insights to the study of new and unfamiliar diseases.[114] The range of possibilities can be seen in the publications of two German physicians, Thomas Jordanus and Johannes Lange.[115]

Originally from Transylvania, Jordanus (1540–86) (Figure 1.4) obtained a medical degree in 1562 at the French University of Valence (at the same time as the botanist Leonhard Rauwolf) before returning East. He served for a time in the Hungarian army in the Turkish campaign of 1566, describing an outbreak of disease in the army, the so-called *lues Pannonica*, the Hungarian pestilence (probably exanthematous typhus), before becoming Chief Physician, *Protomedicus*, of Moravia in 1570.[116] He was in close contact with the doctors at the court of the Holy Roman Emperor, corresponding with Johannes Crato von Crafftheim (1519–85), one of the Emperor's chief physicians, and dedicating his second book, *Luis novae in Moravia exortae descriptio*, *A Description of an Outbreak of a New Pestilence in Moravia*, to another, Julius Alexandrinus (1506–1590). In it he described at length the localised outbreak of a contagious skin disease at Brünn, the capital of Moravia, now Brno (Czech Republic), in 1577. After a lyrical account of the beauties of the city and region, a second Eden, were it not for the high mineral content of the local streams, which encouraged the inhabitants to eschew water in favour of wine and beer, Jordanus uses the events there to advise how best to deal with an apparently new disease.[117] Not only was he familiar with the literature on syphilis (which he calls the disease of the Indies), the English Sweat and other diseases, but, while a schoolboy, he had seen his teacher fall ill with a new disease which subsequently spread from Transylvania to Austria, Germany and, briefly, Italy, but not to France.[118]

Most of the book deals in lively Latin prose with the circumstances of the outbreak and with his ultimately successful attempts to restrain it in the face of unlicensed practitioners "crowding in like vultures around a corpse", Paracelsians, Anabaptists and recalcitrant patients.[119] The disease, which manifested itself quickly in the form of sores and purulent ulcers, joint pains and sometimes serious prostration that might last for weeks, affected all classes of society. Although it resembled syphilis in many ways and could be cured similarly by sweating and the use of guaiac wood, Jordanus was convinced that it was not the same disease. Given that his patients included

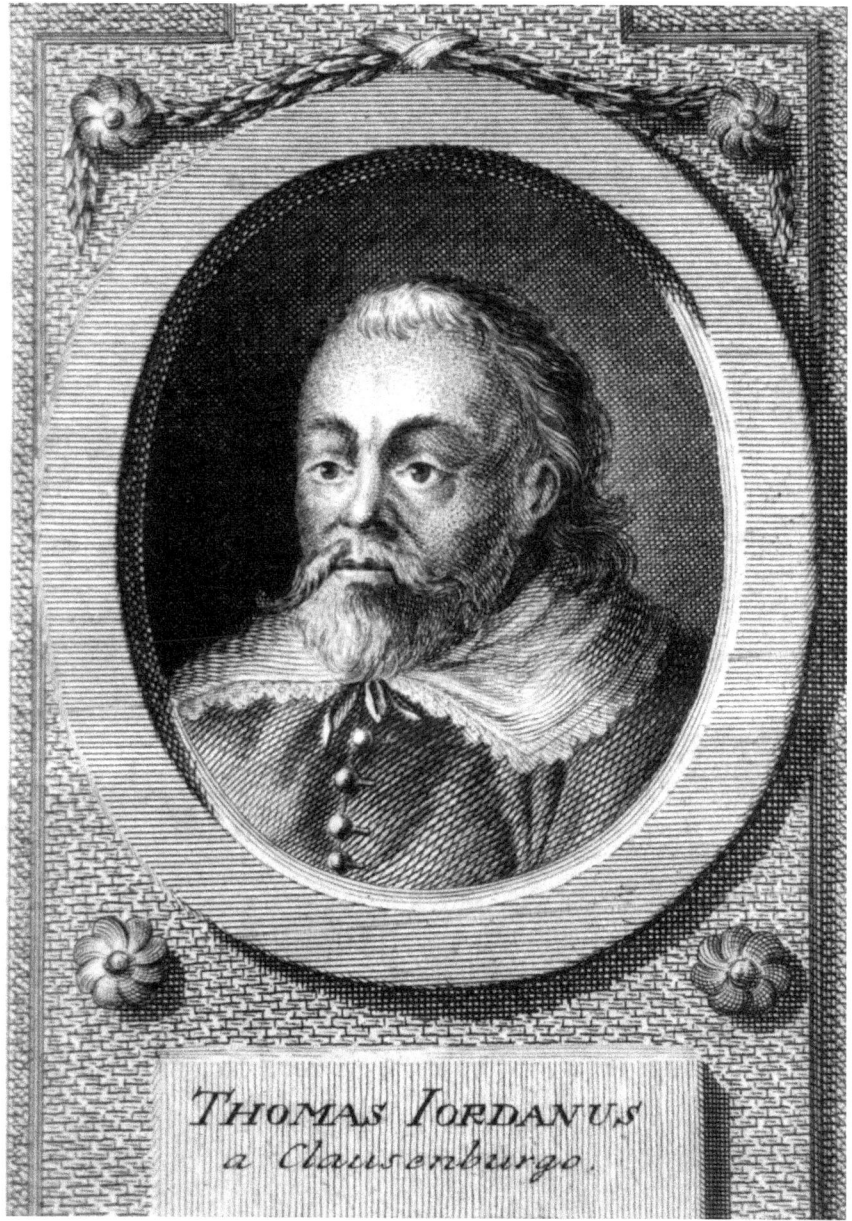

Figure 1.4 Thomas Jordanus (1540–86), chief doctor of Moravia. Copyright The National Library of Medicine, Bethesda, MD. Public Domain Mark.

old ladies and the wives and virginal daughters of highly respected citizens, the disease, as he put it bluntly, did not emerge from the vulva to be spread by sexual intercourse.[120] Even if he was wrong in his diagnosis, his observational skills and his arguments are remarkably acute for their day.

Brno had at least three bathing establishments, one just outside the Jewish or Green Gate and frequented by the upper classes, and two others at the foot of the castle hill, fed by a chalky mineral spring with a reputation for whitening the skin and "favoured by those who prefer pleasure to utility". It was during the holiday that followed St Lucy's Day, 13 December 1577, that the disease broke out among the crowds who came to bathe at the Green Gate Baths and to be bled to improve their health in preparation for Christmas. Many became infected, 80 from the town, 100 from the suburbs and an unknown, and almost certainly larger, number from the countryside. The immediate conclusion was that they had been poisoned by the owner of the establishment. But after Jordanus had persuaded them that the unfortunate owner was not to blame, and that neither the buildings nor the instruments used for bleeding were poisonous, the angry crowd turned on his young assistant who had performed the bleeding. Suspected of being the source of infection, he fled to Germany, but despite searches for him in Wrocław, Nuremberg and elsewhere, he was never caught. The baths were reopened after the owner had thoroughly cleaned them and, indeed, rebuilt parts, but they had to be closed again when new cases began to reappear. To Jordanus's annoyance, the owner, whom he had done so much to defend, soon afterwards began a new business there as a specialist in the treatment of this new disease. Only after several weeks did the outbreak come to an end, and, even then, some of its consequences in individuals continued much longer.[121]

Jordanus instructed his readers what to do if they were faced with a similarly new disease. Their first task was to decide whether it was indeed previously unknown, something which required delving into the literature, both ancient and modern and, for Jordanus, the writings of Fracastoro. Only then could one proceed to the next stage of classifying its type, and then to identify its cause or causes and an appropriate therapy.[122] Jordanus argued that the cause of the outbreak in Brno was some 'seed' of the disease that had been brought in by one of the filthy peasants who came in from the countryside at weekends. The poor standards of hygiene in the baths allowed the contagion to spread, particularly in the cooler rooms, and the infection was spread still more by the fomites adhering to the cupping glasses and scalpels that were used in bleeding and had not been sufficiently cleaned.[123] This explained why most of those who fell ill had also been cupped there, some in many places at the same time, since this created openings in the body and allowed the 'little seeds' to pass easily under the skin. Individual balance of humours further explained why some suffered more severe reactions than others.[124] Although he had been concerned initially about people wandering away from the city on public business or going to a horse fair, the cleaning and subsequent closure of the baths prevented the disease from spreading widely beyond Moravia.[125]

Many other doctors faced with an unfamiliar illness had recourse to their classical texts to find precedents. Johannes Lange (1485–1565), the long-serving professor at Heidelberg and physician to the Elector Palatine, was perhaps the first to deal in detail with the so-called *scherbock*, or land-scurvy (caused by the lack of vitamin C), which he had heard was endemic in Norway, Denmark and other Baltic regions.[126] He was particularly interested in the ancient question, discussed by Plutarch, as to whether new diseases could exist. Like Leoniceno, he believed that all known diseases had long been discovered, asking whether the 300 diseases affecting mankind in Antiquity were not sufficient. Sure enough, he found ancient precedents in Pliny, Strabo and Galen in their descriptions of similar diseases that had caused teeth to fall out and limbs to become weaker. But he was also aware of recent literature, praising Fracastoro's book on contagious diseases and drawing attention to the prevalence of 'sporadic' diseases that, like the Sweat, appeared to come and go at irregular intervals.[127]

A second, and much more problematic, identification by Lange of a modern disease with an ancient one proved more influential, for it led to the creation of a possible imaginary disease entity that had a long life of its own: 'green sickness' or 'chlorosis'. Writing in response to the letter of a father about the illness of his nubile daughter, who was wasting away with a pallid complexion, palpitations, depression, shortness of breath and oedema in the legs after sleeping, Lange asserted that this was no new condition: it was, he had been told, already familiar to women in Brabant who called it 'the white sickness' or even 'the love sickness'.[128] He found a precursor for his treatment of what he called '*morbus virgineus*', 'a disease of young girls', in the Hippocratic treatise *The Diseases of Girls*, where a similar condition was associated with a failure to menstruate. The consequent blockage of blood produced harmful changes within the body, visible particularly in digestive disorders and increasingly poor health. This consultation with Lange was typical in being made at long distance by letter. Here, because the information was solely provided by the father, eager to secure a good marriage for the girl, one cannot be sure that he had disclosed all relevant symptoms. Helen King has shown how much Lange manipulated his Hippocratic text to fit the symptoms: one may suspect that he was equally concerned in his publication of the letter to fit the symptoms to his ancient text.[129] But even if his diagnosis was correct, others, not only in Brabant, were commenting on similar conditions. In England, women of various ages had been said to be affected by a 'green jaundice', a disease of the liver and stomach. By 1557 this 'green sickness' was being termed a new disease and had lost the connection with jaundice, although it was not yet specifically associated either with young women or menstrual disorders. But Lange's association of it with young women was soon widely accepted among learned physicians, aided by the publication of his letter in two large collections, one exclusively devoted to women's diseases. The amalgamation of his 'disease of young girls' or, on another translation 'disease of virgins', with the 'green sickness' was also helped by the presence of adjectives signifying a greenish or pale colour in classical and medieval descriptions of lovesickness. By the end of the century, at least one physician was referring to the condition as 'chlorosis', a term coined from the Greek, and its transformation into a specific disease entity was almost complete.[130]

Lange, Jordanus and other sixteenth-century writers on new diseases were concerned solely with those that they saw in Europe, whether engendered locally or arriving from outside, and said nothing about the arguably even more devastating diseases brought from Europe to the New World. This was not surprising as the Conquistadors were little concerned with the health of the natives they encountered, and it is largely modem historians basing themselves on archival and archaeological data who have revealed the enormous extent of the epidemic catastrophe there. Famine and disease are estimated to have reduced the native population of Santo Domingo (Columbus's first landfall) from a million in 1492 to insignificant numbers 40 years later.[131] Smallpox, brought ashore by the Spaniards from Cuba at Vera Cruz in 1521, helped to facilitate Cortés's capture of Tenochtitlan, the capital of Mexico, and spread as a pandemic throughout Southern Mexico and Central America, killing millions before 1530. Millions more died of measles in Southern Mexico between 1530 and 1534. Typhus, the "great matlazahuatl" followed in 1545. Raging for several years, along with other infectious diseases such as malaria, which became endemic along the coast, it destroyed almost all the remaining Indian population, according to some observers. Even if numbers recovered a little in the third quarter of the century, further epidemics affecting the whole of Mexico reduced the natives to little more than a million.[132] Their harsh treatment at the hands of their conquerors, as well as social and geographical dislocation, added to their difficulties, while the imposition in New Spain of medical controls and organisation appropriate for Europe placed obstacles in the way of traditional *curanderos*.[133] In the mining centres of Northern Mexico it was the Jesuit missionaries who alone provided assistance in major epidemics of smallpox and measles in 1593–4, turning their residences in some of the villages into makeshift hospitals and reaping their reward in ever more converts.[134]

The expansion of the geographical, social, commercial and intellectual horizons in the sixteenth century involved a complex interplay between different types of knowledge and different experiences. It was a long and tortuous process of discovery. Alongside the great voyages of discovery to both East and West can be set the opening up of Northern Europe, to say nothing of publications describing largely unknown or unfamiliar parts of countries further south. But what was found could at first only be understood within older templates. The new natural world, including medicinal substances and new diseases, still required to be interpreted in categories that went back to ancient Greece and Rome and which had gained added authority from the rediscovery and publication particularly of Greek writings unknown or mistranslated for centuries. Garcia D'Orta in his experiences with native healers and native drugs in Goa or the Jesuit missionaries attempting to make sense of Nahuatl medicine in an era of devastating epidemics in Mexico faced severe problems in communicating successfully to Europeans what they had discovered. But by the last quarter of the century, more and more of this new information had become assimilated, despite the dominant institutions in medicine remaining largely wedded to traditional learning. But even traditionalists now expected a steady increase in knowledge and consequently a still greater superiority over those less qualified who offered healing to an ever-growing population.[135]

Notes

1 Manardi, *Ep.* VII, 1: 1556: 39–43, written from Buda in 1514. The subsequent doctoral examination itself had to be cancelled because of the outbreak of war between France and Venice in 1509. For his later views on the importance of the Portuguese voyages, *Ep.* XV, 5: 1556: 260–1 (of 1532).
2 Cagle 2018: 31–2, 39–47. For Spain, Huguet-Termes 2001: 359.
3 Manardi, *Ep.* VII, 1: 1556: 42. For some owners of his *Epistulae*, see Figure 3.2.
4 Egmond 2018a.
5 For Russian penetration of Siberia, Darwin 2007: 68–72; Monahan 2016: 43–9, 78–84. For contemporary understanding of Muscovy, Herberstein 1871–2, originally 1549.
6 Grafton 1992: 1.
7 Sanches 1581: 40.
8 Ramusio 1550–9, showing how little of the traditional world picture was now accepted by scholars; Cooper 2007: 3–20.
9 Abreu 2020 discusses the transfer of Portuguese medical institutions to its Indian empire. For Venetian doctors in the Levant, Pugliano 2019.
10 Clark 1964: 126; Goodwin and Bevan 2004; Stone 2004; Stout 2015.
11 Cuspinianus 1553: for the wider background, see Strauss 1959; Hale 1994: 28–38; Cooper 2007: 14–15; and for Cuspinianus as historian, Siraisi 2007: 199–206, although she does not mention his *Austria*.
12 Caius 1574d: 115–35; 1912: 93–109; Grafton 2017; Nutton 2017b; for English topographers, Rowse 1950: 49–86. Caius's lost *History of Norwich* would have similarly combined history and topography.
13 There is a substantial recent literature on Gessner; Serrai 1990 remains fundamental as a bibliography of his writings. His ideas and influence are explored by Delisle 2008; Leu 2016a; Leu and Ruoss 2016; Funk 2021.
14 Aa.vv. 1553: 289r–99r; Stefanizzi 2011; Danzi 2016.
15 Turner 1562, with Dietz Moss 2012; Caius 1570d: 25v, 1912: 100; Nutton 2017b: 77, 101, summarises his own book *On British Baths*, which was substantially completed by 1561 but never published.
16 For the growth of botanical correspondence networks, Findlen 1999, 2017; and the special focus issue of *Jahrbuch für Europäische Wissenschaftskultur* 6: 2011.
17 Bright 1580; Keynes 1962: 3–4; Wear 2000: 65–6, 75–6.
18 Braudel 1972: 543–70 is a classic account of the Eastern spice trade in the sixteenth century.
19 Grunberg 2006: 160–5.

20 Brasavola 1561: 567, 618; Munger 1949; Huguet-Termes 2001: 362–3, lists only six drugs exported to Spain before 1540: guaiac, tobacco, purgative nuts, cannafistula, new balsam and mechoacan root. For syphilis, Baker *et al.* 2020.
21 Fisch *et al.* 1947; Schmaus 1518; Von Hutten 1519, 2015; Moëll 1984.
22 Stein 2009: 147–52, 101–14 demolishes the myth of the Fugger guaiac monopoly.
23 Brasavola 1561: 578.
24 Martínez Navarro 2018, discussing the *Loor del palo de Indias* of Cristóbal de Castillejo (1491–1556).
25 Vesalius 1546, 2015.
26 See pp. 101–3 for the wider significance of this debate.
27 Marcellus 1518: f. 136v. For his dispute with Manardi over Dioscorides, God-man 1998: 228–33; Grafton 2001: 5–9.
28 Manardi *Epp.* V, 5: cf. VI, 2 (of 1504), defending the Greeks against Arabic pharmacologists, but admitting he and they may not have known all the plants the Arabs did; *Ep.* XVII, 6 (of 1533) for its use; Manardi 1556: 27–8, 31, 176.
29 Brasavola 1536: 2r–3v; 99r (glasses); Turner 1551: 121v–2r.
30 Foust 1992: 8–14; for Russian rhubarb, Monahan 2021.
31 Cagle 2018: 87–92.
32 Morel 1528: sig. D i.v.
33 Morel 1528: 240–5.
34 Arber 1986 is still useful; Cooper 2007: 32–8. For Fuchs, see Brinckhus and Pachnicke 2001.
35 London, Wellcome Collection, EPB 2438.
36 Mattioli 1544.
37 Mattioli 1550, 1554.
38 Mattioli 1573, 1583 (Latin), 1562 (Czech); Ferri 1997; Fausti 2004; Preti 2009; Kusukawa 2012.
39 Cibo, London, British Library, Add. Ms. 22332–3; Tongiorgi Tomasi 1989.
40 Palmer 1985.
41 Findlen 1996: 181.
42 Cooper 2007: 21–40.
43 Turner 1562: 41r, 157r; Raven 1947: 162–5; Jones 1988, 2004. For Penny and Gessner, Funk 2021, doubtful of the visit to Majorca.
44 Borgarucci 1566: 182–3.
45 Findlen 1996: 160–5.
46 Rauwolf 1582; Walter *et al.* 2021.
47 Reeds 1991; Grendler 2002: 347–51.
48 Burckhardt 1917: 34, 134; Benkert 2020: 66–7. The reality may have been different: nothing further is known of inspecting apothecaries' shops until 1564, and a herborizing expedition was not until 1578/9.
49 Muratori and Menini 1947: 47, 54.
50 Findlen 1996: 232–61; Egmond 2021.
51 Triebs 1995: 45. For a town's requirement for the civic physician to tend his own herb garden, see p. 47.
52 Benkert 2020.
53 Brunfels 1530: 15, and Appendix, sig. A 1r.
54 Cooper 2007: 21–41, noting also the rhetoric directed by Paracelsians against many of the common remedies sold by apothecaries.
55 Huguet-Termes 2001: 363.
56 Monardes 1580, ff. 100v–1v; for sassafras, Griffin 2020.
57 Emmart 1940.
58 López Piñero and Pardo Tomás 1996.
59 Beecher 2015.

60 Shaw and Welch 2011: 298–300, 305; Roberts 1965: 170. Thurneisser's comparison in 1574 of old and new remedies is silent about exotic imports, Thurneisser 1574: 52–77.
61 Huguet-Termes 2001: 366–75.
62 Garcia D'Orta 1563, 1567.
63 Nobre de Carvalho 2015.
64 Cagle 2018: 86–97; Abreu 2020.
65 Cagle 2018: 135–8.
66 Cagle 2018: 163–4.
67 Cagle 2018: 97.
68 Findlen 1996: 268.
69 For discussions of the non-epidemic disease pattern, see pp. 236–8.
70 Huguet-Termes 2001: 362–3; Stolberg 2021a: 197, 298–302.
71 Baker *et al.* 2020 provide a good overview of the *status quaestionis*, rejecting both the pre-Columbian and evolutionary hypotheses, but suggesting that the disease was already present in Europe (or globally), even if its recorded manifestations might differ.
72 Erasmus *Epp.* 1593: 2209: Allen VI, 135–7; VIII, 266–7. See also notes 114–16; and Stevenson 1965: 1–4 for 'new' diseases.
73 Caius 1552: 14–15, gives an English view of this last outbreak as the result of bodies being buried hastily.
74 Boaistuau 1570: 120–5; Hobart 2020: 537–84.
75 For Augsburg in late 1495; Stein 2009: 1.
76 Arrizabalaga *et al.* 1997: 26–7.
77 Erasmus, *Ep.* 1593: Allen VI, 137.
78 Arrizabalaga *et al.* 1997: 56–87.
79 Leoniceno 1497.
80 Gilino 1497.
81 Arrizabalaga *et al.* 1997: 91–7, 113–44.
82 Arrizabalaga *et al.* 1997: 270–1. For German debates, Stein 2009: 14–34.
83 Arrizabalaga *et al.* 1997: 50–2.
84 Temkin 1977: 472–5; Stein 2009: 24–9.
85 Brasavola 1561: 470, 473, combines both explanations, blaming a single very beautiful prostitute who infected every French soldier who lay with her.
86 Hale 1994: 499.
87 Erasmus, *Ep.* 2285; Allen VIII, 383.
88 Hale 1994: 506.
89 Brasavola 1561: 420–43, a long list of possible combinations of symptoms.
90 Brasavola 1561: 718; Arrizabalaga *et al.* 1997: 267–9.
91 Brasavola 1561: 637; for a change in the disease around 1520, Fracastoro 1546: 49v.
92 Brasavola 1561: 503.
93 Temkin 1977: 520, 477; MacCulloch 2003: 631–2; Stolberg 2021a: 295–302. Stein 2009: 203, points out that the Fuggers' imperial grant of a monopoly over the land where mercury was found provided them with far greater profits than any trade in guaiac.
94 Fracastoro 1530, 1984.
95 Contemporaries would have understood the finder's name as related to the Greek word for 'sore', *helkos*, Latin '*ulcus*'.
96 Fracastoro 1546: 50v takes issue with believers in the American theory, which became widely accepted, e.g. Jordanus 1580: 50, 57, 70.
97 Fracastoro 1984: 20–7; Gigliotti 1990; Cairns 1994. Frank 2003.
98 Wylie and Collier 1981; Carmichael 1993a: 1023–5, 1993b; Dyer 1997; Taviner *et al.* 1998; Heyman *et al.* 2018.

99 Le Forestier 1490?: sig. a iir.
100 Wylie and Collier's 1981 English version is taken from the still unpublished London, British Library Add. Ms 27582, fols. 70r–7v, dedicated to Henry VII. Its date, like that of the printed texts, is not entirely certain.
101 Walton 1981, 1982.
102 Le Forestier 1490?: sigg. a iir, b i v, expanding on his "*opusculum*".
103 Wylie and Collier 1981: 428–9.
104 Wylie and Collier 1981: 433–5, noting the differences between the English and continental data. Caius 1552: 16 has an outbreak on the Continent in 1549, but this is a misprint (or a wrong dating) for 1529.
105 Caius 1552, 1556, both reprinted in Caius 1912. At 1556: 126: he noted that an exodus of foreigners from London was not followed by any major outbreak in Europe or Scotland.
106 Caius 1556: 124; Wylie and Collier 1981: 426–31. The Sweat was included in the public prayers against plague in the English Book of Common Prayer of 1662, which is still in use today.
107 Caius 1552: 19. For an example of the use of the term in rural Devon, Dyer 1997: 365.
108 Caius 1552: 29, 22.
109 Dyer 1997.
110 Müller-Jahncke 1983; Flood 2003.
111 Flood 2003; Clemen 1923 discusses the evidence from Zwickau, which had 14 deaths and over 100 more cases in late July.
112 Müller-Jahncke 1983.
113 Stein 2014.
114 Nutton 1990d: see further, pp. 225–8.
115 Cf. the discussion of 'new' and 'unknown' diseases in Weyer 1567, 1583, with Hieronymus 2005: 3, 1826–33.
116 Győry 1912: 4; Offner 2018. For the earlier disease, Győry 1901.
117 Jordanus 1580 (originally 1578): for excessive consumption of beer and wine, p. 7. But his preface complains of a certain intellectual provincialism.
118 Jordanus 1580: 50–2. What his teacher died of is far from clear.
119 Jordanus 1580: 10.
120 Jordanus 1580: 100; for female patients 46, 57–8; for suspicion that syphilis might have been involved, *ibid*. 21, 84. His friend Andreas Dudith continued to refer to it as the French disease, Crato 1592: 276–9. For syphilis as the probable cause, Győry 1912: 30–5. Jordanus did not allow for any non-sexual method of transmission, which is much rarer.
121 Jordanus 1580: 11–21.
122 Jordanus 1580: 75, 82–4, 89–92.
123 For people bringing their own instruments to the baths to be bled, Hale 1994: 543.
124 Jordanus 1580: 66, 70, 79–80. For seeds and fomites, see pp. 225–8.
125 For Jordanus's plan in 1579 to examine all the spas in Moravia, Crato 1592: 281–2. Cf. also Dudith 2002: 306–7, for some reactions to his book.
126 Lange, *Ep*. I, 42; II, 13–14: 1589: 209–10, 613–21, including information from Johann Echtius of Cologne, to whom is usually attributed the first description of scurvy at sea in 1541. For Lange, Siraisi 2013: 38–60.
127 Cf. Lange's identification of the Sweat with Galen's typhoid, *Ep*. I, 19–20: 1589: 93–9. The anonymous author of a tract on the Sweat, "his first book", whom he calls a pseudo-medic, is probably Joachim Schiller (1531), whose slim tract was followed by a work on plague, rather than Agrippa von Nettesheim.

128 Lange, *Ep.* I, 21: 1589: 100–5; King 2004. The letter itself is undated and has no addressee.
129 King 1998: 188–204.
130 King 2004.
131 Wolf 1997: 133; Livi Bacci 2008: 41–2, 96–9.
132 Ramenovsky 1987; Bray 1996: 123–32; Cook 1998; Reff 2005: 125–7; Wolf 1997: 133; Livi Bacci 2008: 46–63, 140–3. Depopulation in Peru may have involved different epidemiological factors, Livi Bacci 2008: 186–91. For possible similar depopulation from plague in Western Siberia at the same time, Monahan 2016: 58.
133 Slater *et al.* 2014; Pardo Tomás 2012 discusses some cultural interactions.
134 Reff 2005: 167–71; Livi Bacci 2008: 126–38.
135 How this knowledge was communicated is the theme of chapter 3.

2 Protecting the Health of the City

The growing involvement of government, particularly at a local level, in wider matters of public health is one of the major developments in medicine in the Later Middle Ages and Early Renaissance. The public face of medicine in 1600 was considerably different from what it had been in 1400. Except in the British Isles, always slow to adopt continental practices, almost all medium-sized towns, and many smaller ones, now employed at least one town physician. Especially in Italy there were Health Boards, some of them permanent, charged with dealing with medical crises, particularly epidemics, and employing complex and sophisticated measures to prevent them or at least mitigate their severity. Alongside the older, smaller hospitals that provided warmth, shelter and food for the elderly and destitute, there developed others that were larger and more medicalised, sometimes treating only one type of invalid or becoming the focus for medical services throughout a city and its region. There were new universities and professional colleges ambitious to impose the new medical learning on all who might offer some form of medical assistance to their community. In Spain and in Spanish South Italy a royal medical appointee, a *protomedico*, gradually came to take over not only the role of licensing practitioners of various kinds, but also to oversee almost all aspects of medicine, including public health.[1] These developments were made possible by the growing wealth of towns and their increasing civic cohesion, or, as in sixteenth-century England or Germany, by the desire of rulers to emulate what was happening in Italy. This chapter will focus particularly on town physicians, Health Boards and hospitals, for they were often interconnected and co-operated together, particularly in the face of epidemic diseases such as plague, whose frequent ravages affected the whole community, and not just those who caught the disease.[2]

Plague

The major catalyst for all these changes was the arrival of the Black Death in Western Europe in 1347 and its subsequent spread over the next four years.[3] Very few towns in Northern and Central Europe escaped untouched in the first outbreak, and elsewhere over half the population may have succumbed.

DOI: 10.4324/9781003223184-4

Towns and villages were deserted, and the economic consequences lasted for decades. Recent palaeopathological investigations have confirmed that this plague was caused by the *yersinia pestis* bacillus, spread usually by fleas feeding on infected rodents (and even humans) and transmitted by them or, in pneumonic plague, its most serious form, by droplet transmission directly between humans.[4] It is a largely seasonal disease, at its worst in this period in Europe between spring and autumn, but the extraordinarily labile structure of the bacillus RNA, perhaps allied to some form of individual immunity, explains its very varied occurrence, morbidity and mortality. Symptoms differed from patient to patient or might be so slight (or indeed non-existent) that they failed to attract medical attention immediately. Retrospective diagnosis of observations by Renaissance writers is further complicated by their use of a wide range of terms whose meaning was clear only to locals or which were so all-embracing, like 'plague' or 'pestilence', that they cover what today may be classified as different diseases.[5] Plague might appear at first in a locality in an unusual form that defied identification even to those who were familiar with its symptoms. In 1559 a previously unknown 'bloody flux' carried off 168 victims at Dresden, but by 1566 Johann Neefe (1499–1574), doctor to the ruler of Saxony, was confident enough to claim that this was merely one symptom of plague, and thus treatable.[6] But even if its speed and pattern of spread differed considerably from what is found in outbreaks today, Renaissance doctors were convinced that they, and many other people, could identify plague when they saw it ·· or had merely heard rumours of it in neighbouring regions.[7]

They were also far more familiar with plague than all but specialists today, for plague had quickly become endemic in Europe, even if its manifestations varied from year to year and from location to location. Doctors at Nördlingen in Central Germany in 1571 distinguished between two types of outbreak: one, usually occurring after a famine, attacked mainly the poor and malnourished; the other, rare and much more dangerous, carried off the wealthy also. A Nuremberg chronicler of 1544 made a similar social distinction, glossing a "little" plague with "But only the poor died in large numbers".[8] The chronology of plague established by Jean-Noel Biraben in 1975–6, supplemented by a multitude of local studies, suggests that a town of 10,000 or 12,000 inhabitants might see one or two cases most years, a minor outbreak every decade, and a substantial visitation once a generation.[9] The pioneering work of English demographers, exploiting Elizabethan parish registers, allows a more nuanced interpretation. Trading and coastal towns fared badly since they were most open to infection arriving from elsewhere. Colchester in Essex had six major epidemics between 1579 and 1665, the last killing half of the population that had not already fled.[10] Norwich, a little further north, had outbreaks in 1500, 1503–4, 1513–14, 1544–5, 1554–5 and 1579–80.[11] Towns with more than 10,000 inhabitants, with a larger potential reservoir of infection, might fare even worse. London saw epidemics in 1498–1500, 1504, 1535–6, 1543, 1548 and 1563, when there were 17,404 plague burials with over 1,000 deaths a week. There were a further 3,568 deaths in 1578, and 10,675 in 1593.[12] Even remote villages might be affected. Plague in 1546 ravaged Devon widely, and was back the next year, again moving inland from the coast. Similar outbreaks in 1577 and 1579 seem to have been more localised but a decade later 53 out of 89 parishes show evidence of the disease in 1589 and 1593. In most villages three or four times as many people died in a plague year, and exceptionally even ten times, as in a normal year, and bad harvests only added to the death toll.[13]

In Italy, the carefully compiled records of the Health Boards of major cities show that many plague outbreaks were confined to a region or even a district. One in 1555–6, restricted to Friuli and the Veneto in Northern Italy, was especially severe in Padua and Venice. Others raged more widely. That of 1522–4 spread through almost the whole of Italy, from Caltanissetta in Central Sicily to Rome, Sardinia and particularly to Milan and the Po valley, but without afflicting seriously either Venice or Genoa. In Milan 2,900 deaths from plague are recorded in the years 1523–4, a significant number but still far smaller than the 100,000 in 1523 alone suggested by a local chronicler. Most devastating of all was the plague of 1575–7 which ravaged the whole of Italy. In Milan in 1576–7, 17,239 died, Venice lost over 50,000 inhabitants, Brescia between 16,396 and 20,677, Padua some 10,000. On Sicily Palermo lost roughly 3% of its large population but many smaller towns and the port city of Messina fared much worse.[14] Similar figures have been obtained from France. Poitiers lost a third of its population in 1512–13, Angers between a quarter and a third in 1593–4. Usually an outbreak was relatively local, but in 1585–6 and 1596–7 there was a veritable pandemic throughout France.[15]

Some of those who had lived through an epidemic sought to describe its effects on their locality as precisely as possible for the benefit of succeeding generations. The Basle physician and professor Felix Platter (1536–1614), who had experienced seven epidemics in the city, in 1539–41, 1550–3, 1563–6, 1575–8, 1582–3, 1593–4 and 1609–11, listed the names of many leading citizens who had died of plague in a substantial volume that culminated in a detailed account of the plague of 1609–11 that was, in his view, "at least as deadly as the 'Great Plague' of 1563–6". Platter meticulously recorded which inhabitants of each house, including children and servants, had caught the disease, and whether or not they died.[16] A humbler but no less striking representation can be found in the church in the village of Grossrückerswalde in the Erzgebirge, south of Dresden in Germany. Above a memorial inscription naming the 72 individuals who died in the plague of 1583, a local artist depicted the angel of plague striking them as they stood outside their homes in the village, while other angels protect the survivors. None of its 14 houses was untouched. Everyone at Jorg Neuber's farm died, and a lame boy called Jakob Meyh was discovered out in the fields, while at Bastian Besch's only a brother and sister-in-law out of the 16 members of the household survived. In none of the houses do the living appear to outnumber the dead.[17]

But to get a true picture of plague at a local level, one must forsake numbers for the observations of those, both medical and non-medical alike, who had experienced its full horror.[18] Only then can one begin to get a sense of what it was like to live in a town in time of plague, to hear of the almost inexorable approach of a disease whose deadly consequences were well known, or to see friends, neighbours and family fall ill and die. One can only sympathise with the doctor Simone Simoni in 1568 when his wife, who appeared to have recovered from a fever, suddenly became delirious as they were eating together. Within an hour she was gone. One can feel the pain in Simoni's words. One moment she was alive, the next she had gone, "giving me almost no time to notice that she was ill". Remaining cheerful under such circumstances, as Simoni recommended to his readers, was indeed a counsel of perfection.[19] Descriptions of life in time of plague by non-doctors are rare until the last quarter of the sixteenth century. This period has no Boccaccio, no Defoe, no Manzoni to set a major work of fiction in a time of plague, although Francesco Sanseverino opened his re-publication of an earlier novelle by placing his interlocutors in Venice during the plague of 1556.[20] A more famous writer, Niccolò Machiavelli (1469–1527), has also been credited with a short essay in which he imagines a day in Florence during a plague when corpses littered the deserted streets. The narrator plucks up courage to speak to a newly widowed young woman, and fantasises about marrying her, her beauty contrasting with the stench and horror of the plague-filled city.[21] In contrast, medical accounts and discussions are common, and the plague of 1575–7 produced a new genre of plague writing, called by Cohn the '*successo*' literature, that aimed to describe in some detail how a community managed to withstand the epidemic. These accounts were written, usually in the vernacular, by a broad variety of the literate population, ranging from a bishop and a priest through civic officials to merchants, humanists and lawyers. Some writers had been heavily involved themselves in fighting the plague. The Jesuit Paolo Bisciola's account of plague in Milan emphasised the activities of Cardinal Borromeo and other clergy, while the notary and gate-guard Giacomo Filippo Besta described in substantial detail the administrative procedures there during the same epidemic.[22] Poets, particularly in Northern Italy, also joined in to welcome the ending of the epidemic, often praising the herculean efforts of doctors or government officials.[23]

Doctors naturally also put pen to paper, explaining, advising and, occasionally, as with Mercuriale's own tract on plague, justifying their own failures to prevent disaster.[24] Few of them, however, go into the same level of detail as non-doctors, largely because of their over-riding concern to provide guidance in a present or, still more, a future epidemic. One of those who did manage to combine academic discussion with insights into everyday life was Pieter van Foreest, Petrus Forestus, 'the Dutch Hippocrates'

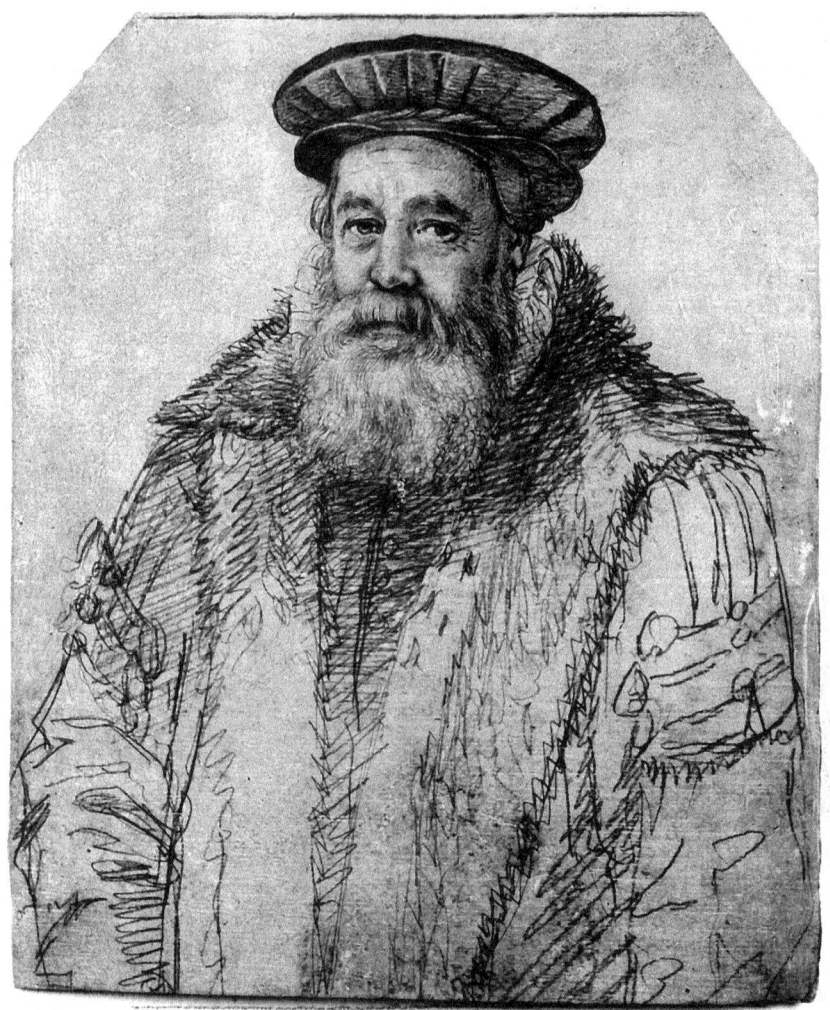

Figure 2.1 Pieter van Foreest (1522–97), the Dutch Hippocrates, served as a town physician at Pithiviers in France and from 1557 to 1596 in Delft. Drawing by Henrik Goltzius 1586.

(1521–97), whose 32 large books of *Medical Observations and Cures*, and a further nine on surgery show not only his great learning and sympathy for patients but also a keen eye and a vigorous Latin style.[25] Van Foreest (Figure 2.1) was well acquainted with plague. He mentions 16 different outbreaks between 1546 and 1597: some very local, like that in Haarlem in 1581; others more widely dispersed (that of 1566 affected Kennemerland in

North Holland and Waterland many kilometres away, but not Amsterdam); others, like that of 1573–4, affected most places in the Netherlands.[26] Book VI of the *Observations*, on "public fevers, epidemic diseases, malignant, contagious and pestilential fevers and plague" occupies some 238 pages in the edition of 1591, and is organised along the lines of a commentary on the Hippocratic *Epidemics*. Each case history, whether Van Foreest's own or provided to him by his friends Livinus Sanderius and Johannes Tyengius, is accompanied by a lengthy commentary, *Scholium*, explaining the case and its treatment, sometimes with reminiscences of other cases. The 1570s and 1580s were harsh years in the Netherlands, and Van Foreest was only too aware of the baleful consequences of war and famine. The moving pages devoted to the siege of Haarlem in 1573 testify to his understanding of the human misery visited on all those, both soldier and civilian, caught up in the fighting.[27] Although his experiences at Delft in 1562 form the centrepiece of his discussions of plague, he is aware of the perpetual problems of peasants, living in close proximity to their beasts, and always in danger from polluted drinking water. This happened in 1562 at Nootdorp and Pijnacker when, in his view, cattle that had died of plague from standing in long-flooded fields might have transmitted it to the villagers.[28] Delft was at first fortunate because the water in its canals and dykes had not risen so high as to putrefy the air, but once it did, disease broke out, and famine, bad and overcrowded housing and general poverty ensured that the poor constituted the majority of victims. Their children were most affected because they had the poorest diet, and Van Foreest remembered them in the street singing to accompany the corpses of their playmates before dying themselves. He saw similarly shocking deaths in 1573, when the weakened survivors of the siege of Haarlem quickly succumbed to plague, which swiftly spread to Rotterdam, Brill and Delft. At Delft it was starving peasants who were the first to die, crammed with their animals into religious buildings whose air was thick with the stench of animal dung. Six hundred died at the convent of St Clara alone.[29]

Plague spared no one, neither rich nor poor. Van Foreest had to fight valiantly for a whole week to cure his wealthy neighbour Clara van Meer, "a bilious lady", the wife of the Town Clerk of Delft.[30] Many of his cases end with a brief "died as I had predicted". Failure by others to act in time often led to disaster. A woman too frightened to show her husband her plague bubo infected him despite, or because of, his confidence that she was not a sufferer. She lived, but he died. Self-medication might prove fatal; home remedies, such as ice-cold cloths, added to the torments of one of his neighbours and ensured that there was no possibility of recovery.[31] At Schoenreloe in 1558, a village of a mere 40 houses, 150 sufferers died within a week. Those who tried to cool their fever by drinking water died within two days, and beer only prolonged their agony. Medical expertise did not always prevail. Plague carried off the wife, daughter and maidservant of his friend, Peter the surgeon of Brill, and, in all likelihood, him as well.[32]

But increasingly plague became a disease of the poor. The rich left town as quickly as possible, their cleaner and better-built houses were less hospitable to rodent vectors, and in many cities their preference for living on a *piano nobile* acted as a barrier to fleas and rats who could find sufficient hosts far more easily at ground level.[33] Huddled in tenements, frequently malnourished, shopping in crowded markets or forced to meet the general public in the course of their work, the poor were more likely to catch the plague than the wealthy, and to suffer the consequences of seclusion and loss of earnings.[34] As such, they often fell below the horizon of civic administrators, and their care was left to neighbours and other charitable members of the community, not least the church. The handbook provided by Cardinal Borromeo for his clergy in the Milanese plague epidemic of 1575–8 is remarkable for the detail it gives of the lives of the poor and of the many ways in which he expected his priests to intervene; other clerics elsewhere in Italy were acting along similar lines.[35]

Civic Doctors

Van Foreest's involvement with Delft lasted from 1557, when he answered the call of the Mayor to become a civic physician, until 1596, when he retired to his native Alkmaar. The institution of civic doctors, whose roots can be traced back to Classical Antiquity, was revived again in Western Europe in the early decades of the thirteenth century with the appointments of doctors by Reggio and Bologna in the Po valley. By the end of the century *medici condotti*, medics hired by a community, were found in most major Italian cities, and by 1450 this system of medical hiring was almost universal in the peninsula. A small town like Sacile in Friuli offered 300 lire a year for a doctor in 1426; the little neighbouring towns of Cherso and Osso in Istria paid jointly for a doctor, a surgeon, an apothecary and a schoolmaster in 1440.[36] By 1400, larger towns in Germany, France and Switzerland were employing civic doctors, and in 1436 the Emperor Sigismund ordered all towns in the German Empire to hire a *Stadtarzt*.[37] Similar doctors appear at Gouda and Kampen in the Netherlands shortly afterwards, and were commonplace in Western Europe by 1550, even if, as the Sicilian doctor Giovanni Filippo Ingrassia (1510–80) complained in 1577, not every town employed one on a permanent basis.[38] In France, the position of civic physician was mainly connected with outbreaks of plague, and, except in the south, temporary.[39] There was one notable exception, the British Isles. Here, well into the seventeenth century, only a few towns bothered to create such a post, whether held by a physician or a surgeon, and those that did were usually those with trading connections like Southampton, Norwich, Ipswich and Newcastle.[40] Even in times of plague, most towns did not trouble to employ a civic doctor or surgeon. A Parliamentary proposal in 1535 for physicians and surgeons to be paid to treat the sick poor who would be able to return to work after being given medical attention found no place in the 1536 Poor Law Act as it was passed and was quietly forgotten.[41]

To attempt to describe the duties of a town doctor is almost impossible, since beyond the most obvious, ensuring the presence of a competent healer, there are objections to almost every generalisation.[42] Sometimes the doctor provided free treatment for all, or only for those in the city itself as opposed to the countryside. Sometimes only the consultation was universally free, sometimes the doctor's charges were to be on a sliding scale related to the patient's income. In some towns, as in Delft, the town physician occupied the highest place in the medical hierarchy and, like Van Foreest, thought it right to oversee and give orders to surgeons. In Zurich in 1536, the town doctor was expected to act in all cases of obstetrics, presumably working with and supervising some of the town's official midwives. In St Gallen, the council agreed to ban all competition with the town doctor except from those medically qualified that it had already approved, but in return the doctor was advised against supplying drugs himself, as this was the role of the apothecary. In Spain and in Spanish, and later papal, Italy, the *protomedico*, the chief physician, had oversight of all healing services, including laying down qualifications for practice, a task that elsewhere was more often left to local guilds or colleges.[43] In many Dutch towns, the town doctor was also the chief medical officer for its hospitals, but elsewhere the choice was left to hospital boards and administrators. Above all, the town doctor was there to give advice to his employers, the town council, in times of plague, cases of wounding and homicide, and whenever it was required of him.[44]

Remuneration depended, like some American professorships, on negotiation. The doctor or surgeon appointed was sometimes paid partly in kind (grain, wine or wood) or by granting privileges of citizenship to an outsider. Usually it included a house, with or without a supply of fuel. When Dr von Hertenstein was appointed at St Gallen in 1551, he was given a suitable, quiet and sunny house with a little garden where he was to plant medicinal herbs, not onions and cabbages. At other times the physician had to pay for some of the medicines he used out of his own stipend. At Gouda in 1582, the town council paid the doctor for visits on a sliding scale: a night visit was paid at twice the rate, and a uroscopy one and a half times the rate of a day visit. But much depended on the circumstances of the appointment, and the age of the appointee. Should it be a young man, "the mere shadow of an experienced doctor", too quick to rush to judgement and ambitious to succeed, but unable to bear "the laborious exercise of healing"? Or should it be a senior man, even though the laziness of elderly doctors was proverbial? It might be good if the senior doctor took the younger under his wing but having two doctors was an expense that the community might not be able to afford, and the two might not always hit it off.[45] A dispute between an older and a younger doctor at Viadana in the Po valley in 1569 ended in the imprisonment and exile of the older man, driven to the angry posting of libellous notices by the high salary and poetic pretensions of his younger colleague as well as his family connections with the court at Mantua and the *podestà* of Viadana.[46] At Nördlingen in Southern Germany, the town council had to intervene in a row between the two town physicians which escalated to the point where one tore up a medical certificate issued by the other.[47] Other doctors soon found that the post was far from what they had hoped for. The Leipzig graduate Antonius Niger in 1537 bewailed his mistaken acceptance of the post of *Stadtarzt* at Braunschweig, where his meagre stipend could not compensate for working in a city that preferred old wives' medicine and the ministrations of "ignorant Jews", herbalists and stupid empirics. The same complaint about the Brunswickers had been made earlier in 1523 by another more famous holder of the post, the doctor-poet Euricius Cordus (1486–1535), who lamented the competition from beggars, monks and travelling mountebanks.[48] This was only one of the woes of Theodore Eccombertus who wrote to a medical colleague in 1583 from the mining town of Schlaggenwald in Bohemia (Horni Slavkov, Czech Republic). He found it hard to live on his salary even with a house included and was waiting for a reply from an otherwise friendly council to his request for a higher stipend and fuel as well. He had expected to make money from private practice but, surrounded by believers in uroscopy and old wives' tales, he had made only 44 thalers, most of it from outsiders. Besides, he needed a wife, and the local girls were all haughty bumpkins with no money to their name (the richest had only 100 florins a year). He had had hopes of finding a wife elsewhere, but no one wished to live at Schlaggenwald. If he had known all this, 20 horses would not have dragged him there. But there was a chink of light. Relatives had told him of a post with excellent prospects at Gotha which came along with the very wealthy widow of the local doctor. But he doubted whether this would work out, and, besides, he much preferred a young girl to a widow who had already buried two husbands. No wonder that his congratulations to his friend on his forthcoming marriage sound a little forced; although, were he to be invited to the wedding, there might be someone there who. . . .[49]

In almost all towns the authorities, when asked to choose between the financial demands of the doctors and surgeons with whom they contracted and the need to preserve the health of the community by having a resident practitioner, preferred to yield to the medics, no matter how sceptical they might be about their morals and their greed for money.[50] Even a small town had also to bear in mind the loss of prestige in the neighbourhood if it failed to appoint someone. In their turn the authorities might offer incentives, such as allowing the doctor to keep a larger proportion of the fees he gained from wealthy citizens or, in contrast, impose strict conditions to get the most value from their civic doctor: Giambattista Fabi, the physician at Argenta in the Po valley in 1590, was forbidden to spend even a night away without permission of the *consoli*.[51] Balancing the expectations of both sides was always tricky. When the town of Auray in Southern France increased the doctors' fee for curing a sufferer from plague to a gold coin, as opposed to a silver florin for a failure, their insatiable greed, so the lawyer Francesco Ripa claimed, drove them to greater and more effective efforts to cure.[52]

One consequence of the *condotta* system was that there were plenty of opportunities for doctors and surgeons in Italy and Germany to find appropriate employment. By 1630 in the Grand Duchy of Florence, there were on average two physicians and two surgeons to every 10,000 people, with smaller towns like Montepulciano, Volterra and Poggibonsi having a proportion far higher than Florence itself.[53] But considerations of cost always weighed heavily.[54] Udine in 1451 had abolished, at least temporarily, the salaries of two of its civic doctors and diverted the money to a worthier cause – the erection of a civic campanile. At Chalons in France in 1483 the flight of a doctor at the approach of plague led the council to decide to employ a town physician only in emergencies.[55] Major Italian towns like Venice, Milan or Pisa from the mid-fifteenth century onwards began to doubt the value of paying outsiders (the majority of those appointed) to come and treat their citizens for nothing when they were apparently glad to do so without this inducement simply because of the profits that could be made from practice there. But these councils were the exceptions, and even here other groups in the community, particularly confraternities, were quite prepared to pay doctors to attend their members.[56]

The problems of supply and demand, not to mention finance, were even greater in times of plague, when the town physician was often the main or only source of help and advice. The title of the plague tract written in 1561 by Johann Ewich (1525–88) for the magistrates of Bremen is explicit: *The Duty of a Faithful and Wise Magistrate to Preserve and Free His Community in Time of Plague*. Its advice was highly valued, for the Latin text was republished in 1582, a German translation of 1583 was reprinted in 1584, 1597 and 1608 and it appeared in Latin again in 1656. There was also an English version made in London by John Stockwood in 1583.[57] Ewich emphasised that, in times of plague, it was not the doctor but the magistrates and other officials who were in charge. Plague was something that involved everyone and decisions needed to be taken locally by appropriate members of the local community, for it was they who had to issue and implement regulations that would impact severely on all daily life.[58]

There was no shortage of guidance for the lay magistrate from both doctors and lawyers on how he should proceed if plague was thought likely.[59] He needed to ensure beforehand that there were sufficient funds available, for this was likely to be the largest item of expenditure in his period of office, find a suitable treasurer and define the financial contribution of each citizen, both then and for long after the epidemic. A city like Pistoia, which spent in 1630–31 over 40% of its revenue in dealing with the plague, without taking into account indirect losses, might take many decades to recover from a major epidemic and might not have paid off its debts after one episode before the next arrived.[60] In Venice officials of the Health Boards negotiated with some of their employees about the costs of 'secret' remedies that they were assured would quickly put an end to the outbreak.[61] Another duty of the magistrate was to produce plague passes, which his officials should know how to check against fraud or misuse, and prepare an appropriate number of plague notices for public display. In Florence, as well putting up written notices, the town crier proclaimed the onset of plague and the imposition of regulations at 40 selected spots within the walls. The magistrate had to enforce quarantine and house-confinement, trying where possible to separate men and women, for plague, wrote one lawyer, was a source of innumerable carnal sins, and newly widowed ladies were often seduced into a hasty marriage with men beneath them in status and wealth. Finally, the magistrate had to set up a hospital in a remote and healthy place ("for a change of location is the best medicine") and ensure that the town had the services of an appropriate number of doctors.[62] After the problems of sorting out wills, contracts and the property of those who died, one question seems to have exercised the lawyer most of all. Who should serve as a plague doctor? Preferably only an MD, but the great medieval professor of law Bartolo had accepted surgeons, although appointing a mere barber-surgeon might seem to some to undermine "the dignity of the doctorate". But in a real emergency even a medical student might prove useful, or indeed anyone with healing skills, such as a pharmacist, but one should draw the line at enchanters, wise-women, magicians and, above all, Jews.[63] But if there was no other choice, then a Jew would be preferable to an evil and godless Christian, for a true *meditatio mortis*, thinking about death, was the best philosophical, or psychological, defence against plague, a message repeated at length by Lorenzo Condio in 1581 in his *A Philosophical Medicine against the Plague*.[64]

Quarantine and Health Boards

How a city dealt with plague was also an indication of the strength and sophistication of its civic cohesion. While almost everywhere from the fourteenth century onwards, councils and magistrates had organised street cleaning, it is no coincidence that the first place to introduce quarantine was Ragusa (Dubrovnik), a town dependent on trade and run by a close mercantile oligarchy.[65] In 1377 34 of its 44 councillors voted that anyone coming from a plague-infested area by sea should spend a month on an isolated island; travellers who were trying to reach Ragusa overland from the south had to stay in a designated frontier town. Residents of Ragusa could not visit those in quarantine without specific authorisation, and any breach of the regulations was punishable with a fine. The council and citizens were aware of the consequences of plague for the city, much of whose food had to be imported. Either in 1377 or shortly afterwards they appointed a committee of patricians to implement the plague regulations decided upon by the two Councils, a committee that became permanent in 1398, and whose members also received a salary from 1457. It was a position of honour but also of danger: in 1437 nine of the ten patricians who stayed behind to run the city died of plague within a fortnight, and in the great plague of 1526–7 only one patrician remained alive in the town to open the gates when the plague ended.[66]

The role of the doctor was to advise these men, to act upon their instructions and to carry out diagnoses and post-mortems. Perhaps surprisingly, the *cazamorti*, as the Board members were called, expected that the official town physician and surgeon might wish to depart at the onset of plague, and were even happy to allow them periods of leave. In February 1527, one doctor and one surgeon were allowed unpaid leave, while Dr Muzi was given a month's leave with pay. He returned in late March, only to resign in April, but he was rehired in August, remaining in post until 1536. In December 1526, he was joined as a plague doctor by a native of the town, Ivan Mednic, at a salary of 200 ducats, plus 3 ducats a month for life for his sons, provided he remained in post after the plague. It is unclear whether this unusual contract shows the weak bargaining position of the council or not. Certainly, his salary was larger than that of a second appointee, Jacobus Rizo, who was paid 160 ducats plus lodging for him and his servant in February 1527. This proved not to be a wise appointment. Rizo was accused of theft and robbery, and, after an official investigation, was allowed to disappear quietly in September 1527.[67]

Although by the sixteenth century, every feature of the plague precautions of medieval Ragusa had been adopted and developed further by towns in Italy, and often beyond, this was a very slow and sporadic development, and it is wiser to see Ragusa as an anomaly rather than a catalyst. Cities like Genoa, Messina and Lucca had occasionally resorted to armed force to keep foreigners away during the Black Death of 1348, but this did not amount to a total ban on trade and economic activity. By 1400 only two cities had banned all outsiders from entering the city in time of plague and imposed severe restrictions on their own citizens. Milan in 1374 removed sufferers outside the city, while Mantua introduced plague passes for travel. These measures were extended further by other Italian cities from the mid-fifteenth century and the period of isolation often extended to 40 days, the *quarantina*, as in Venice in 1448, becoming the first line of defence.[68] These measures were supported by extensive networks of communication giving early warning of potential outbreaks. Venice used its colonies in the Eastern Mediterranean to report on outbreaks there (a common occurrence throughout this period and well beyond), while Milan's listening posts extended north of the Alps. In Italy travellers had to provide a certificate declaring that they were free of plague, an irksome imposition but one that, according to Montaigne who had experienced it, was also easily evaded with a little *douceur*.[69] This still struck the English traveller Fynes Moryson in the 1590s as something worth explaining to his English readers, as it was imposed, he thought, not only for reasons of health, but as a way in which the authorities could discover "the quality of all marchants and of all goodes before they be admitted to free traffique in the cittyes".[70]

It took much longer for Health Boards like that of Ragusa to become established in Italy. Milan set up a temporary Health Board in 1424, but it was not until many years later that other cities followed its example. Pavia did so in 1450, Venice in 1459, although it took a further two years before the decision was implemented, Siena in 1462, Florence probably in 1464. Despite the frequency of plague, it took many years before the Boards were made permanent, by Venice in 1486, but by Florence not until 1527. Some cities never took that step: Cremona and Lucca, which had created temporary Boards in 1480 and 1481, never made them permanent. These Boards were set up initially to ensure that the regulations introduced by the authorities were being followed, but they more and more directed their attention to dealing with undesirable groups such as 'ruffians', beggars, prostitutes and foreigners without licence to travel, who were considered likely to spread the disease by contagion.[71] They also became responsible for all aspects of dealing with plague, from finance and arranging for doctors to attend the sick (often designating particular quarters of a city in which they were to do their work), to organising gravediggers and guards on the gates and establishing emergency hospitals where those infected, and their families, might be sent.[72] As members of the elite, and with their decisions backed further by the town council, the Board members had the authority to order and enforce regulations that had the potential to arouse opposition. These included burning houses and goods, banning public meetings and religious processions and services, an affront to those who believed not only that plague was in some way sent by God, but also that only a religious response would put an end to the outbreak. Not that divine intervention was unnecessary or unwelcome – both Ragusa and Venice at the end of the outbreaks of 1533 and 1576 erected large churches as thank offerings for their deliverance – but preventing transmission by avoiding contagion through gatherings had in the past proved effective.[73] What might happen when authority was lost is neatly illustrated by the events at Montelupo in Tuscany in 1631, where the orders of a callow young *podestà* appointed by Florence were opposed among others by local priests, and led to the breaking open of the town's gate and processions with the crucifix to pray for divine favour. The young man was swiftly replaced by an older and more experienced magistrate who firmly enforced the plague regulations in this poor rural community. Both parties could, in the end, claim that it was their actions that had brought the plague to an end shortly after the new man had imposed his authority.[74]

Cities north of the Alps were much slower to adopt these Italian practices, and specific Health Boards were rare.[75] However, detailed ordinances in times of plague were regularly introduced throughout the sixteenth century, preventing circulation of people, ordering infected bedding to be burned and prescribing the cleaning of streets and elsewhere of rubbish that was believed to be a cause of the plague. England in general took no public precautions against plague, apart from street cleaning, occasionally banning travellers from nearby infected places or killing cats and dogs. The first official plague order in 1518 (perhaps developed from a 1517 regulation introduced by Henry VIII for the canons of Windsor) made it compulsory to identify houses of plague sufferers, and for their inmates to carry a white stick while outside, and these minimal rules were repeated for the next four decades.[76] Only in 1563 was further action taken by the government, prompted by a memorandum from Cesare Adelmare, an Italian graduate of Padua and a Royal physician, who stressed the superiority of continental models. William Cecil, the chief minister of Elizabeth I, drew up in 1564 a more detailed order for the city of Westminster that required all those infected to be shut up in their houses for 40 days. But not until 1579, following a summer of intermittent outbreaks, was wider action taken on the authority of the Queen and implemented by local justices of the peace. These new orders introduced most of the rules that had been adopted on the Continent and that were made known more widely in 1583 by John Stockwood's translation of Ewich's German advice for magistrates (see earlier, p. 49). They emphasised the need to shut up infected individuals, along with their whole family, in their own home, a far more stringent measure than in Italy, which preferred a move to a *lazaretto*. Secondly, they enjoined that the expenditure on guards, gravediggers and the like as well as any provision made for supporting the sick was to be paid for out of a special tax. Such taxes had occasionally been levied in Italy, but this was the first permanent such regulation in any city, and one that applied nationwide. It was, however, far from a comprehensive plan for dealing with the plague, which was not improved upon until 1604 and had to be voted upon annually until it was made permanent in 1641.[77]

But did these plague regulations have any effect in ending, or at least in mitigating, plague? Modern scholars remain unsure, but apart from those who believed that only appeals to God would work, most contemporaries believed that such policies were effective.[78] Santorio Santorio (1561–1636) had experienced disastrous plagues in Venice in 1576 and again in 1630, and believed that, once it arrived, plague would run its course like clockwork until, like a clock, something broke in the chain of infection. But nonetheless he was able to commend at least some of the Health Board's rulings, despite believing many to be useless or even, like incarceration, counterproductive compared with being out in the good fresh air.[79] Many contemporaries pointed to the heroic efforts of individual doctors and administrators in the struggle against plague. Simone Simoni credited the firm intervention of Leipzig's Mayor Rauscher in introducing strict controls with bringing the epidemic of 1575 to an end, when doctors had failed (and most, including Simoni himself, had left).[80] Others sought, and usually found, scapegoats. Oxford University reported in 1519 that it was obstacles in the Thames that were causing flooding that left stagnant pools to pollute the air. It could do nothing itself as the nuisances were on private lands but hoped that the

Chancellor (Archbishop Warham) or Cardinal Wolsey might intervene.[81] The "epidemic pestilential fever" identified by the doctors at Padua in 1541 was credited with a similar cause. New locks on the river, being more efficient than the old leaky ones, held back for longer the mass of stinking and putrefying rubbish, particularly from the town's tanneries, that floated in the water and attracted an unprecedented mass of harmful insects.[82] Sometimes, blame was directed at outsiders or a specific individual. At Ragusa the disastrous plague of 1526–7 was believed to have been caused by a local tailor returning from Ancona who had disregarded the plague measures. His punishment was to be tied to a cart and dragged through the city while being tortured with hot irons until he died.[83] In 1575 rumours spread in Palermo that the plague had been brought by a "cursed galley" that had briefly arrived from Messina and the Barbary Coast, or by a Maltese prostitute working there who had died of "pestilential fever".[84] Others, particularly doctors, placed the responsibility on their fellow citizens. Georg Sturtz put an outbreak of plague at Erfurt down to the inhabitants' "negligence" and "foolhardiness", while Simoni went even further in 1576.[85] In his view, patients were to blame. They were always eager for novelty, believed kin charlatans, lacked patience to follow a course of treatment through and expected to live forever. They, like the authorities, were mean, unwilling to pay a doctor properly, and rarely called in medical assistance until it was too late. They would rather have death in the house than the doctor.

On one notorious occasion, the plague of Venice in 1575–6, it was not the system under which they worked, but doctors themselves that were held to blame. Plague had arrived in Venice in August 1575, killing 3,696 persons between August and February, and then dropping away until only eight deaths were reported in the last week in May 1576. Then numbers suddenly shot up again, there was a mass exodus of the wealthy, and by 9 June, 850 Venetians were quarantined in the two *lazaretti*. Girolamo Mercuriale, who headed the team of medical professors from Padua called in to advise the Health Board, did not believe this was an outbreak of true plague but only pestilential fever, an opinion he defended before a meeting of the Board and the Doge. Against the advice of the Health Board's physician and other Venetians, he demanded the ending of all the Board's restrictions and offered, along with his Paduan colleague Capodivacca, to examine possible plague sufferers himself. After a few days back in Padua, the two professors returned to Venice to the cheers of the crowds, and by 16 June they had gained almost all their demands. Venice was open again, despite the increasingly strong objections of the Health Board. But as the month went on, the numbers of dead mounted, including a Jesuit priest who had accompanied the professors on their visits to the sick. Criticism of the professors grew, and they retreated to Padua, having given further advice to the Heath Board, but still believing the disease was not true plague and did not require the imposition of the strictest controls. The disease quickly proved them wrong, and controls were reimposed. But before December, tens of thousands had died in Venice, and 10,000 in Padua itself, where the university had to be closed. Undeterred, Mercuriale repeated his initial diagnosis in his lectures on plague when the university reopened in January 1577, arguing that the disease had changed at the beginning of July to become true plague. Not everyone was convinced by this special pleading and the two professors continued to be held responsible for the worst epidemic in the history of Venice. Not only had they given the wrong diagnosis, but they had undermined the authority of the Health Board at a time when the disease could have been kept within normal bounds.[86]

Hospitals

Ragusa in 1377, Marseilles in 1383 and Venice in 1423 were all fortunate in having an abundance of neighbouring islets on which to establish an isolation hospital. The first Venetian plague hospital, the *lazaretto*, was small, some 20 rooms, and intended above all for outsiders, refugees, migrants and beggars, provided they gave their consent.[87] It gradually took in more inmates, and in 1471 was supplemented by the Lazaretto Nuovo on an adjacent islet, built at huge cost and capable of housing tens of thousands of the infected and their families.[88] Other towns for a long while made do with transferring the infected to part of a larger hospital, a convent, as at Delft, or often to a leper hospital, now, for reasons that are still unclear, frequently occupied by only a fraction of the many patients who had been living there two or three centuries earlier. In Florence the new hospital of S. Maria Nuova had been the preferred place for housing the plague victims in 1448, although it was quickly acknowledged that its location in the heart of the city was far from ideal, and in 1464 another hospital complained about the costs of having to care for over 100 extra patients displaced from S. Maria to make room for plague sufferers. Nor did increased funding and staff for S. Maria Nuova help to resolve the problem when plague struck again, and in 1479 permission was given to use another hospital, S. Maria della Scala, which was primarily an orphanage, while discussions began about creating a proper *lazaretto*. The new Spedale di S. Bastiano, when it did open on the Prato della Giustizia, was a small affair with only 26 beds, far less than the 200 in Milan's new *lazaretto*, and in 1495 some of the lesser Florentine hospitals were instructed to transfer some of their beds, mattresses, linen and all, to the new hospital. Even so, in the plague of 1497 sufferers were once again being treated in numbers at S. Maria Nuova, and 20 years later S. Bastiano had to be greatly enlarged, and a temporary encampment of huts set up outside the walls for those who had come into contact with plague victims. But this hospital and its buildings did not last long, being destroyed in 1529 during the siege of Florence, and two convents of nuns took its place on the site.[89]

In both Florence and Venice the civic authorities tried their best to provide those sent to the *lazaretto* with both nourishing food and appropriate

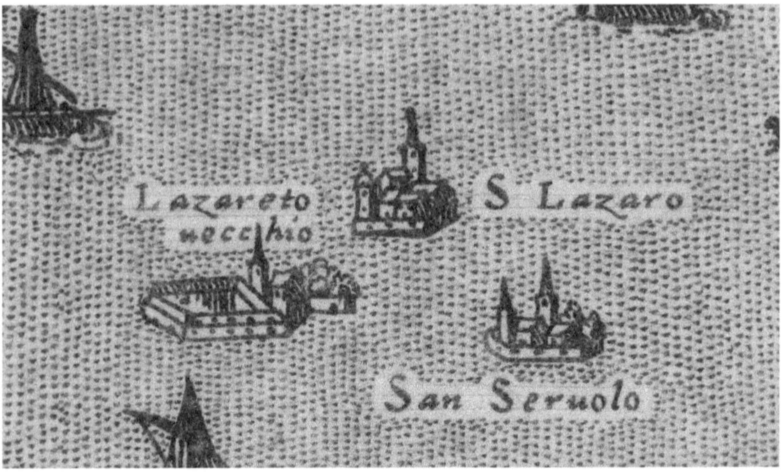

Figure 2.2 The Old Lazaretto in the Venetian lagoon, 1572.

religious sustenance. The administration at S. Bastiano was handed over to the religious confraternity of the Misericordia, and provision was made for religious as well as medical services. Similarly, at Milan in 1576 daily celebrations of the mass and sessions of prayer took place in the temporary huts that surrounded the plague hospital of S. Gregorio, now no longer able to cope with the numbers envisaged in its 388 rooms.[90] Often the sheer numbers overwhelmed even the best provided *lazaretti*, which quickly became places to be feared and avoided at all costs. One writer compared the Old Lazaretto of Venice to Hell, the afflicted stacked three or four to a bed, lacking attention of every kind, and awaiting an inevitable death, after which they were thrown unceremoniously into ditches. By contrast the much larger New Lazaretto was merely Purgatory. Some food and medicines were available, and only 10% of its inmates died, despite lying on smoking, stinking beds.[91] Such stories were repeated across Europe, only adding to the fears engendered by plague itself.

The plague *lazaretti* represent only one of the many forms that 'hospitals' took in the sixteenth century, and, indeed, had taken from their very beginning in the mid-fourth century. They had been originally instituted by Christians endeavouring to fulfil the commandment of Jesus to provide aid and succour to all in need. The main beneficiaries were the poor and those bereft of protection in an increasingly harsh world – widows, the elderly, travellers and the sick for whom proper treatment at home was difficult, if not impossible. This multiplicity of possible functions continued throughout the Middle Ages and the sixteenth century. Few hospitals were founded with a specifically medical purpose; many, indeed, actually banned the admission of the sick, especially those with loathsome or infectious diseases, such as leprosy and plague. Most served a similar function to today's old folk's homes, and indeed some survive today as such still under their old title. London in the early sixteenth century had some 34 hospitals and almshouses, in addition to the ten leper hospitals scattered at intervals outside the walls. Most catered for the poor and elderly either from London in general or for members of certain confraternities or trade guilds. A few were founded specifically for the sick poor. Some, like St Bartholomew's and St Thomas's, came over time to concentrate on the sick, and St Mary Bethlehem (Bedlam) had from the end of the fourteenth century taken in many of the insane. But there were other hospitals originally founded to treat the sick that abandoned that role: St Anthony's became an educational establishment, and the leper house of St Giles, which was founded in 1101 for the support of 40 lepers, housed no more than 14 paupers by the 1530s.[92] A similar pattern prevailed for Florence in the early 1500s. Of its 60 or so hospitals, many offered shelter for pilgrims passing to and fro on the way to Rome, others were old folks' homes, and few offered medical services to the community in general.[93] In both London and in Florence not all the institutions whose statutes declared that they were founded for the benefit of the poor and sick even had a physician or a surgeon on their staff. Some may have had a regular contract with a medical man to come and examine anyone sick, but they tended to rely on barbers rather than on expensive physicians, and in many the arrangements appear *ad hoc*. But the food and shelter they provided were a contribution to health, and one should not underestimate the abilities of the nursing staff to deal with some common conditions. Smaller towns display a similar variety, depending in particular on their location. Those near a pilgrimage route catered primarily for pilgrims, but they might also take in the sick or infirm from the locality, or even beyond. Ospringe in Kent, near to the main road from London to Canterbury and a well-endowed hospital, received a series of elderly men and women who had become too old or infirm to continue in royal service, such as Juliana, "damsel to Queen Eleanor [of Provence]", and Robert of Langley, another royal attendant. They and the staff will have been the prime beneficiaries of the almonds, pullets and fresh goat's meat purchased for the foundation.[94] The Holy Ghost Hospital at Markgröningen, near Stuttgart in Germany, was similarly wealthy. It had been founded by the Order of the Holy Ghost to serve the poor, the sick and pilgrims. Its financial accounts from 1445 to 1448 show that most of its expenses went on its buildings (a common experience) and on providing for the members of the Order, some of whom travelled widely to raise money in alms, and for the wealthy aged who had paid to reside there. The sick, who numbered a mere two in 1445, are hardly mentioned. No wonder that the Duke of Wurtemberg decided to take over the running (and the estates) of the hospital in 1471, or that the town should have earlier set up its own leper house and a small old folk's home.[95]

The history of the S. Maria Nuova hospital in Florence also testifies to another development in the Late Middle Ages and Early Renaissance, the creation and growth of a major hospital which dominated the medical scene in the town. This type of hospital was already familiar in Constantinople and in the Muslim world at the time of the Crusades and can be seen particularly in France in the erection of so-called Hôtels-Dieu, of which the most famous is that in Paris. S. Maria Nuova was founded in 1285 by Folco di Ricovero Portinari, the banker-father of Dante's Beatrice, for the "hospitality and sustenance of the poor and needy". Unusually, it was erected in the very centre of Florence and was originally provided with 17 beds. Within 30 years it had already expanded with a larger ward for men and a second for women. Further expansion followed over the next 20 years, including a change of shape to a T-shaped (later in 1575 a cruciform) plan with the chapel of St Luke at the crossing, so that the daily celebration of the Mass was visible to patients in all the wings. Its purpose also changed. The statutes of 1330 restricted its services to the sick poor, forbidding anyone who was not sick to stay in the hospital for more than three days without the consent of the Portinari family. The hospital by now used a variety of medical specialists, including surgeons and an oculist, some on long-term contracts, others called in when need arose, to treat ever-increasing numbers – by 1347 it housed over 220 sick poor. Its wealth increased along with the size of its buildings. In 1430, its capital was around 42,587 gold florins, three or four times more than that of other hospitals in the city, and its income was increased by gifts and, for a while, by its acting as a bank and as a safe deposit. Around 1480 the Portinari temporarily deposited there the crown jewels of Maximilian, the Archduke of Austria. The hospital's role in the city continued to expand, as well as becoming the main centre for plague victims before the creation of S. Bastiano. New wards continued to be built or enlarged, with major building work taking place in the early sixteenth century and again in 1575. The male ward alone would then have been able to take in up to 320 sick patients, assuming dual occupancy of beds as was normal. But by then the finances and administration had been taken over by the Medici rulers to ensure the hospital's stability in times of crisis.[96]

The mid-fifteenth century was a time of major expansion in Italian hospitals, as well as of their medicalisation, sometimes directly modelled on S. Maria Nuova and on S. Maria della Scala at Siena. In 1456 Francesco Sforza, Duke of Milan ordered his ambassadors there to provide him with detailed information on these two hospitals. The report on Siena survives, giving a short description of the plan but concentrating on its administration, finances and personnel. That hospital emphasised its treatment of acute conditions, excluding those with chronic conditions such as lepers and cripples. It also took in foundlings, as did later the Ospedale Maggiore in Milan and S. Spirito in Rome, another hospital that underwent major changes in this period, evolving from its original role as a pilgrim hospital to become the major medical resource for the city of Rome.[97] Another large

Roman hospital, that of S. Maria della Consolazione, formed in 1506 from the merger of two smaller 'guild' hospitals, was headed from 1536 to 1556 by a Dutch physician Gisbert van der Horst, who used to take northern students, including Pieter van Foreest, around the wards with him to give them practical experience at the bedside.[98]

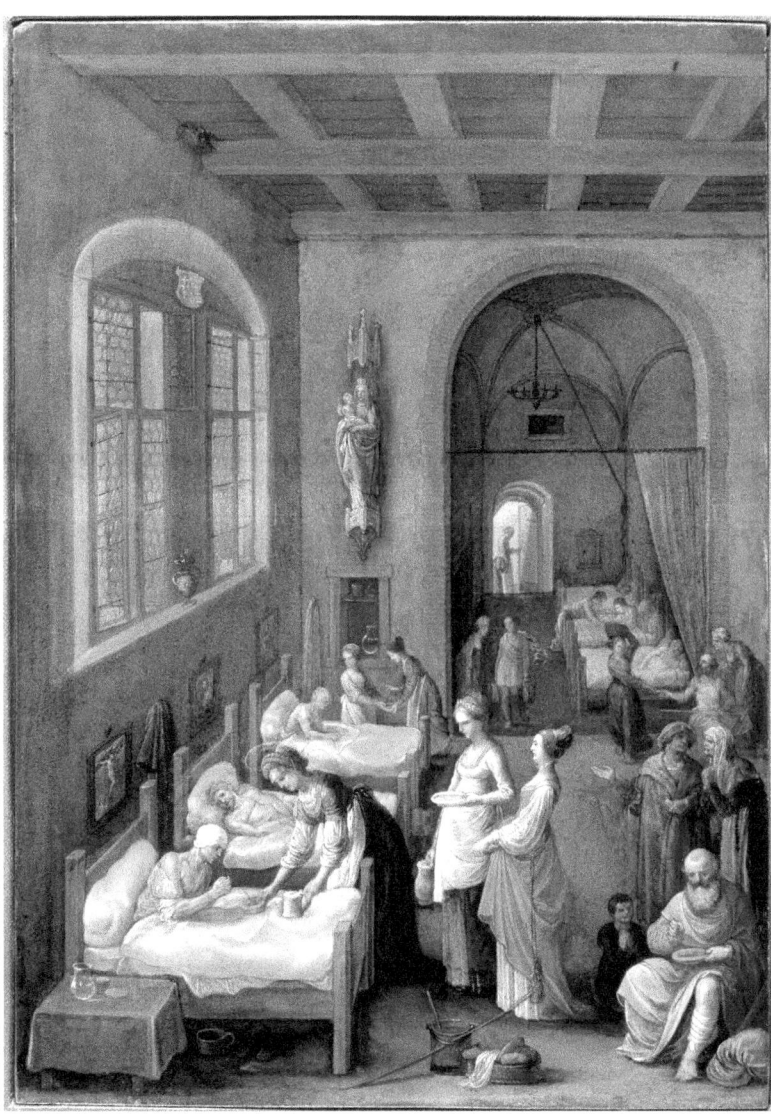

Figure 2.3 Saint Elizabeth of Hungary bringing food for the inmates of a hospital. Oil painting by Adam Elsheimer (1578–1610). London, Wellcome Collection.

These Italian hospitals, with their impressive size and wards frescoed with religious scenes by distinguished artists, were a source of civic pride. Giovanni Giacomo Gilino's detailed description of the Ospedale Maggiore at Milan in 1508 was not intended solely for the Milanese authorities.[99] Nor was Francesco Sforza the only ruler to consider external models for his new foundation. Around 1500 Henry VII of England, arguably the first modern English monarch, asked Francesco Portinari, the son of a late Florentine ambassador to England, to provide him with plans and a detailed account of S. Maria Nuova in preparation for the creation of his own hospital at the Savoy in London. Portinari's list not only deals with the arrangements for the appointment of the Master of the Hospital and the Treasurer but itemises much of the daily life of the hospital. Four barbers attended on Thursdays to shave and cut the hair of its residents, and the butcher slaughtered each month 1,200 rams, 700 lambs, 500 young goats, 400 calves and 100 pigs, most reared on the hospital's own farm. Three junior doctors and the infirmarer dealt with normal cases, reporting in difficult cases to six other doctors, "the best in the city". During meals, which ranged from chicken soup to something more substantial, the infirmarer and his assistants were to note who had failed to eat and provide them with a more suitable repast, as well as reporting this to the other doctors. The arrangements for feeding are at least as good as those in a modern hospital, and the attention to failure to eat arguably superior. How much of this remarkable document was followed by Henry's executors when the Savoy Hospital was opened in 1517, eight years after Henry's death, is far from clear, although its cruciform plan does correspond in many details to that of Florence. No other British hospital of this date was so ambitious, but, as we shall see, it did not flourish for long.[100]

Whether large or small, catering for the elderly or foundlings, concerned with general medical care or concentrating on specific groups such as lepers, plague victims or, a sixteenth-century innovation, syphilitics (called in Florence and elsewhere "the incurables"), all these institutions were united by a religious aim: to secure the well-being of the soul as much as that of the body.[101] Whether founded by a religious group, a confraternity or a religious Order like the Order of the Holy Ghost, a bishop, a nobleman or a wealthy merchant anxious to demonstrate his Christian concern and to secure privileges in Heaven or Purgatory through his good works and the intercessions offered for his soul at the daily mass in the chapel, they took the religious obligations in their statutes very seriously. At S. Maria Nuova, according to Portinari's report, all members of staff had to go to confession three times a year and take communion at Christmas and Easter. The hospital sacristan oversaw 12 other chaplains and six clerics, as well as acolytes, and foreign priests were to be called in to attend sick travellers from England, Spain, France and Germany. Meals were to be eaten in silence while passages from scripture were read out, just as in a monastic refectory.

The religious upheavals of the sixteenth century, which affected all of Christian Europe, brought far more changes to hospitals than did warfare, which was confined to a small number of areas along well-travelled routes. Counter-Reformation clerics continued the practices of their predecessors but on a more lavish scale. The Julius Hospital at Wurzburg, founded by its Prince-Bishop in 1576 on the site of a Jewish cemetery and from the endowments of an abandoned monastery at Heiligenthal, bespeaks by its huge size and splendid architecture the triumph of a resurgent Catholicism.[102] On the other side of the religious divide, Evangelical rulers and wealthy cities took over many sites for their own purposes. Zwickau in 1519/20 transferred the small number of inmates in the leper house to two other hospitals outside the walls and turned it into a hospital for syphilitics.[103] At Markgröningen in 1543 the Duke of Wurtemberg took over the hospital completely from the Order of the Holy Ghost, leaving its last Master, Johannes Schanz, for the moment only with his clerical duties and handing over its administration to the town and its Steward. Similar arrangements were put in place in other hospitals of the Order in Memmingen, Wimpfen and Pfortzheim.[104] In Hesse its newly Evangelical ruler, the Landgrave Philip, used the revenues of some dissolved monasteries to found in 1533 four hospitals deep in the countryside to serve a scattered rural population.[105] Relatively little is known of the hospitals at Hofheim and Gronau, but the substantial archives at Haina and Merxhausen show that he had planned to create his hospitals along the lines of a monastery, where godliness and health went hand in hand. Haina was originally intended for men and Merxhausen for women, but in the course of time both sexes were admitted to both. Haina, in particular, developed a reputation for treating the insane that extended far beyond the boundaries of Hesse. The original regulations said nothing about medical treatment for the sick beyond the need to keep them well fed and warm but a good deal about the sins that might be found among them and would be eliminated by Christian advice and instruction. The men at Haina were warned against luxuriously lying in bed, while the women at Merxhausen were considered prey to more evil habits – arguing, cursing, envying, grousing, gossiping and, even worse, clambering over each other to get to food at mealtimes and refusing to stay silent.[106]

It was England that saw the greatest change in the fortunes of hospitals as a result of religious developments that were not primarily concerned with them. In 1534 Henry VIII broke with Rome and became head of the Church in England. One of his first acts was to draw up a list of clerical holders of religious benefices who could then be taxed, including those associated with hospitals. This affected two kinds of hospital, the larger ones, like St John's in Exeter, with a staff of clerics that resembled monasteries, and smaller ones which had been reclassified as chantries. Two years later, a new statute ordered the abolition of all monasteries with yearly incomes of less than £200, which would have included almost every hospital if it was classed as a monastery. Many were immediately closed, especially those linked with monastic houses and considered a part of them. Gradually over the next few years larger monasteries surrendered themselves to the king, as did chantries and even large hospitals. Some provision was made for the replacement of almshouses, but there was no consistent policy, and many smaller foundations were never abolished. Cities fared worse than smaller towns. York lost the major hospital of St Leonard's, which had employed a physician, and 13 other smaller institutions.[107] In London, despite appeals from the Mayor, most of the hospitals dispensing medical aid were suppressed, including St Thomas's and St Mary Bishopsgate in 1540. St Bartholomew's was reduced in numbers, and in 1547 its government, like that of St Mary Bethlehem, was handed over to the City. The rich Savoy Hospital was dissolved in 1553, and much of its property transferred to the City to maintain three new hospitals, Christ's Hospital, for poor children, Bridewell for poor vagrants and a revived St Thomas's. The Savoy Hospital was re-founded by Queen Mary in 1556, with ladies of the court subscribing towards new bedding and equipment, but it never recovered from the loss of its extensive properties.[108] In 1570 the Master, Thomas Thurland, was dismissed for abuse of office after removing the hospital's treasures, selling its beds, burdening it with a private debt of £2,500 and engaging in sexual relations with the staff. Although it survived as a hospital to the end of the seventeenth century, its buildings were increasingly used as private houses and even a military barracks. It was not until the mid-eighteenth century that London regained the level of medical provision within hospitals that it had had before the Reformation.

The impact of royal intervention can also be seen in another capital, Madrid, which had expanded massively in size in the sixteenth century from a small town to become the centre of the Spanish kingdom. Its 11 hospitals in 1516 were all small, and, in the words of a report of 1532, the sick in them "were not treated or cared for as they deserved". There were also hospitals run by confraternities, and, over the next few years, some new institutions, including a hospital devoted exclusively to caring for members of the court. The report of 1532 recommended that there should be only one general hospital in every town, into which all the others should be amalgamated, and two in major cities, one for contagious, the other for non-contagious diseases. But this plan was a long time in coming to fruition. Philip II began the process of amalgamation in Madrid in 1566–7, but it was not until 1581 that the General Hospital was set up under the protection of a Royal Councillor, and it never seems to have taken in vagrants and beggars but only the sick poor. In 1587, apart from a few hospitals that dealt exclusively with foreigners coming to the capital, Madrid was left with four hospitals: the court hospital; La Latina, an old and wealthy private foundation; Antón Martín, which treated contagious diseases under the oversight of the new General Hospital; and the General Hospital itself. But even here medical provision was limited to one or two physicians, one surgeon, a barber and a bonesetter.[109]

Neither in London, Madrid nor Markgröningen was the provision of strictly medical assistance given priority over the general provision of food and shelter for those in need. But it was not entirely neglected, and, apart from plague hospitals, hospitals were not the portals of death that some traditional accounts and some contemporary opponents suggested. They may not always have lived up to the wording of their statutes, beacons of hope in a naughty world, and much depended on the type of inmate admitted (or excluded). Short stays, from a week to a fortnight, were the norm, but at S. Maria Nuova women stayed for on average twice as long as men, perhaps indicating a more generous attitude to women, who had fewer opportunities, or less incentive, to return quickly to profitable employment than men. Statistics for mortality vary greatly, even without taking into consideration years of epidemics. S. Maria Nuova boasted an average male mortality of 9.7%, half that of the Misericordia at Prato, but substantially more than that of S. Paolo in Florence, a mere 3.5 to 5.2%, although this figure may be explained by S. Paolo's growing function as a place for convalescence. Figures from elsewhere are less cheerful: the general hospital of Santa Creu in Barcelona at the end of the fifteenth century had a mortality rate of 26%, the Hôtel-Dieu in Paris 33%.[110] Some of this discrepancy may be explained by the number of aged staying in the hospital, the type of patient admitted and, at Paris, the custom of having three persons to a bed. A better indicator of attitudes towards hospitals is the willingness of high-status individuals to come and be treated in a hospital. At S. Maria Nuova, eight rooms, complete with hearths, wash basins and toilets, were reserved for the sick of a high social class, including nobles. Between 1513 and 1530 there were at least 17 patients with the surnames of famous Florentine families, few of whom actually died there, probably because they returned home to die.[111] At Haina and Merxhausen potential inmates had to submit a written request setting out why they should be admitted. Analysis of these documents by Christine Vajna and Louise Gray shows that most applicants had continued to live and work in the countryside with a range of what might be termed severe disabilities before they entered the hospital, presumably wishing to remain with, and contribute to, their families as long as possible. But once they had decided that the burden was too great, they willingly applied for this assistance. Indeed, numbers of inmates in both institutions grew substantially during the second half of the century, in part because the provision for the inmates was better than they might have enjoyed at home, to the consternation of the authorities concerned with the hospitals' finances.[112] The strict division between the two hospitals in terms of gender was also modified as couples gained admission. Elsewhere, as in London, hospital provision became more and more intertwined with notions of the poor as sources of pollution, responsible, as one author wrote in 1535, for "sundry and diverse diseases, contagions and infections". St Bartholomew's in 1552 claimed to have cured during the previous five years 800 poor of "the pox, fistulas, filthy blanes and sores . . . which might have . . . stunk in the eyes and nose of the city", and its beadle had the duty of searching the city for vagrants.[113] The growth and better organisation of poor relief in the sixteenth century across Europe turned even the deserving sick poor into a problem that charity by itself was no longer expected to resolve.

The three types of public response to disease discussed in this chapter, Health Boards, public doctors and hospitals, all testify to new ideas about civic and state organisation, whether in an oligarchy like those of Ragusa or Venice or in a monarchy eager to improve the efficiency of its rule like those in England, Germany or Spain. Italy was often seen as the model to which all should aspire, and the facilities in its hospitals, even including their painted bedposts, were widely admired by many travellers.[114] But implementing these aspirations took time, and there were vast discrepancies between countries and regions, Britain lagging far behind other areas of Europe in its localised system of parish poor relief and its late adoption of even minimal plague regulations or publicly paid physicians.[115] Public health in this period involved more than medicalisation and the concentration of important decisions in the hands of a few doctors or learned surgeons, who, despite the impression given by their writings, were viewed far more often as subordinate employees than as crucial decision-makers. Plague control above all was a matter primarily for lay authorities who might or might not choose to follow medical advice, and hospitals placed far more emphasis on the cure of souls and on caring for the elderly and the needy than on curing disease. If the development of institutions to protect the health of the community may be judged an index of modernity, their successful implementation was also a mark of civic cohesion, at its most fragile when faced with epidemic disease.

Notes

1 Lanning 1985; Gentilcore 1994; López Terrada 2007.
2 For theories of plague, see pp. 225–30.
3 For public health arrangements in Italy before the Black Death, Geltner 2019.
4 Benedictow 2004; Nutton 2008a; Green 2014.
5 Carmichael 2008; Cohn 2010: 43–54. Unless otherwise made clear, I use 'plague' to mean the disease caused by *yersinia pestis*.
6 Clemen 1928.
7 Walloe 2008.
8 Dross 2020a: 198.
9 Biraben 1975–6, esp. I: 377–449; Central European epidemics are listed in Eckart 1996.
10 Moote and Moote 2004: 202 (major outbreaks in 1579, 1603, 1626, 1631, 1644 and 1665–6).
11 Slack 1990: 141; Fay 2015.
12 Slack 1990: 61, 151; Harding, also noting numbers of plague deaths in the early 1580s and 1592. The figure for weekly deaths in 1563 is given by Prospero Borgarucci 1565: 32.
13 Slack 1990: 84–5, 90.
14 Cohn 2010: 20–2.

15 Brockliss and Jones 1997: 38, suggesting a slight drop in the regularity of major epidemics at the end of the century from one in 11 to one in 15 years. A similar fall is suggested for N. Italy by Stevens Crawshaw forthcoming.
16 Platter 1987.
17 Wear 1995: 222. Only the dead are listed for the last four houses, probably because of lack of space.
18 Coste 2007; Montagne 2017 discuss the ways in which French doctors described plague.
19 Simoni 1576: 48; Stevens Crawshaw forthcoming, gives similar examples from Venice.
20 Sanseverino 1561: Day I.
21 Machiavelli 2019. The traditional title *Descrizione della Peste di Firenze dell'anno 1527* (Cohn 2010: 96–7) is shown by the latest editor to be misleading. This Defoe-like story was probably written in 1523.
22 Bisciola 1577; Besti 1578.
23 Cohn 2010: 100–60; some non-medical French reactions in literature are discussed by Hobart 2020.
24 For plague theories, including Fracastoro, see pp. 225–30.
25 Houtzager 1989; Bosman-Jelgersma 1996a, 1996b.
26 Bosman-Jelgersma 1996a: 70.
27 Forestus 1591: 132–3, 137; 1653: 229–30.
28 Forestus 1591: 70–1; 1653: 209.
29 Forestus 1591: 133–7; 1653: 229–30.
30 Forestus 1591: 134–40; 1653: 229–31.
31 Forestus 1591: 118–19, 133–4; 1653: 226, 229.
32 Forestus 1591: 125–6, 148–9; 1653: 227, 233.
33 Cohn 2010: 218–29, although major epidemics ran through cities indiscriminately.
34 Crato 1611: 78, a reflection by Donzellini.
35 Cohn 2010: 229–37.
36 Nutton 1981: 28–9.
37 Park 1992: 84.
38 Cohn 2010: 246. Mendelsohn *et al.* 2020.
39 Brockliss and Jones 1997: 14.
40 Pelling 1985: 122–3.
41 Elton 1953: 59 prints the relevant clause.
42 Pomata 1998 is a detailed study of medical contracts in Bologna, although most of her discussion concerns surgeons in the seventeenth century; for Germany, Kinzelbach 2020a; Stolberg 2021a: 402–9, emphasising the poor pay for some positions. Stolberg 2019 is a study of the casebook of one such German town physician, Hiob Finzel, in Zwickau.
43 Gentilcore 1994; López Terrada 2007; Clouse 2011.
44 Nutton 1981; Palmer 1981a; Van Lieburg 1989; for Zurich, Russell 1981: 146; for Nuremberg, Dross 2020b; for St Gallen, Milt 1959: 46–7.
45 Milt 1959: 46; Ripa 1538: f. 32r; Carrarius 1581: 186–7, 191–2.
46 Nutton 1974.
47 Kinzelbach 2020a: 168–71.
48 Clemen 1903.
49 Clemen 1907b.
50 Ripa 1538: ff. 32v–33v; Carrarius 1538: 95, 120–1, 198.
51 Pomata 1998: 48, 216.
52 Ripa 1538: f. 35r.
53 Cipolla 1976: 80–3.
54 Blazina Tomic and Blazina 2015: 80–2, 87–92, list and discuss payments to Ragusan civic doctors and surgeons from 1500 to 1588.

55 Nutton 1981: 34, 177.
56 Palmer 1981a: 47; Pomata 1998: 215.
57 Nutton 2014: 212.
58 For a doctor's proposal for greater medical involvement in health regulation, Kalff 2018: 243–51.
59 Ascheri 1997; Pastore 2007.
60 Cipolla 1981: 75.
61 Stevens Crawshaw 2014; for 'secret' remedies, see pp. 171, 199–200.
62 Ripa 1538: ff. 22v–6v, 29r–31v, 32r–5r. Cf. Previdelli 1524: ff. 28v–34v.
63 Ripa 1538: ff. 32v; Carrarius 1581: 164–5. But not a woman, Stevens Crawshaw 2014.
64 Ripa 1538: ff. 35r–9v; Previdelli 1524: ff. 34r–v.
65 Blazina Tomic and Blazina 2015: 106–9.
66 Blazina Tomic and Blazina 2015: 164–82. Possibly a quarter of the population died in this outbreak.
67 Blazina Tomic and Blazina 2015: 175–6.
68 The period might vary from place to place, as Sam Cohn tells me: by 1574 it had been reduced to eight to 12 days.
69 Montaigne 1955: 68, 79; Villamont 1600: fols. 4v–5r; Bamji 2019.
70 Moryson 1903: 260.
71 Carmichael 1986: 122–5.
72 Palmer 1978; Cipolla 1981 (mainly dealing with the next century); Carmichael 1986: 116–20; Cohn 2010: 238–63. But there seems to be no indication of special clothing to be worn until the seventeenth century, Ruisinger 2020.
73 Blazina Tomic and Blazina 2015: 181. Venice commissioned Andrea Palladio to build the church of the Redentore in a prominent position on the Giudecca.
74 Cipolla 1979.
75 Lindemann 2010: 199–203.
76 For Windsor, Roger 2020.
77 Slack 1990: 44–8, 207–11.
78 Simoni 1576: sig. A2r.
79 Nutton and D'Alessio 2021.
80 Simoni 1576: sigg. A2r–v: Ludwig 1909: 239–41.
81 Mitchell 1980: 87–9.
82 Da Monte 1583: 1106–20.
83 Blazina Tomic and Blazina 2015: 163.
84 Cohn 2010: 85.
85 Clemen 1907a: 6; Simoni 1576: sigg., A2–3r, 4r–v.
86 Mercuriale 1577; Preto 1978, 1979; Palmer 2008; Cohn 2010: 162–92; Celati 2021. For a student comment on Mercuriale's change of mind, see p. 83.
87 The word has nothing to do with Lazarus, the New Testament beggar, but is a corruption of the name of the island, S. Maria di Nazaretto.
88 Stevens Crawshaw 2012.
89 Henderson 2006: 93–7, 101, 354.
90 Cohn 2010: 108.
91 Cohn 2010: 127, noting that the poor may have had a better chance of survival here than in their own homes.
92 Rawcliffe 1984.
93 Henderson 2006: 340–55.
94 Orme and Webster 1995: 62, 112–4.
95 Militzer 1975: 104–5, 27–32; for a leper house in S. Germany, Kinzelbach 2020b.
96 Henderson 2006: 19–23, 52–60, 153.

97 Henderson 2006: 152–3.
98 Forestus 1591b: 80, 179; 1591: 54; 1653: 4, 27, 53, 264. For other northern students associated with Horst, see O'Malley 1964: 405 (Wolfgang Meurer) and the anonymous visitor to Rome in 1536 (Margócsy *et al.* 2018: 309). For his role in medical botany, Andretta and Pardo-Tomás 2019: 20–1.
99 Gilino 1937.
100 Park and Henderson 1991.
101 MacCulloch 2003: 631–2; Henderson 2006: 98–104: for he Fuggerei, the pox hospital at Augsburg, Stein 2009: 91–9.
102 Sticker 1927: 54–8; Lindemann 2010: 126.
103 Karant-Nunn 1987: 219.
104 Militzer 1975: 21, 27; Scott 2002: 140. For the Calvinist example of Groningen, see p. 318.
105 Midelfort 1980.
106 Midelfort 1999: 329–34.
107 For an exemplary account of the closure and reopening of the Great Hospital of Norwich, see Rawcliffe 1999: 198–239.
108 Orme and Webster 1995: 159–65; Schen 2002: 91–6, 238.
109 Huguet-Termes 2009.
110 Henderson 2006: 262–7, 281.
111 Henderson 2006: 270–1.
112 Midelfort 1999: 335–53; Gray 2001, 2002, 2007; later, pp. 202–4.
113 Wear 1995: 244–5.
114 Chaney 1981: The bedposts were admired by Luther 1967: 296.
115 Wear 2000: 275–349; Lindemann 2010: 198–208.

3 Medical Communication: Print and the Post

Few changes have been so enormous and so all-embracing as the introduction of the printing press to Europe around 1457. The new geographical horizons were matched by the new intellectual horizons opened up by the availability of books of all kinds in a variety of languages (for the learned world principally in Latin). The time-consuming process of copying documents singly by hand was superseded by the production of multiple copies at one time which circulated far more quickly than before, thanks to improved methods of transport, including a postal service. New centres of book production sprang up, and, with a growth in literacy, particularly encouraged by an Evangelical insistence on reading and understanding the words of the Bible, the reading and possession of books were no longer confined to a tiny elite or to a mainly religious setting. The exaggerated claims of the American historian Elizabeth Eisenstein for the impact of printing as an agent of change have been modified and many of her misunderstandings corrected by subsequent scholars without overthrowing her overarching thesis.[1] Indeed, they have only confirmed it by showing the many ways in which new ideas and new forms of communication came to coexist alongside the older traditions, and were allowed to flourish precisely because of the opportunities provided by the new technology in introducing illustrations or in creating indexes.[2] The impact of these developments on the world of medicine has been largely neglected until recently, and attention has been focussed, following Eisenstein, on the major publications of the 1540s, Fuchs and Vesalius to the fore. Adrian Johns, the severest critic of Eisenstein's views on medicine and science, has concentrated on the period after this date, and, with a few notable exceptions like Ian Maclean and Sam Cohn, medical historians have been slow to exploit the abundance of material now available on the web and accessible through major cataloguing projects around Europe.[3] But to focus entirely on printed literature is to miss another major feature of the intellectual world of the sixteenth century, the exchange of information between doctors and scholars by letter, often preceding its appearance in print. Nancy Siraisi in her 2013 Singleton Lectures discussed three letter collections, those of Mercuriale, Johannes Lang and Orazio Augenio (1527–1603), focussing on the selections that appeared in print.

DOI: 10.4324/9781003223184-5

The unwary might be misled by her final observations to underestimate the size and geographical extent of the collections that are not mentioned in her book or lurk unnoticed in archives.[4] Doctors were at the very centre of many European networks of information, and few modern libraries are without examples of the academic and medical epistles which circulated alongside the printed book in the transmission of knowledge.

But the most extensive method of communication is also the hardest for historians to penetrate. Medical information was transmitted most frequently by word of mouth accompanied by gesture, almost invisible to historians reliant on written material. This was a crucial component of what Pamela Long has termed artisanal relations, and to leave it out, whether in the classroom or at the bedside, is to misrepresent much of the healing process in the sixteenth century.[5]

The Printed Word

Paradoxically, there have been remarkably few studies of matters medical among the very many histories of the book, and those that exist tend to focus either on bibliography or on the more famous productions.[6] There are also substantial gaps. The bibliographies of medical imprints before 1501, the so-called incunabula, are now more than 50 years old, and Durling's pioneering census of Galenic printings remains 60 years after its publication unsurpassed in its listing of the libraries that hold copies of individual items.[7] Its Hippocratic successors are all unsatisfactory in different ways, and only Dioscorides and Paul among less familiar authors from Antiquity have been made the subject of detailed discussion.[8] More modern writers fare even worse. Although there are several useful bibliographies of individual authors, from Karl Sudhoff's remarkable investigations into the writings of Paracelsus onwards, very few researchers have investigated who owned and used them.[9] Even the major survey by Stephen Joffe and his team into the surviving copies of Vesalius's *Fabrica*, a resource that will continue to be mined for many years to come, is limited to the two editions of 1543 and 1555.[10] The great national catalogues of Italian, French, German and English imprints are now available online, but cross-checking is not always easy. Surveys of Renaissance medical and scientific holdings in individual libraries also can trap the unwary, for both terms are fluid and the catalogue of a medico-historical library, like that of the Wellcome Collection, may contain a much greater variety of books than its title suggests. There is as yet nothing to rival Frank Hieronymus's catalogue of Basle printings in medicine and science, with its substantial translations, many illustrations and comprehensive listing of ownership and use, that throws new light on the role of Basle as an intellectual forum.[11] To mention these gaps is not to belittle the work of librarians and cataloguers, or to deny that during the last 20 years, thanks to the internet, an abundance of new material has been placed at the disposal of historians. Rather, it is to reiterate that we are still far from being able to gain a comprehensive vision of the impact of medical printing across Europe in this century, and that we are forced to proceed by means of pointilliste examples and general impressions.[12]

Two related generalisations need always to be borne in mind. The books that were most often printed and reprinted are largely not those familiar to most historians of medicine. *Practicae*, short guides to medicine, often written in the vernacular, far outnumber theoretical discussions and academic works, and even if they were (or purported to be) composed by a distinguished professor, such as the Viennese Puff von Schrick or 'the most celebrated physician' Magninus or Maino de' Mainieri, doctor to the bishop of Arras, they have been little studied.[13] Secondly, printers were concerned to make a living and to publish what would sell. An unwary choice of title or a misjudgement of the market could lead to bankruptcy. The last years of one of the most famous of all Renaissance publishers of medicine, Johannes Oporinus, were a constant struggle to keep afloat, not least because, despite a substantial loan and assistance with production costs from its author, the second, 1555, edition of Vesalius's *Fabrica* did not sell as well as the first and many copies remained unsold when Oporinus handed over his business.[14] Vesalius may have wished to bring out a third edition, but if his corrected version ever arrived in Basle, the sheer costs of printing another edition of so large a book would have been a strong deterrent to its appearance in print.[15] As Sachiko Kusukawa has brilliantly shown, illustrations, to say nothing of the top quality paper required, added enormously to the costs of production. Not surprisingly, Fuchs's and Matthioli's illustrated herbals, alongside the *Fabrica*, were among the most expensive of all Renaissance printings, far beyond the resources of a local printer without access to an international market or the pocket of most potential purchasers.[16]

Medical printing expanded steadily from 1470 onwards and it is not easy to decide on a suitable periodisation. Books printed before 1500 were almost all produced in Italy, reflecting both the burgeoning Latin book culture of Northern Italy as well as a market of wealthy students coming to study from beyond the Alps. Parisian printers are almost entirely absent, Lyons and Basle enter in the 1490s, but Basle does not become an international centre for medical production outside its region for a further 30 years.[17] The favourite authors were the medical standards rather than any novelties, and perhaps not until the 1510s did living authors begin to outnumber the dead. Two authors of books dealing with problems at both ends of life stand out. The Paduan teacher Gabriele Zerbi (1445–1505), published in Rome in 1490 his *Gerontocomia, Looking after the Elderly*.[18] Far more striking because of its theme and origin is a small book on children's diseases, *Opusculum de aegritudinibus infantium, A Little Book on the Diseases of Infants*, produced at Louvain in 1486–7 by a local doctor, Cornelius Roelants (1450–1525). Most early medical books were produced in large folios, with margins, like those in manuscripts, wide enough to take many annotations, and containing a compilation of texts.[19] The 1473 Milan edition of the *Aggregatus, Supplement*, of the twelfth-century Arabic pharmaceutical writer Serapion the Younger also contained the (pseudo-) Galenic tract *De virtute centaureae*, *The Property of the Century*. Subsequent editions in the fifteenth century added the *Breviarium* of Serapion the Elder and the *Practica* and *De simplici medicina*, *Simple medicines*, by Johannes Platearius, and other works were added in the next century to make it a valuable compendium of simples and their use.[20]

A similar pattern of expansion can be seen in printings of the staple of university teaching, the *Articella*, *The Little Art*, from 1476 to 1534, which contained a variety of texts from Byzantium and Classical Greece. Over time new and more accurate Latin versions taken from the Greek were printed alongside older ones coming via the Arabic, Hippocratic texts were replaced by different introductory material, such as Mesue's *Aphorisms*, and yet more material continued to be added until the final edition of 1536.[21] Studied by first-year students across European universities, this was an obvious early candidate for profitable printing, as were some of the short compendia from the Arabic like the *Ad Almansorem*, *A Book for al-Mansūr*, of Rhazes, published in Milan by Pachel and Scinzenzeler in 1481. Bigger works were at first avoided, except for sections of Avicenna's *Canon*, and particularly its opening chapters, with 14 printings between 1472 and the end of the century. Academic commentaries come a little later, mainly by Italian authors: there was no printing of the Parisian teacher Jacques Despars (d. 1465) until 1498 and only one by a Montpellier professor, Jean de Tournamire (1325–96) in 1490. Some works were printed only in Italy, while others never crossed the Alps. The popular compendium of Ortolf von Baierland circulated in a variety of forms, titles and German dialects, each within its own geographical and linguistic area.[22]

Until the 1550s printing in the vernacular languages was confined to short texts of practical medicine for use in the home, advice on distillation, herbals and plague tracts, as well as smaller numbers of works on surgery. Most were published in German dialects, followed by French and, far fewer, English and Italian.[23] Translations of academic texts or the ancient Classics from Latin are very rare; the few in English were usually made from a French intermediary. Vesalius's simultaneous production of a Latin and German version of his *Epitome* of the *Fabrica* in 1543 and Estienne's of his anatomy in Latin and French in 1545 and 1546 helped strengthen the move towards the use of the vernacular. But it is not until the flood of Paracelsian tracts in German from the late 1550s that learned medical books are published first or only in the vernacular, testimony both to the emerging wider readership in German and to the German focus of Paracelsus and his immediate followers. The first publication of Latin versions of many Paracelsian treatises did not appear until 1575, when it was swiftly bought by non-German speakers.[24]

By the 1520s humanist productions began to circulate more widely beyond Italy, and a growing number of medical students and practitioners, together with their wealthy patrons, provided an expanding market for printers. Booksellers such as Garrett Godfrey in Cambridge in 1527–32 were able easily to make available foreign books to their university customers.[25] Lyons and, from the 1520s, Basle began to compete with the Venetian presses in the international market, sometimes by a direct take-over of Italian books but in a different format, sometimes by deliberate competition.[26] Rouille's Lyons imprints of individual Galenic treatises in a small format, aimed at a student market, exemplify the first, the Basle printer Froben's participation in what John Caius called an 'honourable rivalry' with two Venetian presses to produce the first and most accurate edition of the complete new Galen in Latin, the second.[27] Booksellers sprang up as intermediaries between printer and reader, and wealthy patrons expected friends and protégés to provide them with news and copies of the latest publications. In 1567 Johannes Neodicus, a student in Padua, purchased a variety of medical books in Venice for his patron, Thomas Rehdiger (1540–76), in Wrocław. He was particularly pleased to have bought a complete Averroes for 25 lire, far cheaper than the 32 for which it was being sold in Padua.[28]

The format of books also changed. Although the stately folio still commanded prestige, particularly for collected works or titles with a similar content, such as the collection on baths, *De balneis*, published by Tommaso Giunta at Venice in 1553 or the *Epistolae medicinales*, *Medical Letters*, published in 1556 at Lyons by the heirs of Giacomo Giunta, handy manuals and compendia in smaller formats spread this learning to a wider readership both professional and lay. Disgruntled professors warned that they were a snare and a delusion, to say nothing of a waste of money.[29] The writing of books was also coming to be a sign of both the author's intellectual and social standing. By 1564, when the first catalogue of the Frankfurt Book Fair was published, the world of academic printing resembled our own in many respects. Books were printed in a variety of formats – the Paracelsians generally favoured octavo and quarto editions – and places. University towns increasingly came to have one or two presses who issued the offerings of local professors, and the list of authors and their works grew ever longer. When Conrad Gessner produced his *Bibliotheca Universalis* in 1545, he intended this massive volume of 631 folios to be a catalogue of everything in print.[30] Ten years later it had to be supplemented by a slightly smaller *Appendix*, which added the names of 3,800 new authors. By the end of the century, two medical scholars, Paschasius Gallus in 1590 and Israel Spach the following year, independently thought it worthwhile to produce a list of all medical printings divided according to their subject area as an aid to physicians who needed a guide to this ever-burgeoning literature.[31]

Printing also made the dissemination of illustrated books, pamphlets and so-called fugitive sheets much easier. At one extreme of the financial spectrum it allowed the publication of large-scale images of plants, animals and the human body in lavishly illustrated collections from 1542, when Fuchs's herbal first appeared, followed the next year by Vesalius's *Fabrica*. Gessner's books on animals, birds and fishes performed a similar service for natural history, the images being copied from specimens or pictures sent him by friends such as Caius, some of which have been only recently rediscovered (Figure 3.1).[32] At the other end were the fugitive sheets, sets of images of

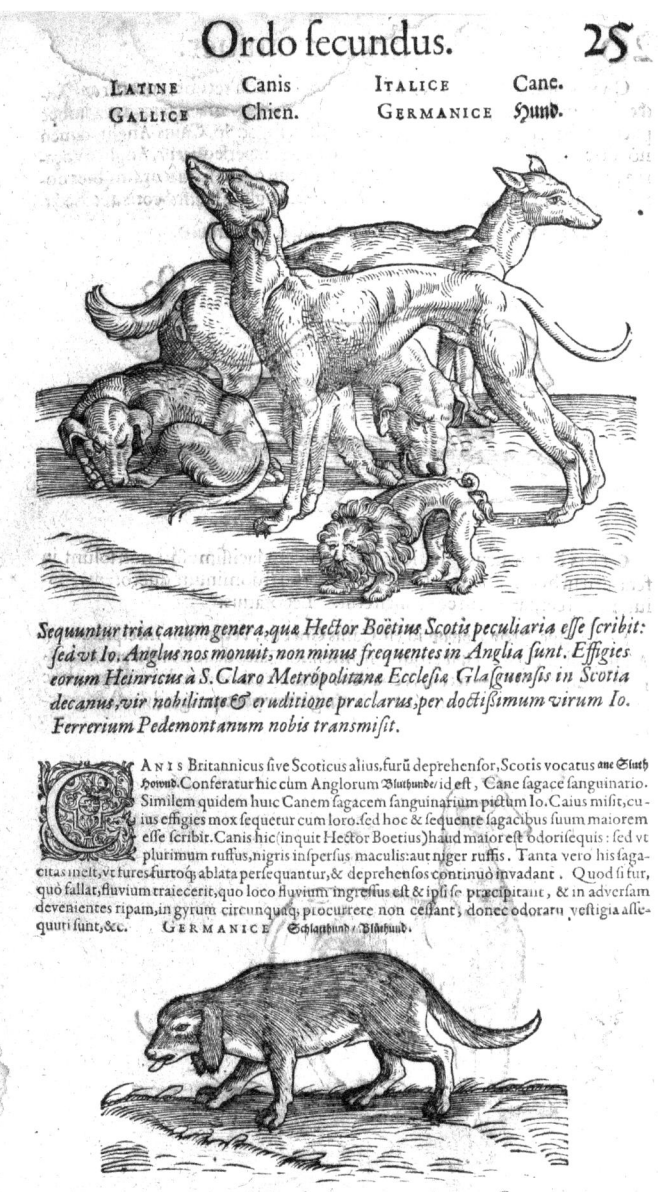

Figure 3.1 Conrad Gessner (1516–65), *Icones animalium*, Zurich: C. Froschover, 1560, p. 25. In his description Gessner explains that Hector Boece (d. 1536) had written about three native Scottish dogs, including the bloodhound, but his friend John Caius had complained that they were also English. Henry Sinclair, Dean of Glasgow 1550–61, had this drawing made for him, which was sent to Zurich by the learned Giovanni Ferrerio from Piedmont (the author of the continuation of Boece's *History of Scotland*).

a male and female body, usually with a short verbal exposition, and with representations of the internal organs of the body that could be cut out and stuck down as flaps.[33] Beginning around 1538, and possibly linked with the six anatomical sheets put out by Vesalius for his Padua students in that year, these were the successors of medieval schematic representations of the body and circulated widely around Europe in a variety of languages, including French, Flemish and English as well as Latin and German. Some, particularly those printed in Wittenberg (see Figure 9.2), were designed as memory aids to accompany university lectures, but others were aimed at a much broader audience, being available cheaply in many centres that lacked a university. Their overall message was to extol the wonders of the human body, and they often had headings with a religious tone. They thus echoed many of the introductory prefaces of leading anatomists justifying their activities as a necessary part of a Christian education.[34]

Plague Tracts

Far more widespread were tracts on plague. Figures are hard to determine, but Cohn calculates that before 1600 at least 378 had appeared from Italian presses and 778 from German ones.[35] Figures from France are lacking at present, but a total approaching 1,500 separate printings across Europe over the century is not unlikely. They were overwhelmingly in the vernacular, some 60%–70%, although there seems to have been an increase in more academic writing on plague in Latin in the third quarter of the century. They were produced steadily throughout the century, with major peaks around plague years, and, in Italy, with a massive leap in numbers in the plague years of 1575–8 that coincides with a drop in the production of other medical literature, including practical handbooks. Very few of these plague books contain more than 64 pages: the *Gewisse unnd erfahren Practick . . . vor der Pestilentz, A Practical Guide against Plague Based on Learning and Experience*, of Jacobus Theodorus Tabernaemontanus (c. 1525–90), written in 1551, was unusually long for a book in the vernacular, some 381 *sedicesimo* pages in the Heidelberg edition of 1564.[36] Some, particularly plague orders, are only a page long, and most could have been printed on one or two folio sheets before they were folded over into a book, something that could be done in a day or two. They were printed on cheap paper, one of the reasons for their poor rate of survival, since many are found today in only a handful of copies. Several were printed in towns without a medical school or a tradition of medical printing – Asti, Carmagnola or Macerata in Italy, Neisse, Unna, Schmalkalden or Neustadt an der Hardt in Germany. Medieval authors of plague tracts, such as Johannes Jacobis and Benedictus Kanuti, who dominate printings before 1500 were quickly replaced by a huge variety of authors, very few of them from the scribbling classes. Two-thirds of them are known only by a single tract: that of Caspar Kegeler, printed with two revisions in seven different places between 1521 and 1600,

is unusual in its longevity and geographical range of presses. Most authors were local physicians writing for their own community in an emergency to be read either individually or aloud to those who were illiterate. Only one author of a plague tract published in England was a member of the London College of Physicians, William Bullein (d. 1576), and he lived and practised 100 kilometres away in Suffolk. His co-writers included clergymen, school-masters, a translator and a lawyer, Simon Kellwaye (fl. 1593), the author of *A Defensative against the Plague*.[37] These few English examples are all relatively short, and the only exception from England that resembles learned continental tracts was written in French by a former student at both Paris and Cologne, Janus Julius Monacius, for the benefit of the exiled French Protestant community in London in 1560.[38] Most plague tracts concentrated on advice on prevention and on preparing the body to resist disease by means of diet and, in one instance, on explaining at length how to obtain the necessary state of mind to avoid disturbing the body.[39] Such precautions were rudely dismissed by Simone Simoni, who affirmed in his title and text that he had devised a scientific method of cure that he had successfully employed, although its immediate use in the Leipzig plague of 1575 was prevented by a shortage of printers to publish his volume.[40]

Who read these largely ephemeral productions and how they were used is hard to determine. Kellwaye's book was owned and read by one of his neighbours, and most physicians would have owned a selection of them.[41] They formed about 10% of the large library of the Nuremberg physician Georg Palma (1543–91), including one in manuscript, and several were annotated by him.[42] Another physician, Pierre Costan (fl. 1550–70), a Montpellier graduate, included corrections and reminiscences of his experiences at Rodez in Central France in a collection of five small tracts he had bound together. Two of them are unique: a tract written by an otherwise unknown Guillaume Dassonville at Béthune in 1546 and published at Paris, and a collection of proven remedies put out by the bishop of Rodez to help his flock and printed at Toulouse in 1558, and only one, by Jacques Daléchamps, is at all widely preserved. But such detailed annotations in plague tracts are rare, for in general their small size and poor paper quality made them inhospitable to notes.[43]

Books, however, are no use if they are not read, and the growth of publisher's networks, numbers of booksellers, sales catalogues and, in the last third of the century, book fairs, of which that in Frankfurt was the most important, speeded up and extended the transfer of knowledge by this route. In 1558 the university of Heidelberg decided that the senior professor of medicine should visit the Frankfurt fair each year and bring back anything of interest.[44] The town school at Zwickau seems also to have had bought each year small practical guides to medicine that might be used in the school. School versions of Melanchthon's *De anima, The Soul,* were produced for use in Lutheran schools in Central Germany and beyond.[45] Larger works, particularly those on plants and natural history, also had a market all over

Europe that extended beyond the medical profession. Matthioli claimed to have sold 30,000 copies of the first ten editions of his commentary on Dioscorides, and Vesalius's *Fabrica* was being read around Europe within a matter of months by diplomats as well as professors.[46] Authors with good connections and an established reputation could take advantage of the varied regulations between regions and of the different expertise of printing houses to secure publication wherever it best suited them or was most profitable.[47] Publishers too could take advantage of widening markets to issue in almost serial form what might otherwise have been expensive to print at one time. The most remarkable such publication was that of the *Observations and Consultations* of Van Foreest. Some of their contents date back to the 1540s, and almost everything was ready for the press by the 1570s, but the first volumes, consisting of two books only, did not appear till 1584, and it took until 1606 for all of the 32 books to appear. The final selection, the nine books dealing with the physician's involvement in surgery, were not published until 1610, 13 years after their author's death.[48]

Medical Libraries

The growth and development of medical printing is mirrored in the libraries of individual scholars. Before 1500, ownership of medical manuscripts was still common, although numbers were small, and books were rapidly overtaking them. Once a work appeared in print, it was rare for manuscript copies still to be made, with the exception of Greek manuscripts of medicine that continued to be produced (and some forged) until the middle of the sixteenth century.[49] The collection of such manuscripts amassed by Leoniceno, rivalled but not surpassed by those of Bessarion and the Medici, was far more extensive than that collected by John Caius in Italy and England in the 1540s and 1550s, or by Mercuriale a decade or more after that.[50] By contrast, Caius's library is largely composed of books by humanist authors, many of them in imposing folios, and contains relatively few written after 1560 or in the vernacular. The contrast between his library and that of another Cambridge medical teacher, Thomas Lorkyn, in the next generation is marked, not only in size, but also in range, format and use. The posthumous inventory of Caius's library in 1573 lists 126 titles, 43 of them medical; that of Lorkyn in 1591, 588 titles, 400 or so medical, roughly the same as that of his father-in-law John Hatcher, a Cambridge don who died in 1587. While Caius's book buying had largely ended long before his death, Lorkyn continued to keep up to date, specifying in his will that his collection should be placed in the university library for the benefit of staff and students. (He had during his lifetime loaned books to his friends and colleagues and obtained in return others from them by gift or purchase.) Folios were far fewer in his collection and were heavily outnumbered by octavo printings, and although his books were largely in Latin, a small number were in English or French.[51] The library of his Nuremberg contemporary Georg Palma

is even more extensive, with 668 medical titles, many of them bought hot off the press, with a major acquisition of books from Basle printers in 1565. The standard classical and humanist authors are there in numbers, but there are also many writers in the vernacular and on very specific themes.[52] These libraries are exceptional in their size, but by the end of the century most medical men would have owned a library of 100 or so books, perhaps five times more than their predecessors a century earlier.[53]

The cornucopia of information made available even in out-of-the-way small towns as a result of printing not only favoured the spread of new ideas and stimulated debate but also presented new problems in organising and assimilating the knowledge that had suddenly become available. Many solutions were traditional ones transferred to a new technological environment – the production of digests and student summaries, assisted by marginal headings and the new memory techniques popularised by the followers of Petrus Ramus (1515–72) – but others were new and soon became standard.[54] The numbering of pages and, still more, the provision of indexes facilitated consultation even of small books like the 1538 *Institutiones anatomicae* of Guinter and Vesalius.[55] The availability of detailed indexes to larger collections opened up easy access to otherwise complex material such as the 1556 Giuntine collected edition of *Epistolae medicinales*. The massive indexes of plants, remedies, parts of the body, and diseases, over 150 pages long, that open the later editions of Matthioli's *Herbal* almost constitute a guide to Renaissance practical medicine in themselves. If one wishes to investigate Galen's ideas, the single huge volume that contains Brasavola's index to the Giuntine editions of the Latin *Opera omnia Galeni* from 1551 onwards is often more helpful even today than a straightforward word index to a modern edition.[56] Whereas in the Middle Ages academic debate centred on the detailed investigation of a relatively small number of sources, in the sixteenth century learned argument involved the reading, citation and easy availability of a far larger number of titles, which privileged those who could consult and utilise a large library, whether their own or that of a university. Bibliographical rather than philological and textual knowledge was becoming the mark of the expert physician. Footnotes and appendices likewise established the importance of medical erudition among practitioners. But this was also made available to non-professionals through large compendia or encyclopaedias like the 29 volumes of the *Theatrum humanae vitae*, *The Theatre of Human Life*, of the Basle professor Theodor Zwinger (1533–88).[57]

Case Histories and Medical Letters

Two related genres that straddle the boundary between manuscript and print become ever more important as the century progressed: namely collections of observations and of medical letters, both of which had precursors in the *consilia* literature of the Later Middle Ages. It was common then,

and for centuries after, for advice to be sought from a distant practitioner who would then reply with a letter setting out what should best be done. A recently discovered *consilium* by Vesalius for a sufferer with a urinary tract problem was sent in reply to a request from three doctors in Naples who had provided him with details. He expected it to be sent on to others, and it survives, along with another epistolary contribution to the case by a Paduan colleague, in a later copy that had reached Germany.[58] Such cases, *consilia*, like similar cases in law, could then be used in teaching to suggest general rules for effective practice.[59] Substantial collections of these *consilia* were made in the mid-fifteenth century, and two were among the earliest medical literature to be printed, evidence for their value to the learned doctor. Both those of Antonio Cermisone (d. 1441) and Bartolommeo di Montagnana (d. 1470), appeared in 1476, the latter a massive 354 folios long, which increased to 396 in the Venice edition of 1497.[60] Other *consilia* appeared in print within collections of more general medical letters, and the bedside consultations of Giambattista da Monte with his colleagues were dutifully recorded by his pupils and published from their notes in many editions from 1554 onwards.[61] Of greater importance as a model for some of the later *Observations* were the 700 case histories assembled by the Portuguese Jewish doctor Amatus Lusitanus (1511–68) which were published in a series of volumes in many cities around Europe from 1551 onwards and told of his experiences in places as diverse as Paris, Antwerp, Ancona and Thessalonica.[62] His case histories furnish extensive descriptions of the case and its context, and many are then followed by a, usually brief, *scholium* or commentary, adding further learned comment to what has just been expounded. This organisation emphasises his own singularity, for Lusitanus is using his own text for comment in the same way as a Renaissance philologist would have interpreted Homer or a doctor dealt with Galen in his commentaries or as some put it, observations. In this way, Amatus not only established his account as a true record of the case, but, via the *scholia*, displayed his own considerable learning, including, for example, a quotation from a Byzantine poem on gout in Greek.

By using the title 'cures' Amatus stressed that he had been successful in his cases. Later writers modified his egocentric approach by either adding or replacing it with the words *Observationes*, Observations. In so doing they shifted the emphasis away from the individual patient to the diseases and symptoms they were describing, sometimes, like François Valleriola (1504–80), saying plainly that this was something remarkable, *mirabilis*, and out of the ordinary.[63] It is not clear why the early books with this title all come from north of the Alps, with one exception, the book of *Medical Observations* by the papal physician, Marsilio Cagnati (1543–1612), which in fact contains only philological emendations and elucidations of a wide variety of ancient and medieval texts on medicine and science.[64] But the emphasis on the importance of the individual case can be found in various genres of medicine across Europe by 1600 and mirrors the earlier discussions of individual

plants and animals by the naturalists who commented on Dioscorides and shared their findings in letters.[65]

Many observations of this sort can also be found in collections of medical letters.[66] The earliest such printed collection contained those written by Giovanni Manardi, whose first volume, divided into six books, appeared in 1521. Six more books followed in 1532, and the posthumous edition of 1540 added a further eight. He explained that many medieval *consilia*, like those of Di Montagnana and Cermisone, had been originally sent as letters, and that two Roman predecessors of Galen, Themison and Archigenes, had composed some of their major medical works (alas, now lost) for circulation in that form. Classical scholars with medical interests such as Ficino and Politian were familiar with the Latin *Letters* of both Cicero and Seneca (c. 5 BCE–65). Those of Cicero resembled modern letters in usually recounting the writer's reactions to incidents around him, while Seneca's, which often touched on medicine and natural science, were longer and more akin to short essays.[67] Manardi's example was widely followed throughout the century by other authors with an international reputation, such as Niccolò Massa, Conrad Gessner or Girolamo Mercuriale, and also by some of a merely local fame, such as Giovanni Baptista Teodosi of Parma (1475–1538) and Luigi Mondella of Brescia (fl. 1538). The earliest collections were almost entirely written by Italians and printed in Italy: those of Johannes Lange, printed for the first time at Basle by Oporinus in 1554, were the first to be composed by a German and published north of the Alps (Figure 5.2). Their inclusion in the collected volume of medical letters put out in 1556 by the Lyons branch of the Giuntine Press in a large folio edition stimulated more interest, but Parisian authors such as Fernel preferred to publish in the older and more restricted genre of *consilia*. At the end of the century Lorenz Scholz (1552–99) collected and edited a series of letters originating with the circle around Crato von Crafftheim and originally assembled by Peter Monau (1551–88), Crato's successor as imperial physician. Like the letters of Manardi, publication of individual volumes was slow: Book I appeared in 1591, the last, Book VII, only in 1611. Sometimes the same letters were also included in other selections edited by Scholz and published by the same press under the different titles of *Consilia*, *Medical Advice*, and *Epistolae philosophicae, medicinales ac chimicae*, *Philosophical, Medical and Chemical Letters*.

The contents of published letters are as varied as the book titles. Lange, and later Mercuriale, discussed topics that would interest a wider, antiquarian audience.[68] Some letters, like those of Gessner and Matthioli, focus on material that they later discussed in their major works on natural history and botany, and 14 of the 17 letters included in Mondella's second book could also have been titled *consilia*.[69] Trincavella's son, who edited his father's letters, *consilia* and some *quaestiones* 18 years after his father's death in 1568, distinguished between them on grounds of topic and of length, but admitted that several could have fitted into more than one category.[70] The first six

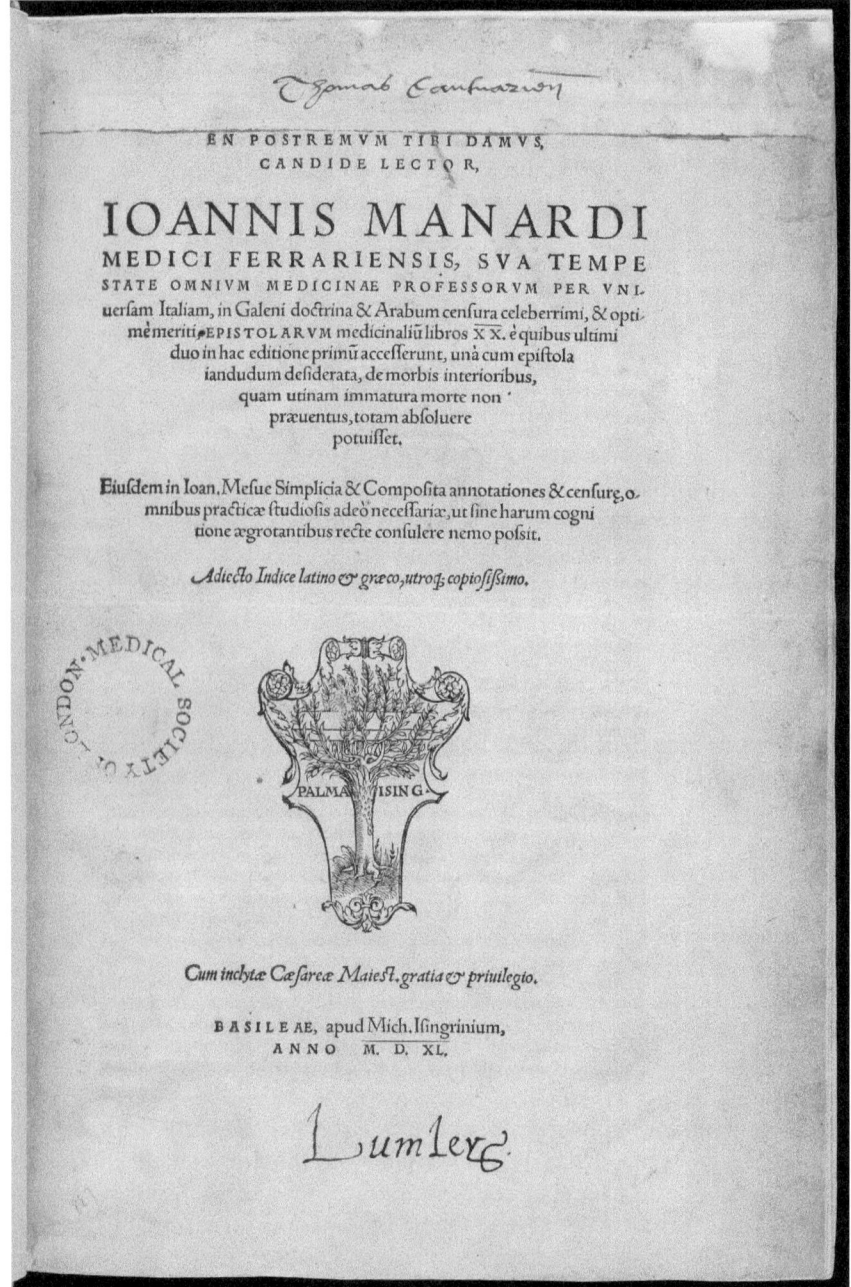

Figure 3.2 Giovanni Manardi (1461–1536), *Epistulae medicinales*, Basle: M. Isin-grin, 1540. This copy, London, Wellcome Collection EPB/D/66223, was owned by, among others, Archbishop Cranmer, the antiquary Humphrey Llwyd (1527–68), the benefactor of the London College of Physicians Lord Lumley (1534–1609) and Henry, Prince of Wales (1594–1612).

books of Manardi's letters typify the range and content of these printed collections. Their 24 letters are addressed not only to fellow doctors but also to non-medical friends and academics such as his Ferrara colleague Calcagnini. One-third deal with diseases and their cures, including one *consilium*, another third with botanical questions, and most of the rest expound difficulties in standard texts such as Avicenna and Hippocrates. Throughout, Manardi emphasises the crucial importance of a correct understanding of terms in trying to resolve medical problems.[71] Some of his letters, especially in Book III, provide important advice to his contemporaries over the classification of internal and mental diseases, but others produce more heat than light. His pupil Brasavola described one such epistolary exchange between Manardi and Leoniceno on the translation of a word in Hippocrates's *Aphorisms* as two old men making a mountain out of a molehill.[72]

The ability to write well on a variety of themes was a mark of excellence among Renaissance humanists, as Manardi explained in his opening letter, but it does not make for easy consultation without the aid of the long index to the 1556 edition. By contrast, Scholz organised many of the letters in the collections he edited at the end of the century thematically, and his juxtaposition of letters by different hands hence resembles an international debate among friends. One of the great medical correspondents, Ulisse Aldrovandi in Bologna, sometimes retained the originals of the letters he had received, but sometimes had more legible copies made and entered into small notebooks. He then organised them by their author, giving prominence to those by "men of distinction" so that he and his students could make easier use of them.[73]

How these collections of letters were put together, usually after the death of their author or authors, can best be shown by the example of the three volumes of medical letters of Conrad Gessner that appeared at Basle in 1577, 12 years after his death. They were edited by his friend and executor Caspar Wolff (1525–1601), who selected and often filleted the original documents to give a more coherent and more elegant appearance. But in this he was only doing what Gessner himself had done. If he received a letter from a correspondent, he often cut it up and stuck it into a letter book, to which he appended his own reply. Sometimes, if he thought it particularly interesting or problematic, he would send it on, often along with his own comments, to another friend for them to comment upon. This was a method he found particularly valuable when attempting to identify plants or animals, to check the truth of what his original informant had told him or simply to have a second opinion on difficult cases. The result in print is at times far removed from the original, but, as Candice Delisle shows, in the process of circulation and ratification an individual and possibly uncertain observation has been turned into a fact that can then be relied upon and utilised by others.[74]

These printed editions of letters constitute only a tiny part of the massive surviving correspondence between doctors that languishes in manuscript in (mainly) European libraries and has yet to be properly investigated.[75]

The art of letter-writing had been appreciated in Antiquity and the Middle Ages, but it had almost entirely been carried on at an official level in government and the church. The massive improvement in communications in the late fifteenth and sixteenth century, as well as the development of postal services, and, one might add, the increasing number of individuals who were able to write and to share their views with others, led to the growth of networks of information both more extensive and more individual than the printed word.[76] There were still the hazards of travel, notably robbers and accidents. The complimentary copy of Vesalius's *Fabrica* sent by Oporinus to his friend Vadianus in St Gallen, was badly damaged when the courier's horse fell into a stream, and the publisher had kindly to supply a replacement, although since the accompanying letter and another book had been returned to him, he suspected that the courier had decided to keep the damaged copy for himself.[77] A friend apologised to Crato in 1580 for a delay in writing because his original letter (and many others) as well as books he had sent to him had been stolen when the courier was ambushed by robbers.[78] But there were also far more travellers to bring letters back from Padua or Brussels for friends of friends, and, despite complaints about costs and delays, the postal system was more frequent and more organised. Although even humble townsfolk could engage the help of a scribe to ask for medical assistance from afar or enquire about a natural curiosity they had come across, these correspondents almost always came from the elite. They can be loosely divided into two overlapping networks, one concerned with the life of the university, the other with the world of nature, and largely centred upon individuals with easy access to postal routes in major cities. Some of their letters today survive in thousands, but those of other correspondents, such as John Caius, are lost except for references in their own printed books or those of others.

University Life and Letters

Just as today, the move away from home to study was an exciting adventure, something to be described to the folks back home to allay any worries they might have. Thomas Platter, for instance, wrote reprovingly to his son Felix at Montpellier that instead of wasting his time in dancing and play he should spend his time dancing with Galen and wandering around the town visiting patients with doctors.[79] Sometimes, as with the letters exchanged between Wolfgang Reichart and his son in Padua, we have both sides of the correspondence, but more often we have only occasional letters from a dutiful son.[80] Far more common are letters between students and their old teachers or friends, eager to hear about what was happening in Italy, France or elsewhere. Sometimes they were sent by a regular carrier, but often students returning home would bring with them letters from others to be delivered en route. Georg Fabricius on his return from Padua to Chemnitz passed on to Georg Agricola a letter from Wolfgang Meurer (1513–85) describing his experiences in Padua, Naples and Rome.[81] Typical are the surviving letters of Georg Purkircher (c. 1533–77), who had studied at Wittenberg and Padua before returning to practise in his home town of Bratislava.[82] While in Padua, where he matriculated in November 1561 and graduated in December 1563, he associated with some old friends from Wittenberg, and especially Joachim Camerarius (1534–98), the son of one of the most eminent professors in Germany, also named Joachim Camerarius. Both father and son were great letter writers at the centre of a pan-European network of scholars, particularly in humane letters, medicine and natural history.[83] Purkircher, who was already famous as a Latin poet before coming to Padua, remained close friends with Camerarius all his life, and wrote gossipy letters to him telling of academic matters both there and in Bologna, especially the problems of finding a suitable anatomist after the deaths of Falloppia and Bassiano Landi in quick succession. He remarks on the curious behaviour of professors, including Cardano at Bologna, whose lectures he attended and found so ridiculous that the audience broke into laughter. He worries about the failing health of Trincavella, who was now becoming a joke among students for his memory lapses. He records the disdain of the keeper of the botanic garden, Melchior Wieland, at the salary he was offered, and reports the rumours in February 1563 that Vesalius might return as Professor. But he also reveals something of the rowdiness of student life, with constant fights between Germans and Poles, sometimes ending in serious injury. A few years earlier Camerarius himself had described to Crato similar brawling over the election of a student Rector in 1560–61 and feared for the future of the university since its teachers were very negligent and, with one or two exceptions, unkind. There had scarcely been 30 days of poor lectures in the whole year, and Falloppia and Bellocato scarcely took anyone with them on their busy practice visits.[84] Camerarius was more sympathetic to Trincavella, whose lectures he had found valuable, even if his method of delivery was off-putting at first, and only two or three students stayed to the end of his course, preferring those of Fracanzano. He thought Falloppia second to none as an anatomist, although his contentious divergences from Galen and Colombo made Camerarius wonder whether certainty could ever be obtained about many bodily particulars. But he was already concerned that Falloppia's health might prevent the annual dissection from taking place, as indeed it did.[85] The letters of Purkircher and Camerarius deal with much besides medicine. They are filled with stories of what is happening at the Council of Trent, in the French struggles over religion, or simply the weather. Spring 1563, wrote Purkircher, had been so bad that the plants in the botanic garden were extremely late.[86]

Thirteen years later another student, Peter Monau, reported back to his friend Crato von Crafftheim on the Paduan anatomist Fabricius's vivisection of a pregnant sheep which revealed things never previously observed. A similar letter to Joachim Camerarius tells of the unfortunate interventions of Mercuriale and Capodivacca in the plague of Venice.[87] Monau's later letters include several to his former teachers asking for their advice about contagion and the role of sympathy in spreading disease, or simply for news of their forthcoming publications. In 1584 he gently enquires when Mercuriale will publish his long-awaited edition of Hippocrates, a "true storehouse of medical information", and whether it will include a Latin translation alongside the Greek.[88] Other teachers kept up a long correspondence with their pupils. Bartolommeo Maranta, asserting his claim to be the literary executor of his Paduan teacher Luca Ghini, claimed that he had received a letter a week from him on botanical matters.[89] Students might also transmit their own transcripts of lectures they had heard at Padua to help remoter colleagues across the Alps keep up to date, as well as sending them lists of their own libraries in case they might wish to borrow from them.[90]

The subjects in Monau's letters range widely, from a report of a cure of the King of Poland's scabies in 1578 by a mysterious John of Piedmont and complaints about slow-moving rivers in Bratislava filled with faeces, muck and even dead animals to comments about the failings of other doctors.[91] Mercuriale's letters from Italy to Theodor Zwinger (the son-in-law of Oporinus) in Basle enquire about northern scholars and the progress of their books, as well as attempting (in the end successfully) to have some of his own writings published there. In turn Zwinger recommended to Mercuriale students from Basle who were travelling to Padua and provided a channel of communication between the two men. Some of Mercuriale's letters to other correspondents deal with such disparate topics as the effects of dysentery on the liver and the possible use of love philtres, something "not to be considered by prudent medical practitioners". The best philtre, in his view, was a similarity of manners, education and age, combined with honourable behaviour.[92]

All the letter writers so far mentioned in this chapter were interested in plants and other aspects of the natural world. Their letters are filled not only with recipes but with arguments about identification and reports of new substances that were unknown or unavailable to the recipient. Purkircher not only provided Camerarius with a list of seeds given him by Wieland but offered to forward to Camerarius examples of whatever he wanted. He himself wrote to the Imperial botanist Carolus Clusius (1526–1609) in 1577 for him to pass on a request to another royal doctor, Aichholz, to send him some aquatic plants or just their roots to plant in the moats around his estate.[93] Sometimes seeds were sent by the normal courier but often friends or mere acquaintances brought them along in their luggage. In 1537, Michael Throckmorton, one of Cardinal Pole's circle in Padua, sent a collection of seeds to Edward Wotton in London via another friend of Pole, Henry Cole, who sent them on from Paris to London with another colleague, Mr Leyton.[94] Thirty years later, Clusius having ascertained that his patron Thomas Rehdiger was in Padua, recommended a meeting with the distinguished local botanist Cortusio and also asked him to persuade Wieland to send him seeds of rare plants for, he averred, in tumultuous times botany provided appropriate leisure for a gentleman.[95] Correspondents were often concerned about costs: seeds were easy to send, but couriers drew the line about cumbersome minerals. If specimens were not available, one could always send drawings, especially of birds and animals, such as those John Caius passed on to his friend Gessner for inclusion in the massive volumes of his enquiries, *Historiae*, into plants, animals, birds and fishes.[96] Books seem to have been regularly sent long distances. Caspar Peucer (1525–1602), for example, a student at Padua with Camerarius and Purkircher, and later a significant figure in medicine, ethics and religion at Wittenberg, where he married the daughter of Melanchthon, sent Camerarius copies of his publications as soon as they appeared.[97] But even transport of books by the equivalent of the diplomatic bag might cause problems. The English Ambassador in Paris in 1542, Sir William Paget, had to apologise to Henry VIII for opening a package sent from Italy that contained a presentation copy of Brasavola's edition of the Hippocratic *Aphorisms*. It is not known whether the king was satisfied with his excuse that Italy was full of poison, and since traitors there might be sending almost anything, he had felt it best to check before sending the substantial volume on. He concluded that the book's author was "well-minded" but left any judgement on his learning to King Henry's "excellent wisdom".[98]

These correspondence networks, the Renaissance equivalent of Facebook, covered the whole of Western Europe from the Baltic to the further shores of Spain. They involved a huge number of individuals, not all of them physicians, across boundaries of politics and religion. The Evangelical Gessner, for example, was equally in touch with Catholics like Aldrovandi and Matthioli (never the easiest of colleagues) and with Evangelicals like William Turner, twice exiled from England for his extreme religious views. John Caius, in theology very much a high Anglican, corresponded frequently with Gessner, and wrote a long and moving eulogy of a friendship that must have been almost entirely conducted by letter.[99] Even if by the end of the century one had to be careful about what one said to members of a different Christian belief, that did not prevent Mercuriale from frequently corresponding with the Evangelical Zwinger, or from helping Protestant students.[100] He had provided Christoph Schilling (1534–83) with letters of introduction to colleagues in Rome, Florence, Bologna and Ferrara, and Schilling's list of those he met on his travels in Italy and South France rivals that of Gryllus in its enumeration of the good and great.[101]

The Crato Circle

Although recent years have seen a renewal of interest in the networks of natural history, in France, with Daléchamps and Rondelet, in Switzerland, with Gesner and Zwinger, and particularly with Aldrovandi, Matthioli and other scholars in Northern Italy, research into similar medical networks in the German-speaking world, with a few exceptions, such as Johannes

Lange and Joachim Camerarius, is still in its infancy.[102] This is in part the result of the dislocations of war over the centuries which have dispersed the letters of one of the greatest networkers of them all, Johann Crato von Crafftheim, the selection of whose letters and *consilia* by his friend Leonard Scholz covers only a tiny fraction of his output.[103] Modern scholars have not entirely forgotten him, but they have concentrated either on his role in the religious debates of the time as one of the leading proponents of the humanist, eirenic Christianity favoured by Emperor Rudolf II or on his strong opposition to Paracelsianism.[104] Robert Evans's enlightening few pages on Crato's place in the intellectual coteries at the Prague court give only a tantalising glimpse into his role within the wider medical world, but his suggestions have not been followed up.[105] Crato was in many ways a typical academic physician of the period, and, were it not for his role at the Habsburg court, he would merit no more than a footnote for his achievements. Neither his medical ideas nor his therapeutics were particularly novel, and he made no great discovery, but through his correspondence he was able to keep himself informed and to inform others about almost everything that was going on in the world around him. When the publisher Wechel in 1572 was forced to flee as a Huguenot from Paris after the St Bartholomew's Day massacre, it was Crato and his friends who helped to set him up in business in Frankfurt by sending him some of their works to publish.[106]

His talents were spotted at an early age. The son of an artisan and town councillor at Breslau (modern Wrocław), he was proud of his centuries-long roots in the community there. After completing his studies at the Latin school, he was given a grant by the town council (and later by some wealthy citizens) to go to Wittenberg to study arts, on the understanding that he would come back and serve the town and his old school.[107] He lodged with Luther and his family as a paying guest for six years, during which he made a complete change of career. At first he decided to study arts and philosophy, but after several bouts of illness it was Luther himself who warned him against such a physically demanding career as that of a clergyman, suggesting instead that he become a physician.[108] A further grant from Breslau, still hoping for his return to work there, allowed him to continue in Wittenberg, but he had higher ambitions, and it was Melanchthon's intervention on his behalf with the city Council that made them grant him a further subsidy to travel for study, necessary since both Luther and Melanchthon were aware of his abilities and his straitened circumstances. He began his medical studies in Leipzig, where he met the young Camerarius, but soon moved on to Padua in 1546.[109] He immediately became a close friend of Da Monte, editing some of his lectures, and defending his teacher against what he saw as an unjustified plagiarism of his ideas on 'method' by John Caius. Caius's response is a half-hearted apology at best.[110] After a brief spell of practice in Verona, he returned to Breslau as second town physician, serving with distinction in two outbreaks of plague and gaining a large increase in salary

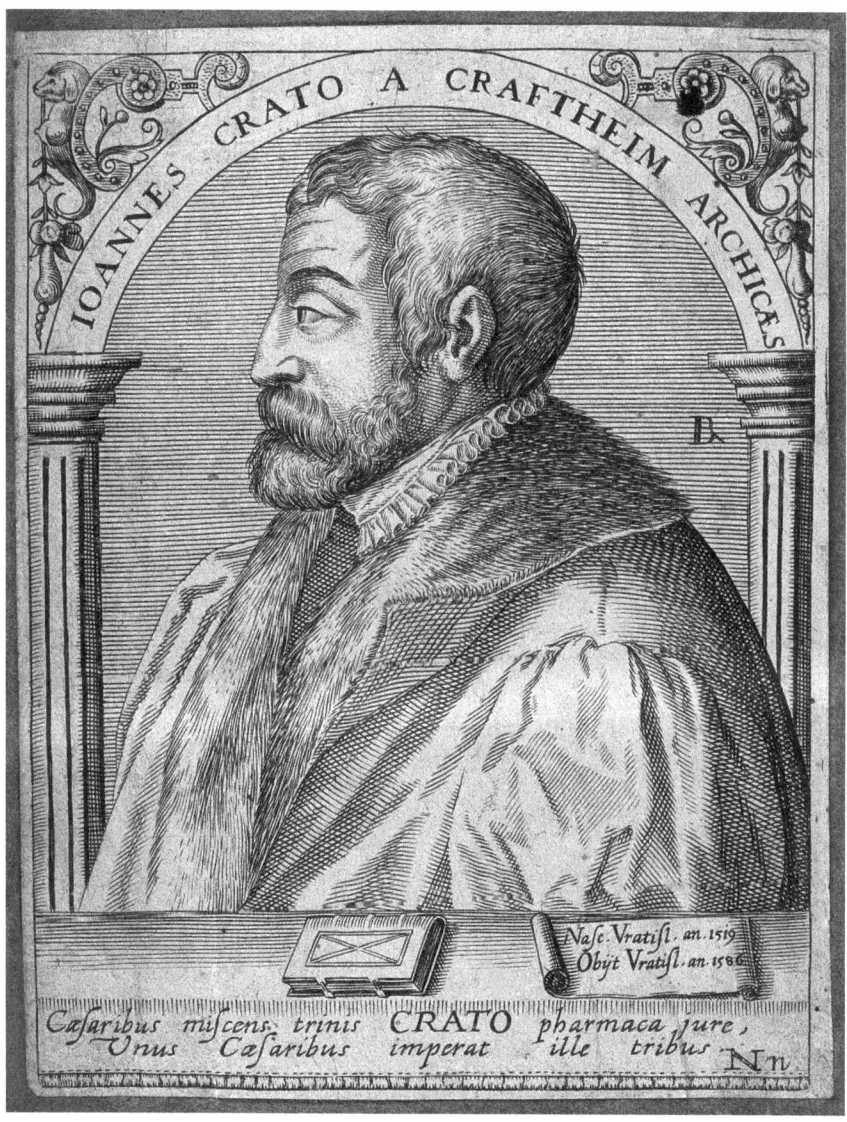

Figure 3.3 Johann Crato von Crafftheim (1519–85), imperial physician. Line engraving by T. de Bry, 1650.

for his efforts in 1554, but he was suspected of Calvinism and dismissed from his post (he had earlier converted from Catholicism to Lutheranism). This did not prevent him from being picked in 1560 by Emperor Ferdinand I to become one of the imperial physicians, a post which he held, with short intermissions, until 1581, when he retired briefly to his Bohemian estate. He later returned to Breslau and continued in active practice there until his death in 1585.[111]

What stands out in Gillet's biography is Crato's gift for friendship, and the way in which, from his earliest days in Wittenberg, he remained in close contact with some of the leading figures in Germany, Italy and beyond.[112] Some, like Caspar Peucer and Joachim Camerarius the younger, he had known since his Wittenberg days when he had become acquainted with all the leading Evangelicals in Germany through his stay in Luther's house, personal contacts that become immensely important as he and the Emperor tried to find common ground in the religious upheavals of the 1560s onwards. His position in Breslau, a major commercial city, and then at court allowed him access to an even wider group of correspondents, including the imperial botanists Clusius, Mattioli and Dodoens, the physician-astrologer Thaddeus Hagecius, younger doctors like Peter Monau, Georg Purkircher, Wenceslas Raphanus and Thomas Jordanus, and, over the Alps, with Mercuriale, Donzellini and other Paduans. One of his closest friends and regular correspondents was the Hungarian cleric and later free-thinker, Andreas Dudith (1533–1589), who, although not a doctor himself, was deeply interested in natural philosophy, and keen to participate in medical debates within the Crato circle.[113] This was a group of scholarly individuals that, like other intellectuals, flourished in the relatively open atmosphere of the imperial court of Rudolf II.

These networks, whether of Italian botanists or of German physicians, were more than avenues for professional advancement, and, equally significant for historians, they give a sense of what topics were of great immediate interest. Correspondents pass on details of what they have read, and particularly of new books and of others they are expecting. A typical letter of Crato mentions books by Mizauld, Cornelius Gemma of Louvain, Valleriola, Rondelet and the surgeon Alfonso Ferri.[114] Nancy Siraisi has neatly described the debates about contagion among the Crato circle, and one can find equally vigorous correspondence there about syphilis, gout, catarrh and many other diseases.[115] Writers summarise information they have gained from new books, recent letters and their own or others' experiences of treating diseases with a variety of drugs, including chemical ones. But they often also include details of their own personal lives. Caspar Wolf, the editor of Gessner's letters, in 1581 blames his delay in replying to Crato because of the demands of the Zurich printer Froschover on him to provide yet more material from what Gessner had left behind, while at the same time constantly failing to print his own studies of Dioscorides and Athenaeus.[116] At almost the same time Peter Monau complains about the difficulty of working when his library has had perforce to be split between houses in his home city of Breslau and the two imperial cities of Prague and Vienna. He also muses on the advice he received when he was a student in Padua that, when discussing a possible outcome in a case of gout, no doctor tells the truth, for it is so depressing to learn that one's condition can be palliated but not cured.[117]

The Didactic Word

Such letters have one advantage for the modern historian, even if their details are not always easy to understand in the absence of a context or, with Scholz's selections, an index. In their immediacy, they take us close to the individual doctor and his concerns, only surpassed in this by casebooks, marginal notes and annotations that were always intended to be private and where we can observe directly the writer at work, emphasising, interpreting, correcting and pondering what was on the page before him.[118] But letters, particularly those that have not gone through a process of redaction, can also mimic the most common of all methods of communication, the interplay of voices. Of course, we can no longer hear the actual voices of Renaissance practitioners and their patients, but several medical writers have a talent for conveying conversations, particularly when describing incidents in their own practice. Van Foreest regularly included reminiscences of conversations with patients and colleagues, while another vigorous stylist, the English surgeon William Clowes (1544–1604), frequently inserted long stretches of dialogue into his case histories, which, at the very least, are modelled on his own manner of speaking to patients and colleagues.[119] But one may get even closer to reality by examining the notes taken down by students in their lectures or, occasionally, at bedside consultations that are preserved in libraries and archives. Most, like those of Baldasaer Heseler recording the confrontation between Corti and Vesalius at a Bologna dissection in 1540, or those on later Paduan anatomy teaching studied by Michael Stolberg, are, like modern student notes, a mixture of summaries and occasional phrases copied verbatim.[120] But others, particularly those associated with Da Monte at Padua, appear to be word-for-word transcripts with little or no editorial intervention.[121] In his manuscript *Consultationes* we can listen to a dialogue between Da Monte and his colleagues at the bedside as they offer opinions as to what should be done, while some of the copyists of his academic lectures were so diligent that they included his opening and closing remarks as well as his verbal mistakes.[122] Copies of the same set of his lectures by different students confirm their general accuracy, as well as suggesting that the copyist, whether student or professional scribe, tried to take down everything exactly as it was spoken. This is as close as we can get to being in the room with the master, although we cannot hear his voice and few today are so fluent in Latin as to be able to understand an hour or so's Latin lecture in every detail. But this is a useful reminder that communication depends not only on what is said but also on the participants' ability to hear, see and understand, and, most essential of all, the ability to access the relevant material, particularly once it had been written down. Printing widened this accessibility, libraries and personal collections of letters conserved it, and contacts, whether in person or by letter, helped to create and sustain an international medical republic across countries and creeds.

Notes

1 Eisenstein 1979; Grafton 1980, 1992; Johns 1998.
2 Panse 2012 is exemplary in considering the cultural aspects of printing.
3 Jones PM 1996; Frasca-Spada and Jardine 2000; Maclean 2002; Cohn 2010, 2018.
4 Siraisi 2013; for a more local example, Siraisi 2016.
5 Long 2011, although she is scarcely concerned with medical practice. See also for surgeons as artisans of the body, Cavallo 2007; Kinzelbach 2014a; and the essays in Brendecke 2015: 78–121.
6 Earlier, notes 1 and 3. The useful *Cambridge History of the Book in Britain* divides its volumes at 1550, which hampers comparison between both halves of the century.
7 Klebs 1938 (partly supplemented by Stilwell 1970); Durling 1961.
8 Riddle 1980; Rice 1980.
9 Sudhoff 1894–99.
10 Margócsy *et al.* 2018.
11 Hieronymus 2005; Leu 2014.
12 Cf. Frasca-Spada and Jardine 2000.
13 Nutton 2019: 79–80.
14 Steinmann 1967.
15 Nutton 2012a.
16 Kusukawa 2012.
17 Leu 2014.
18 For the development of ideas on healthy living, Cavallo and Storey 2013, 2017.
19 For the advantages of wide margins in which to copy notes, Ludwig 1999: 265–9.
20 Nutton 2019: 78.
21 Arrizabalaga 1998.
22 Nutton 2019: 80.
23 For England, Slack 1979, Nutton 1999; for France, Davis 1975: 190–226; for Germany, Panse 2012; for Italy, Cavallo and Storey 2013: 14–47; for Czech Republic, Zemla 2016.
24 Paracelsus 1575: see also later, pp. 281–2.
25 Jones PM 1995: 161–4; 1996, for non-medical owners.
26 Hieronymus 2005; Leu 2014.
27 Durling 1961: 300, although many students seem to have opened only the first pages, or none at all; Caius 1570c: fol. 6v: tr. Nutton 2018a: 58.
28 Wrocław, University Library, Rehdiger MS 472, fol. 160r; *Ep.* 121.
29 Rinaldi 2006.
30 Gessner 1545, 1555a; Serrai 1990: 89–202, 220–1.
31 Gallus 1590; Spach 1591; Nayar 2019: 61–63 discusses the massive boom in publication from 1550 and the turn towards inventories rather than invention.
32 Caius 1570a,b, 1576, 1912; Egmond 2018a, 2018b.
33 Carlino 1999b. Not all the copies I have seen were correctly stuck down by their owner.
34 Helm 2001.
35 This section is based on Cohn 2010: 22–32; Nutton 2015: 431–7.
36 Tabernaemontanus 1564.
37 Bullein 1559; Kellwaye 1593; Slack 1979: 243.
38 Monacius 1560.
39 Condio 1581.
40 Simoni 1576; Nutton 2008b.

41 Kellwaye's neighbour owned London, Wellcome Collection EPB/B/3537.
42 König 1961; Murphy 2019: 97–121.
43 Nutton 2005: 436, citing London, Wellcome Collection EPB/A/7429.2. For prayers in time of plague, Cyrus 2021.
44 Maclean 2000: 109; 2009: 82.
45 Nutton 1990b: 136; 1993: 24–5.
46 Findlen 1999: 374; Margócsy *et al*. 2018; for Pa'ez de Castro in 1544–5, and doubtless also his master, the diplomat and book-collector Diego Hurtado de Mendoza, Hobson 1999: 81.
47 Maclean 2002: 48.
48 Details in Bosman-Jelgersma 1996b: 28–87.
49 Savino 2019.
50 Mugnai-Carrara 1991; Grierson 1978; Agasse 2002–3.
51 Jones PM 1995: 166–77; Kusukawa 2012: 252–7.
52 König 1961; Murphy 2019: 104–8.
53 Maclean 2002: 63–6, 2017; for German doctors, Lorenz 1983; for Paris, Lehoux 1976.
54 Yates 1992: 228–38.
55 Guinter 1536, 1539; Guinter and Vesalius 1538.
56 Brasavola 1551.
57 Zwinger 1586–7.
58 Steeno et al. 2020
59 Agrimi and Crisciani 1994.
60 Cermisone 1476; Di Montagnana 1476, 1497.
61 London, Wellcome Collection, WMS 567; Da Monte 1554b; Clbabritto 2012.
62 Amatus Lusitanus 1551: 387 (the poem); Ventura 2009–10; Lopes Andrade *et al*. 2015.
63 Valleriola 1573; Nance 2005. For the *Observationes* of Pieter van Foreest, see pp. 239–40.
64 Cagnati (1581): cf. earlier philological works, e.g. N. Burtius, *Observationes in Virgilium*. Bologna, 1489.
65 See earlier, pp. 13–4, 20–1. For training in writing 'scientific' letters, Ogilvie 2011.
66 Maclean 2000: 103, 2009: 59–86; Siraisi 2013; Walter 2020.
67 Siraisi 2013: 8–9.
68 Lange, *Ep*. 1.68: 1556: 537–40, with Siraisi 2013: 42–6; Mercuriale 1571 (with later enlarged editions in 1576 and 1585) with Nutton 2008c.
69 Mattioli 1561; Gessner 1577.
70 Trincavella 1586.
71 Manardi, *Ep*. II.1: 1556: 6.
72 Manardi, *Epp*. I.2, IX.1: 1556: 2–3, 95–9 with Brasavola 1541: 407 (lit. 'making an elephant out of a fly').
73 Marcus 2020: 28.
74 Delisle 2006, 2008.
75 Nothing on medical correspondence in the useful Bethencourt and Egmond 2007. The Munich BAW database of medical letters, www.aerztebriefe.de, analyses 70,000 letters written to and from German correspondents, but many more are still to be added; see Walter 2020.
76 Caplan 2016.
77 Arbenz 1891: 247. The lost book, however, may have been the predecessor of the *Epitome* now in the Vadianus Library in St Gallen.
78 Wrocław, University Library, Rehdiger MS 243, fol. 152r; *Ep*. 96/94.
79 Burckhardt 1917: 65.

80 Ludwig 1999.
81 O'Malley 1964: 405.
82 Purkircher 1988; brief biography in English in Birnbaum 1983: 306–8. For rumours that the poet and medical student Lotichius Secundus had been poisoned in Padua, Clemen 1929: 26.
83 Murphy 2019: 123–46.
84 Gillet 1860–1: II, 461–2, 484–5; Wrocław, University Library, Ms. Rehdiger 243, fol.72v; *Ep.* 59/57.
85 Camerarius, Wrocław, University Library, Ms. Rehdiger 243, fol.105r: *Ep.* 80/78 (of February 1560).
86 Purkircher 1988: 149–6.
87 Crato 1619: 432, 572 (see above, pp. 54–5).
88 Crato 1592: 484–92 (to Capodivacca), 493–4, 526 (to Mercuriale).
89 Findlen 2017: 153–4.
90 Crato 1592: 268–9, for discussions of plague.
91 Crato 1611: 67, 53, 63 (Dudith to Monau).
92 Siraisi 2013: 28–9. This book examines in detail the letter collections of Johannes Lange, and Orazio Augenio.
93 Purkircher 1988: 150–2, 176.
94 Gairdner 1891: 16. For the Paduan links, Woolfson 1998: 225, 276, 287.
95 Wrocław, University Library, Rehdiger MS 242, fol. 204r: *Ep.* 156.
96 Earlier, pp. 72–3; cf. also for drawings and seeds, Egmond 2018c; Funk 2021; for Basle at the end of the century as the centre of a network of botanical correspondence, Benkert 2020: 165–86.
97 Purkircher 1988: 154–5, 159; Peucer 1554a, 1554b, 1557, and probably 1555, London, Wellcome Collection, EPB 4964–7. The first three bear Peucer's autograph dedication to Camerarius.
98 Nutton 1990c: 240–1.
99 Caius 1570c: 21r–4v: Roberts 1912: 94–8; Nutton 2018a: 73–5.
100 Nutton 2017a: 15–17; Siraisi 2008, 2013. But cf. the unfortunate end to the career of Donzellini, later, pp. 316–7.
101 Dudith 2002: 284–7.
102 Findlen 1996, 1999 is fundamental for Northern Italy. See also, for Daléchamps, Schmitt 1977; for Lange, Siraisi 2013; for Camerarius, Murphy 2019; for the Roman circle of Hurtado de Mendoza, Andretta and Pardo-Tomás 2019. Information on much primary material is becoming available online at www.aerztebriefe.de.
103 Many unpublished letters survive in the Rehdiger collection in his hometown of Breslau (modern Wrocław or Bratislava as he called it in Latin), and 1271 letters to Joachim Camerarius in the Sammlung Trew in Erlangen. Some letters to him from Clusius and other Flemings were published in 1847 (Ram 1847) and one must often have recourse to the footnotes and appendices in the remarkable biography (Gillet 1860–1) by J. F. A. Gillet (1804–79) the leading cleric at the Hofkirche in the city centre.
104 Louthan 1994, 1997; Fichtner 2001: 102–3; for his anti-Paracelsianism, Bröer 2002; Gunnoe and Shackelford 2009; Murphy 2019: 126 mentions him briefly as a correspondent of Camerarius.
105 Evans 1984a: 98–100, 118–23.
106 Maclean 2009: 169.
107 Gillet 1860–1: I, 52–5.
108 For a sketch of Luther in a book owned by Crato, Hieronymus 1991.
109 Gillet 1860–1: I, 58–63.
110 Nutton 2018a: 39.

111 Gillet 1860–1: II, 1–39, 206–55. The manuscript of his *Historiae Urbis Vratislaviae synopsis*, 1584, seems to have been destroyed in 1945, Lambrecht 2002: 253, note 41.
112 Gillet 1860–1: I, 61–76; II, 40–95, 303–90.
113 Evans 1984a: 98–100, 105–10, 117–20, 203–4; Agasse and Pennuto 2016. For Dudith's interest in medicine, Fossel 1913. For Purkircher and "noster Crato", Purkircher 1988: 177.
114 Wrocław, University Library, Rehdiger MS. 242, fol. 39r–v; *Ep.* 37.
115 Siraisi 2013: 20–3.
116 Wrocław, University Library, Rehdiger MS. 248, fol. 54; *Ep.* 36. None of these works ever appears to have been printed.
117 E.g. Monau in Crato 1592: 298–300 is a typical miscellany: books, 319; gout 317–8.
118 E.g. Vesalius's annotations, Nutton 2012a, 2017a; Hieronymus 2005 is a fascinating treasure-store for the note-hunter. Stolberg 2021a is an exemplary study of one set of casebooks.
119 Clowes 1602: 51–61, 1588: sig. vii.4v–viii.4r: 1948: 59–70, 107–18.
120 Eriksson 1959; Stolberg 2018a, b.
121 A complaint made by J. M. Durastante about Valentin Lublin's editions of Da Monte's lectures and consultations, Da Monte 1558b: pref., 4v–5r. They brought Da Monte to life, but Durastante felt it essential to improve their ungainly Latin.
122 For transcripts of consultations, London, Wellcome Collection, WMS 567. Cf. Da Monte 1583. Cf. also the essays by Sabine Schlegelmilch and Michael Stolberg in Brendecke 2015: 100–21.

4 The Rediscovery of Ancient Medicine

Writing around 1518 in the preface to his *Discorsi*, his *Commentary on the First Ten Books of Livy*, the Florentine administrator and writer Niccolò Machiavelli justified his decision to draw appropriate lessons for contemporary politics from the Roman historian Livy by comparing his project with what had long been the case in medicine. When men fall ill, he explained, "they always have recourse to diagnoses and treatments that have been approved and codified by the ancients . . . medicine is nothing more than the experiences of ancient doctors which form the basis of the notions of modern doctors".[1] Machiavelli's assertion that the learned medicine of his day was founded on classical principles was commonplace. But his formulation conceals the fact that it was precisely at this point, in the first 30 years of the sixteenth century, that what was understood as ancient medicine, and in particular the ancient texts that constituted it, was undergoing a considerable change. In these years Latin Europe rediscovered Classical Greek writings on medicine that had been known at best indirectly before and transmitted them to a wider audience through new Latin versions. The immediate beneficiary of this Hellenic renaissance was, paradoxically, Galen of Pergamum (129–216?), who had for more than a thousand years, since at least 400 CE, been acknowledged as the most authoritative promoter of that most effective of medical theories, the doctrine of the four humours. But the reappearance in Western Europe of his texts in their original Greek, many of them long forgotten because they were never translated into Latin, challenged traditional ideas about his beliefs by revealing a much more experimental and less dogmatic physician. This new Galenism at first strengthened his authority, even if it also soon revealed errors and inconsistencies that led to rejection or to a variety of compromises as doctors attempted to fit new information and new diseases into the old template. Even if faith in Galen himself diminished somewhat, learned physicians, excluding some followers of Paracelsus, continued to believe that what had been written in Antiquity still contained much of value, and that no medical practitioner could afford to neglect the Classics.

DOI: 10.4324/9781003223184-6

Galen of Pergamum

The son of a wealthy architect, Galen had studied in several of the leading intellectual centres of the Greek world, notably Alexandria in Egypt, before making his way to Rome where he served as an imperial doctor for almost 40 years.[2] His judicious observational skills, whether of the world around him or of the human body, allied to a coruscating rhetoric and a devastating ability to see the weakness of his opponent's case, went far towards convincing those who knew him that he was a supreme exponent of the medical art. He also appeared to know more than most physicians. He had amassed a remarkable library including, he believed, the greatest collection of medical recipes in the world, and, even after much of it was destroyed in the Great Fire of Rome in 192, he could still recall or obtain afresh many of the books that he had read. He had been trained in a tradition of medicine that he and his teachers believed went back to Hippocrates of Cos at the end of the fifth century BCE, and he asserted that he was largely repeating the ideas and practices of this long-dead master that ignorant or mischievous commentators had neglected or misinterpreted. It was a powerful claim, even if one disputed by today's historians, for he could appeal to centuries of apparently effective practice whose rare failures were, he alleged, the result of others' mistakes. His success in his lifetime was aided by his reputation as a philosopher, and particularly a logician, and, still more, by his enormous output of writings on a wide range of subjects. Within a generation of his death, his books were being read in Egypt and Latin Africa as well as Rome, and he influenced Christian theologians as well as pagan philosophers and elite physicians.[3] Over the next three centuries, the multitude of competing medical theories and practices in Rome and the eastern half of the Empire of Galen's day was gradually replaced by a more unified culture of medicine in which his ideas came to dominate. Alternative views were pushed aside and in handbooks and medical encyclopaedias the name of Galen largely subsumed those of other writers in the same Hippocratic tradition.

The Galen of the sixth century was something very different from the Galen of the second, and the presentation of his ideas took on a form remote from the way he had wished his books to be read. The need to constantly copy and recopy by hand manuscripts of his writings, together with the irrelevance to medical practice of most of his philosophical and non-medical writings, meant that many were quickly lost and others survived only in isolated copies. His larger compositions were in particular danger of disappearing. Only fragments remain of the fifteen books on *Demonstration*, which he considered his most important contribution to philosophy, half of *Anatomical Procedures* is preserved today only in Arabic, and medieval Europe knew only a shortened Latin version of *The Usefulness of Parts* (see later, p. 248). By 500 CE there had been developed a short and coherent syllabus of 16 or, on a different calculation, 20, books, that followed the model of an earlier selection of writings bearing the name of Hippocrates, with associated lectures, commentaries and student summaries. Often linked with Alexandria, this syllabus in turn was translated into a variety of vernaculars, first into Syriac and then into Arabic, Hebrew and other oriental languages.[4] A shorter series of texts by Hippocrates and Galen was being lectured upon in Latin at Ravenna, the outpost of the Byzantine Empire in Northern Italy, from which copies circulated a little later among Benedictine monasteries such as Nonantola or Monte Cassino.

In the first third of the sixth century, the philosopher, doctor and priest Sergius of Resaena in Syria translated into Syriac the everyday language of the Christians of the Middle East, at least 26 treatises of Galen, a number substantially increased three centuries later to over 125 by the great doctor-translator Hunain ibn Ishāq (809–77) and his family in Baghdad. They and their competitors also made versions in Arabic for their Muslim sponsors, thereby extending the readership and influence of what can be termed Galenism to the entire Islamic world. Not only could scholars like ar-Rāzī (Rhazes, d. 925), al-Majūsi (Haly Abbas, d. 994), Ibn Sīnā (Avicenna, before 980–1037), Ibn Rushd (Averroes, 1126–98) and ben Maimon (Maimonides, d. 1204) pursue the Galenic ideal of the philosopher-doctor, but in their medical treatises in Arabic they produced massive syntheses of Galenic doctrine far superior in quality to anything available in Byzantium, let alone in the contemporary West. They had access not only to more works of Galen in Arabic translation than became available to the West in their original Greek after the fall of Constantinople in 1453, but also to a smaller selection of other Classical Greek authors, notably Rufus of Ephesus (fl. 120 CE), the pharmacologist Dioscorides and a variety of shorter writings attributed to Hippocrates.

Galen had declared that the body was made up of the four Aristotelian elements, earth, air, fire and water, and their four qualities, cold, dry, hot and wet. These formed the basic individual parts of the body, such as bone and flesh, as well as the four fluids or humours – blood, yellow bile, black bile (or melancholy) and phlegm – whose balance and proportion, constantly changing with the seasons, determined one's good or bad health. Within the body there were three near-separate systems of conduits. Food from the stomach passed to the liver where it was turned into venous blood that circulated via the veins to distribute nutriment to each part of the body, however small. A tiny amount of venous blood was transformed in the heart along with the admixture of *pneuma*, spirit or air, to create arterial blood that circulated in the arteries to provide a sort of energy, the vital spirit. A third transformation within the so-called *rete mirabile*, a vascular network at the base of the brain, turned a small amount of this arterial blood into psychic spirit, circulating from the brain via the nerves and helping with sensation and movement. Body and soul were closely connected in the living organism, whose physical and mental changes interacted with each other. The aim of any treatment was to remove whatever was causing the problem and to restore the body's balance by diet, drugs or, as a last resort, surgery. Particular attention was paid to what became known as the six non-naturals, six factors that could influence the natural body for good or ill and cause an unnatural condition or illness: food and drink, exercise, sleep, evacuations, the environment and the emotions. Keeping these in balance was, it was thought, an effective way of preventing illness.

Like their successors in the medieval West, the Arabs paid relatively little attention to the structures of the body itself, relying on Galen's own description and eschewing actual dissection, for, in their view, the imbalance of humours was a sufficient explanation for illness. On the other hand, they did improve on the surgical techniques described by Galen, the author of the pseudo-Galenic *Introduction*, and another Greek writer, Paul of Aegina (fl. 610 CE), and, even more so, on Greek pharmacology. Not only did they know and use far more medicinal substances in a greater range of compound recipes than Galen, but they also developed one of his ideas into a major principle of drug classification. He had floated the possibility that the actions of drugs might be located along a scale of a dozen grades, ranging from the almost imperceptible to the enormously powerful, in order to help judge an appropriate and precise response to the severity of any illness. Unfortunately, and typically, Galen never succeeded in providing grades for all the herbs that he described, nor did his twelve-fold scale match any of his various attempts to devise a similar classification for illnesses. This was unfinished business that Arabic writers such as al-Kindi (d. 873) in his *Book of Grades* sought to complete.[5] The result was a much tighter and more dogmatic synthesis than Galen himself ever achieved, logically structured and eliminating many of the inconsistencies that he had introduced over 60 years of writing and updating.

Medieval Latin Galenism

This classical heritage reached Latin Western Europe in three different stages. Early medieval Europe had only a very limited knowledge of the writings of Galen and Hippocrates, who remained little more than names and sources of short and often enigmatic extracts.[6] The initial impulse towards the recovery of this ancient wisdom is associated with the doctors of a small Italian trading city in S. Italy, Salerno, and with a monk, Constantine (d. before 1088–9), a Christian from North Africa who joined the great monastery of Monte Cassino, with which Archbishops of Salerno maintained the closest of contacts. Constantine was a prolific translator into Latin of medical texts from the Arabic, including the major compendium, the *Pantegni* (*Universal Art*) of al-Majūsi (Haly Abbas) and the treatises on fevers, urines and diet by Isaac Israeli, (Isaac the Jew d. c. 932), which were far more detailed and sophisticated than anything previously available in Latin. Constantine was also responsible for some translations of Galen, all taken from the Arabic, including the substantial work *The Method of Healing* and his commentary on the Hippocratic *Aphorisms* which introduced a new technique of medical teaching, the elucidation of a short text by means of a commentary.[7] This method was practised by medical teachers at Salerno from the early twelfth century using a small selection of practical texts, mainly originating in the Greek world and brought together at Monte Cassino. It began with an *Introduction*, the *Isagoge*, by Johannitius, a dogmatic redaction of the *Questions and Answers* of Hunain ibn Ishāq; followed by the *Book on Pulses* by Philaretus (probably tenth century); the *Book of Urines* by Theophilus (seventh or ninth century); Hippocrates's *Aphorisms*, along with Galen's commentary, *Prognostic* and *Regimen in Acute Diseases*; and Galen's *Art of Medicine*, to which, much later, was attached a Latin version of the commentary by Ali ibn Ridwān (Haly Rodoan, d. c. 1081).

This was an effective syllabus, beginning with an introduction to medicine, followed by guides to the two main aids to diagnosis, pulses and urines, and ending with two classic texts on medical practice. All were relatively short, but none was easy to understand without the intervention of a teacher to explain and develop their ideas. The suitability and flexibility of this syllabus ensured its long survival as the basis for first-year medical education in Western universities, where under the perhaps slang title of *Articella* it was still being used well into the sixteenth century, when its original translations were replaced or, more often, supplemented by others more modern and more accurate.

The example of Constantine was soon followed in the twelfth century by other translators from the Arabic. Most notably among the works they made accessible were the *Canon* of Avicenna, and the *Liber ad Almansorem* (*The Book for Al-Mansur*) of Rhazes, both practical compendia of medicine. At Toledo in Spain a major group of Latin translators, headed by Gerard of Cremona (d. 1187) and assisted by Hebrew scholars, embarked on a massive programme of translations of Greek scientific and medical texts. Other translations were made elsewhere in the Mediterranean where Muslims and Christians encountered one another – in Sicily, where around 1270 Faragius translated the *Liber Continens* (*The All-Embracing Book*), a massive collection of extracts made by Rhazes from earlier, often Greek sources, and in the Holy Land with translators like Stephen of Antioch (around 1127). All these translators were faced with the problems of rendering works with a very specific technical vocabulary unfamiliar to those who were not themselves physicians from languages with a very different syntactical and grammatical structure from their own, problems that only worsened as the number of intermediaries between the Greek original and the new Latin increased. Often all that was done was to transcribe the foreign word, sometimes providing it with a gloss, in the hope that, with time, the word would become a recognised technical term in Latin.

The technique adopted by Hunain and his school when translating from the Greek was to make a translation into fluent Syriac or Arabic, concentrating on giving the sense of a passage as far as possible. This, however, was not the method favoured by the increasing number of Latin translators working directly from the Greek, a language which shared many technical terms with Latin and whose syntax was far more compatible. They accordingly preferred a more literal word-for-word approach. Chief among them was a Pisan judge, Burgundio (c. 1110–93), a member of the expatriate community at Constantinople, who translated many of the most important works of Galen. The Greek manuscripts that he used survive, often with his Latin versions written between the lines or in the margins. By the middle of the thirteenth century blocks of Galenic material in Latin were circulating among university students and teachers, and they were supplemented in the early fourteenth century by further versions from the Greek by Pietro D'Abano (d. c. 1316), a professor in Padua, and by a doctor at the court of Naples, Niccolò da Deoprepio da Reggio (fl. 1305–48). Niccolò, a prolific translator, concentrated on Galen's minor works, which proved a handicap to their widespread diffusion, as his versions seem to have been owned mainly by professors or wealthy doctors who wanted a complete Galen. The phenomenal accuracy of his word-for-word technique has been a great boon to modern editors as it enables them to reconstruct his original Greek manuscript even in tiny details, but in his own time it is questionable how far his Graecisms were appreciated outside bilingual Southern Italy.

By 1450 there had developed a standard system of medical education in the Western universities which had sprung up since the mid-twelfth century. From Coimbra to Cracow and from Oxford to Naples, an aspiring doctor would begin with lectures on the *Articella*, followed by sections of Avicenna's *Canon* and Rhazes's Book 9 of the *Almansorem* on fevers. He might own a codex of Galen containing largely the texts familiar from the old Alexandrian syllabus, but he knew little of Hippocrates or other Greek doctors, and his major studies centred upon the classics of Arabic medicine.[8] This was a Latin medicine, whatever its roots. Hieronymus Surianus, the editor of the 1502 edition of the complete works of Galen in Latin, saw nothing strange in describing a nocturnal vision of Galen showing him a large codex of his writings in Latin and indicating his own desired corrections in the form of Latin marginalia.[9] This medicine derived strength from its long pedigree and from the subtlety of argument and range of medical information deployed by its authors. The Galenic knowledge of a professor such as the Parisian Jacques Despars (d. 1465) is arguably superior to that of a modern Galenist, and authors like Ugo Benzi (d. 1448) and Bartolommeo di Montagnana arranged for the circulation of hundreds of their cases, *consilia*, to show the ways in which this learning could be put successfully into practice.[10]

The Humanist Rediscovery of Antiquity

The humanist revival of the Latin Classics which began in the late fourteenth century added relatively little to the available store of medical literature.

Only one Roman author was rediscovered: Cornelius Celsus (around 30 CE), whose treatise on medicine was found at Siena in 1426. Although many copies were made of it and of a second manuscript discovered the following year, and it was printed in 1468, it seems to have been owned and read more by students of Antiquity than by physicians.[11] More valuable to the latter, and the subject of lectures in some universities, were the medical sections in the great encyclopaedia, the *Historia naturalis*, *Natural History*, of the Elder Pliny (23–79), which contained an enormous amount of information on plants and animals as well as on their medicinal uses. Some of it had already been extracted in the Early Middle Ages to form independent treatises under headings such as the *Physica Plinii*, *Pliny's Physic*, but the revival of the Classics gave, at least temporarily, this ancient Roman an added authority, especially as his Latin, like that of Celsus, was far more acceptable than the hispid medieval Latin of most medical translations.[12]

The entire basis of this Western Latin medicine was rudely challenged in 1492 by a professor at the University of Ferrara, Niccolò Leoniceno.[13] Relatively little is known of the first 60 years of his remarkably long life, and the detailed biography by his pupil Antonio Musa Brasavola seems to have disappeared sometime after 1824. Born and educated in Vicenza, where he gained an excellent education in Latin and Greek and a reputation for his linguistic skills and prodigious memory, he went to Padua to study medicine, following in the footsteps of his paternal grandfather. On graduation in 1453, he visited England and Oxford in the company of an English student he had met at Padua, but his only recorded memory of this trip was of being forced to drink wine by the over-exuberant clients of a Dutch bar on his return journey through Holland. He may have taught for two years at Padua before transferring to the University of Ferrara, where, with occasional periods of teaching at Bologna, he remained until his death. He was so much an institution there that it was said that winter began when he put on a cap, and summer when he removed it.[14]

From its foundation in 1391 the University of Ferrara was a pioneer of the new humanist learning, in deliberate contrast to the more traditional Padua and Bologna. The Este rulers were intent on increasing their reputation as patrons of culture and made their city one of the major intellectual centres of Europe for the next century and a half. Leoniceno fit perfectly into this new society. As well as his university teaching, he was paid from time to time as a ducal physician, and between 1470 and 1490 he was occupied in translating for Duke Ercole many of the ancient historians, particularly from the Greek, as well as the *Dialogues* of Lucian and the modern *Roma Instaurata* of Flavio Biondo. Some of these he turned into Latin, but many also into Italian, most, alas, now lost or preserved only in manuscript.[15] He was on friendly terms with leading humanist scholars such as Urceus Codrus in Bologna, Giovanni Pico della Mirandola and Politian in Florence (whose ruler Lorenzo de' Medici made tentative approaches to obtain his services), and, above all, with the printer Aldus Manutius and his circle of Hellenists in Venice.

Venice, with its domination of some of the Aegean islands and trading posts in the Eastern Mediterranean, was an obvious place of refuge for many Greeks who had fled from Constantinople after the Turkish conquest of 1453. Several were distinguished academics in their own right, who found employment teaching Greek in Northern Italy or, like Janos Laskaris, in acting as agents bringing manuscripts of the Greek Classics to Italy to enrich the collections of grandees like the Medici in Florence or Cardinal Bessarion, who had strong links with Venice. Other Greeks worked as scribes, making copies of the Greek Classics for Italian humanists such as Giorgio Valla (1447–1500) in Venice and Politian in Florence.[16] When and how Leoniceno began collecting manuscripts of Greek medicine and science is unclear, but by 1492, to judge from the authors he mentions, he had acquired the largest such collection in Western Europe, part copied from manuscripts already in Italy, part obtained directly from the East. At his death he owned at least 75 Greek codices, many including several treatises, and encompassing works by almost all the classical medical authors known today.[17]

Speaking in 1491 in a debate before the court at Ferrara, he set out a novel manifesto that, when it was published by a local printer the next year, caused a sensation. Its title, *De Plinii et aliorum in medicina erroribus, The Mistakes of Pliny and Others in Medicine*, gave only a slight hint of its power to subvert, for this was a wholesale attack on the basis of all Latin medicine from Late Antiquity onwards. Leoniceno argued that the Latin texts that every modern doctor studied were filled with innumerable errors because of the complex process of their transmission. The multitude of translators, the different routes these earlier texts had taken, and the variety of languages involved, to say nothing of the vagaries of copyists and the misunderstandings of readers, had led to errors of all kinds. The names of plants and diseases were confused. Pliny had thought '*leucographis*' was a plant, although Dioscorides, Galen and Paul had recognised it as a mineral, and he had mistaken the herb '*struthius*' for its homonym, a bird. He identified '*parthenium*' wrongly with another herb '*perdicium*' that he had himself described very differently a few sections earlier in Book XXI. Avicenna and the pharmacologist Sarapion were taken similarly to task for errors whose consequences could be seen in the fallible productions of those who confected pills and other remedies, as Leoniceno did not fail to point out as he walked the streets of Ferrara.[18] These mistakes were not simply the fault of medieval scribes: even the Roman Pliny had made many errors in transliterating plant names from the Greek botanists into Latin. Only by returning to the original Greek of Galen and the botanist Dioscorides could one be sure of the actual meaning of the words that they had used and, consequently, of the validity of the principles that had been inculcated for so long.

Leoniceno's blanket condemnation of the follies of those without Greek and his demolition of the chapters on herbs of the Elder Pliny excited two immediate responses.[19] Ermolao Barbaro, a celebrated Venetian humanist (1454–93), argued that, even if Leoniceno was correct, the fault lay not with Pliny but with ancient and medieval scribes, whose Latin was imperfect and whose knowledge of Greek was non-existent or insufficient to allow them to correct their own mistakes. As a Roman scholar, Pliny would not have made the errors that they had. Pandolfo Collenuccio (1444–1504), a lawyer, introduced a new element into the discussion by emphasising his own personal knowledge of plants which allowed him to discriminate between the disparate ancient sources and which, he argued, made him a much better judge of the plants themselves than the book-bound Leoniceno. Leoniceno, rightly suspecting that his humanist rival Politian was behind Collenuccio, replied with a series of letters and small tracts that stressed his own superior knowledge of plants and the overall value of his studies for doctors.[20] For him there was more at stake than mere words.

He followed this up with a series of short tracts demonstrating how a knowledge of Greek texts could resolve long-standing disputes or point the way to curing new or previously incurable diseases. He showed how an obscure phrase at the beginning of Galen's *Art of Medicine*, which medieval commentators believed referred to types of logical analysis, dealt solely with appropriate methods of teaching, discussing whether one should begin with general principles, examples or initial definitions.[21] A largely unknown Galenic tract revealed that Galen had disagreed strongly with Aristotle about the formation of the embryo. Aristotle had argued that the woman merely provided the matter which was formed by a principle within the seed of the man. Galen, by contrast, believed that both male and female produced seed, and that the principle that formed the embryo was a particular mixture of the four elements present in both seeds and introduced as innate heat into the female matter at the very moment of conception.[22] Ancient therapeutics could also be shown to be directly relevant to present concerns. In a widely republished tract on the French disease, or syphilis, Leoniceno argued that both a true climatic explanation and a valid cure in humoral terms could be found in ancient texts, thereby also showing that this was no new disease.[23]

His methodology of seeking in previously unknown or unstudied Greek texts for solutions to contemporary problems was widely accepted by those who believed that, in some way, Antiquity, and particularly Greek Antiquity, was superior to its medieval successors. But the Greek terminology presented serious problems if these ancient texts were to be properly used. That was why Giovanni Manardi devoted a long letter to a clearer and more extensive classification of skin diseases, utilising Greek sources including lexica, while Giorgio Valla attempted the same task for parts of the body.[24] For a long while the old and new vocabularies coexisted, but gradually the more Classical Latin of the Renaissance superseded the arabised terms of the Middle Ages. In an age when style mattered, the ability to turn a fine Latin phrase served as a social cachet and helped to distinguish the modern physician from those who were content to stick with the old ways or, worse, possessed only a weak grasp of the universal language of scholarship and high culture, humanist Latin.

Leoniceno's clarion call for action, however, could not easily be followed except by the small group of physicians who lived in or, like the Englishman Thomas Linacre (1460–1524), had studied in Northern Italy and who could both obtain and read Greek manuscripts of medicine and science.[25] Some of the major collections already in Italy, like those in the Vatican or at Urbino, were difficult or impossible to access, and Bessarion's bequest of his library to Venice remained in boxes for almost 30 years.[26] Copies of medical treatises in Greek were not easy to come by. The anatomist Antonio Benivieni (1440–1502) did not have any work of Greek medicine among his small collection of Greek manuscripts.[27] Even when manuscripts were available, no printer dare risk his capital on a publication that might not sell unless there was a sufficiently large and interested readership, and that took time to build up.

Waiting for the Greek Galen

It was Aldus Manutius in Venice who was the first to print Greek scientific texts, beginning with Aristotle and Theophrastus in 1497–8, followed by Dioscorides in 1499, all authors with a potential readership beyond the medical profession. Aristotle was required reading throughout the university world, while an interest in plants was not confined to doctors. Besides, compared with Galen's orotundity and wide range of topics, the Greek of Dioscorides was relatively simple and his organisation and focus straightforward. Although Leoniceno at the end of his life acquired a reputation as a 'book burier', presumably because he was reluctant to let others use the rarities in his library, at this point he was certainly willing to allow access to his collection.[28] For the (pseudo-)Galenic *History of Philosophy* in the Aldine Aristotle Aldus depended on a manuscript that Leoniceno had sold at the cost-price of 1 ducat for 32 folios in return for the assurance that it would appear in print.[29] A year or so later, he allowed two other Venetian printers, Zacharias Callierges and Nicolas Vlastos, to use his manuscripts for an edition of Galen's *Method of Healing* and the shorter *Method of Healing, for Glaucon*, which appeared in a beautifully printed edition in 1500 (Figure 4.1). This was the first of a projected series, for their agent, Musurus, instructed to report on the Greek texts in Leoniceno's library, had hinted that he might be willing to help further.[30] Aldus may have been planning a rival edition, for he arranged for at least one copy to be made of Galenic manuscripts in Florence. But all these plans came to an immediate halt, for the 1500 Galen seems to have been a commercial failure. Vlastos went back to his earlier job as a Greek scribe and it was almost a decade

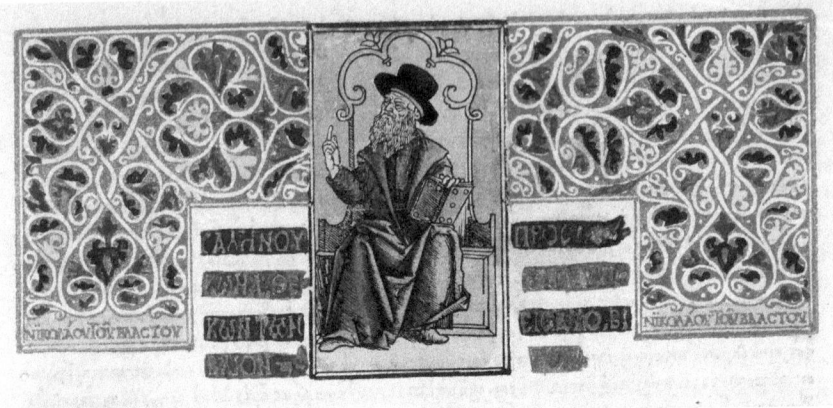

Figure 4.1 Galen in a heading from the first Greek printing of Galen. This edition of his two works on the *Method of Healing* was published in Venice by Z. Kallierges and N. Vlastos in 1500. This copy, London, Wellcome Collection, EPB/INC/2.f.4, was annotated by a contemporary Greek physician.

before Callierges returned to printing. Not for another quarter of a century was the publication of ancient medicine in the original Greek resumed.[31]

Meanwhile, as a frustrated Salzburg doctor wrote in 1519, no matter how much one hoped to see Greek authors turned into Latin and widely accessible, or accepted that one might gain more solid learning from a day reading Galen than a whole week of Avicenna, those without Greek could do little while editions and translations of Galen were few and far between, or available only in a few major cities.[32] War and financial caution also foiled attempts to edit or translate Galen. Until the 1520s publishers and translators were unwilling to go beyond producing new and more accurate versions from the Greek of treatises that were already known through the huge folios that constituted the complete works of Galen in Latin.[33] But many of the treatises found there were not by Galen, and there were major gaps compared with what was to be published in Greek in 1525. Only Giorgio Valla in 1498 broke new ground with a selection of short texts but the final four of those he translated were later discovered to be wrongly attributed to Galen.[34]

Valla's volume also contained a translation of a dietetic treatise, *De victu humano*, *A Universal Dietary*, ascribed to the Byzantine author Michael Psellus (1018–79), which, when reprinted the following year at the German town of Erfurt, became the first newly discovered medical text to be printed north of the Alps.[35] As a short, practical text accessible to the layman, it was eminently saleable, which may also explain why it was chosen in preference to any of the Galenic texts in Valla's volume. The moving spirit behind this was Georg Eberbach, Professor of Medicine at the local university, who had studied at Freiburg and Ferrara, assisted by his colleague in Arts, Nicholas Marschalk. In his commentary Marschalk explained the new 'humanist' terms that Valla had adopted to replace the older arabised vocabulary, and occasionally, particularly when dealing with plants, he gave their original names in Greek. He further praised Eberbach as a scholar familiar with Hippocrates, Galen, Dioscorides, Asclepiades, Celsus and Pliny, although whether Eberbach knew Greek is far from certain. The presence of Asclepiades (none of whose works had survived) in this list also indicates Marschalk's source – none other than Pliny, whose *Natural History* continued to play an important role at Erfurt, a major centre of German humanism, for another 30 years.[36] One of its luminaries, the physician and poet Helius Eobanus Hessus (1488–1540) described in verse the portraits that his medical colleague Georg Sturtz had commissioned for his Museum, the meeting-place of scholars and literary figures.[37] None of those he described in 1524 derive from Greek authorities: his knowledge of such major Greek figures as Herophilus, Asclepiades and Paul of Aegina is demonstrably weak, and his description of Antonius Musa, doctor to the Emperor Augustus, was so flawed that it had to be replaced when he published an enlarged version of the poem in 1531. The nine new names that were then introduced included the medieval pharmacologist Macer, Avicenna "the great glory of medicine", and the late-Latin medical poet Quintus Serenus, while the rest were taken from references in Pliny. The proof is simple: Hessus eulogises one Creon, the name given only in contemporary editions of Pliny to Acron of Acragas, the founder of Empiricism. The teachers at Erfurt may have been aware of the impact of Hellenism, but as late as 1531 their view of medicine still depended on medieval and Classical Latin precedent.[38]

1525 and After

But by this stage things had changed dramatically. The year 1525 saw the publication of the first Latin translation, by Fabio Calvo of Ravenna, of what is today often called the Hippocratic Corpus, and, from the Aldine Press, the first volumes of the edition of the complete works of Galen in Greek. The following year saw the completion of this edition, along with the first edition of Hippocrates in Greek, to be followed in Greek in 1528 by Paul of Aegina, and the first part of another encyclopaedist Aetius of Amida in 1534. But although the Aldine firm promised to publish a complete Aetius as well as an Oribasius, the sheer difficulties and costs of the enterprise were against this, and only the first volume of Aetius was printed.[39] The price of each volume was beyond the pocket of all but the wealthy. A Nuremberg doctor in 1526 paid 30 gulden for a complete Galen, one-third of his annual stipend as a civic physician.[40] Purchasers looking for less familiar ancient authors, such as Aretaeus and Alexander of Tralles, as well as for individual tracts of Rufus of Ephesus, Soranus, Oribasius and the Byzantine author Johannes Actuarius, had to wait until the 1540s and sometimes well beyond. Outside Venice, printers were reluctant to commit themselves to huge tomes in Greek. The Basle printers stayed safe with new editions of Galen (1537–8), Hippocrates (1538) and Paul (1538), while the Parisians preferred single texts and selections which could be sold relatively cheaply or, like Rabelais's 1532 edition of the Hippocratic *Aphorisms*, appended to a more saleable Latin version.[41]

In 1524–5, when Aldus's successors embarked on their momentous editions of Galen and Hippocrates, the situation was vastly different from what it had been a quarter of a century earlier. There were greater opportunities to study Greek at school – it was, after all, the language of the New Testament – many Greek authors, such as Homer, Plato and Thucydides, were being read in the original, and, as we have seen, there was a widespread belief that being able to read Galen and Hippocrates in their own language would allow medicine to progress beyond its medieval heritage. Greek was no longer confined to a handful of scholars in Northern Italy, even if, as one Spanish scholar complained in 1540, knowledge of Greek was grossly deficient elsewhere, and medical faculties preferred their own stubborn ignorance.[42] The fortunate absence of external conflicts meant that there was an abundance of metal available in Venice that could be made into type instead of cannon, and Bessarion's codices in the Marciana Library were finally becoming accessible. One voracious reader of them, Niccolò Leonico Tomeo (1456–1531), boasted that he had read through the whole of Galen and made careful notes on everything relevant to philosophy.[43] The death of Leoniceno may also have made his library at least potentially available to be consulted, and his heirs may have been hoping to sell it, if they had not already done so. There were also talented young men in Venice and Padua from all over Europe with the necessary skills to be employed as editors and printers' assistants.

Giovanni Baptista Opizzoni (1485–1532), Professor of Medicine at Pavia, had long had contacts with the Aldine Press before being engaged in 1523/4 to oversee their programme of editions of Greek doctors.[44] He owned a house in Ferrara, where he was a friend of Leoniceno and Manardi, and often stayed in Venice. His choice of assistants fell, perhaps surprisingly, on five North Europeans from England and Germany. Georg Agricola from Saxony (1494–1555) is famous today as the author of a major treatise on mining and mineralogy, *De re metallica*, but he had been headmaster of the town school at Zwickau before turning to medicine. He was an excellent Hellenist, although nothing remains today of the volumes of corrections and emendations he made to Greek texts.[45] The four Englishmen had all taught at Oxford and were friends of Thomas Linacre, a Greek scholar and translator of Galen with a European reputation. Least is known of William Rose, "astrologer, physician and philosopher", a friend of Sir Thomas More and a Fellow of Oriel who died in Rome in 1525 before he could return to England. Thomas Lupset, who seems to have acted as Opizzoni's deputy because of his experience in seeing through the press some of Linacre's translations, was closely connected with the English cleric and humanist, Cardinal Pole (1500–58), but he too died relatively suddenly in 1530.[46] The two others, Edward Wotton (1492–1555) and John Clement (1500–72), enjoyed similar careers. Both taught Greek at Oxford, before being sent to study medicine in Italy, and both were elected members of the College of Physicians at the same meeting in 1528. They differed, however, in their religious views.[47] Clement married Margaret Giggs, the ward of Sir Thomas More, and went twice into exile in the Catholic Netherlands for his beliefs. By contrast, Wotton, the President of the London College in 1543–44, accommodated himself to all the religious changes in England, serving Cardinal Pole and his household as well as becoming executor to Robert Holgate (1482–1555), the Evangelical Archbishop of York under Edward VI.[48] Clement played the leading role in emending the text of the edition and preparing it for the press, but his involvement with the text of Galen did not stop there. He passed on many excellent suggestions to the editors of the Basle 1538 edition, and John Caius later made considerable use of manuscripts from his library and the emendations he wrote in the margins of his own copy of the Aldine edition, recently discovered in the Leiden University Library.[49]

The Impact of the Aldine Galen

The availability of the complete works of Galen in their original language was greeted with enthusiasm. The Flemish doctor Jan van der Velde (1486–1558) in a treatise on conception and parturition went so far as to declare that without Greek the entire profession of medicine was now simply an imposture.[50] Looking back from the 1540s, Girolamo Cardano (1501–76) rejoiced that medicine had now become an essential part of the education of any man of culture.

> I remember seeing Andreas Alciati, that great luminary of our age, attending to the works of Galen: and what of Erasmus, Budé, Rhodiginus, and the lawyers and theologians, all experts in Greek and Latin and the writers of authoritative works in their own fields?[51]

But criticism was not slow in coming. The whole enterprise had been rushed. Begun in 1524, the first three volumes were available in April 1525 and the fourth by August, although the fifth, containing Galen's Hippocratic commentaries, had to wait until 1526 as it was coordinated with the Aldine Hippocrates of that year. Even the editors admitted serious failings. A gap at the end of *Barley Gruel* had been caused, so John Clement later admitted, when the pressman fell asleep and let his candle fall on the manuscript he was copying.[52] Both Clement and Agricola later made hundreds of corrections that they inserted into their own copies or notebooks. Even those sympathetic to the enterprise had to admit that it was marred by mistakes of every kind. Not even a free copy from the printer could soothe the disappointment of the most influential of all European humanists, Erasmus.[53] Never had he come across a text more corrupt or so full of error. It was a disgrace to scholarship, to the author and to the press. For the sake of the few pounds it would have cost to employ a more experienced and scholarly editor, a great sacrilege had been committed, and the task of correcting left to a man hardly familiar with the rudiments of Greek. It was a harsh, but not unfair judgement. But it should also be noted that, even after the considerable improvements made in the 1538 Basle edition, it was not until the late nineteenth and arguably not until the twentieth century that further substantial progress was made in editing Galen. (The similar big change in editing Hippocrates had come somewhat earlier, with Littré's edition in the mid-nineteenth century.)

Others quickly embraced the new Greek learning. The Basle cleric and reformer Oecolampadius, inviting Simon Grynaeus in 1529 to become the professor of Greek, explained that he wanted Grynaeus to train a suitable successor quickly so that he himself could then become Professor of Medicine and lecture on the original Greek texts of Galen, Hippocrates and other eminent ancient doctors.[54] However, a further plan in 1533 to have someone (possibly Grynaeus) to teach Greek to medical students seems never to have been carried out.[55] Although Manardi claimed in 1535 that there were so many Greek texts available, and so many readers, that he no longer needed to provide translations of his quotations, to focus on the Greek is misleading.[56] The overwhelming majority of medical practitioners continued to gain their knowledge of the ancients through the medium of Latin translations. Even as Grynaeus was being enticed to Basle, his publisher, Andreas Cratander, was preferring to publish Latin translations, since so few doctors knew Greek.[57] Translations of Galen into vernacular languages were infrequent, and were either of works of non-medical interest, such as Tarchagnota's Italian version of some of his moral treatises, or of those thought useful for surgeons, many of whom could not read Latin.[58] French translations of Galen surgery in turn served as the basis for translations into English by and for learned London surgeons. Vernacular versions of Hippocrates were even rarer. One notable exception, the 1597 translation of Hippocrates's *Prognostic* into Scots, was made, almost certainly from the French, by Peter Lowe, the founder of the Glasgow College of Surgeons, who had studied at Orleans (and who may also have been a spy in the pay of France).[59]

It was Erasmus, ever alert to the main chance, who in May 1526 became the first to produce a Latin translation based on the new Aldine material. He chose three short texts, all previously unknown (or neglected) and all with an appeal to a non-medical audience: the *Exhortatio ad bonas artes*, *An Exhortation to the Arts*; *De optimo docendi genere*, *The Best Method of Teaching* (of which an earlier version by Niccolò da Reggio had appeared in the 1490 *Opera omnia*); and *Qualem oporteat esse medicum* (*The Best Doctor Is Also a Philosopher*).[60] A handful of translators, most notably

Thomas Linacre, had been at work before Erasmus to provide more stylish and accurate Latin versions of treatises that circulated widely in the Later Middle Ages, relying on manuscripts they either owned or, like Wilhelm Cop (1460–1532), doctor to the King of France, had access to. Some of these humanist versions found their way into new printings of the *Articella*, where they appeared alongside their more familiar medieval predecessors. But, on the whole, they added little that was new to the stock of knowledge about Galen, 'the prince of physicians'. Leoniceno himself, in an act of sublime optimism, had tried to remedy this, gaining a substantial grant in 1592 at the age of 93 from the authorities of Ferrara to translate the whole Galenic Corpus. Not surprisingly, hampered by increasing ill health, he had made little progress before his death a couple of years later.[61] It was symptomatic of this lack of wider interest in new material that a translation of the previously unknown *Anatomical Procedures* by the distinguished Greek scholar Demetrius Chalcondylas (c. 1424–1511) should have remained neglected for several decades before it was brought to the notice of the Bolognese anatomist Jacopo Berengario da Carpi (1460–1530) around 1523 by his colleague in Greek, Lazzaro Bonamico.[62] Even so, despite encouragement from scholars and patrons alike, it was not until 1529 that this translation appeared in print, shortly before the much more influential version by Johann Guinter (Figure 4.2).

The flood of new Galenic translations that followed those of Erasmus was truly remarkable. Between 1500 and 1525 an average of two or three editions a year had appeared, with a maximum of seven in any one year. Between 1526 and 1561, the average rose to just over 12, with 16 in 1537, 21 or 22 in 1538, 21 in 1547 and 30 in 1549. After 1561 there followed an equally dramatic fall back to no more than three or four printings a year. Leading aside the four major centres of Venice, Paris, Lyons and Basle, editions and translations were published in 42 different places around Europe from Lisbon to Cracow, and from Rostock and Gdansk to Campania. The number of translators is equally impressive, 111 in total, all but a few translating into Latin. Some of them, like Giovanni Baptista Rasario (1517–78) and Johann Guinter, were in effect professionals, responsible for well over 40 separate tracts each.[63] Neither had an unblemished record. Josephus Struthius (1500–68) complained that Guinter never bothered to check his Aldine against Greek manuscripts but rushed headlong, thinking nothing of tossing off 100 pages while standing on one leg. Worse has been imputed to Rasario, who has been rightly suspected of basing several of his translations, particularly of Galen's Hippocratic commentaries, on his own constructions cobbled together from genuine Greek fragments in late encyclopaedias, translations of quotations by medieval authors such as Maimonides, and his own invention.[64]

Other classical authors enjoyed a similar revival to that of Galen. A much older and fallible Latin translation of Dioscorides from the eleventh or twelfth century had been printed in 1478, and around 1481 Ermolao

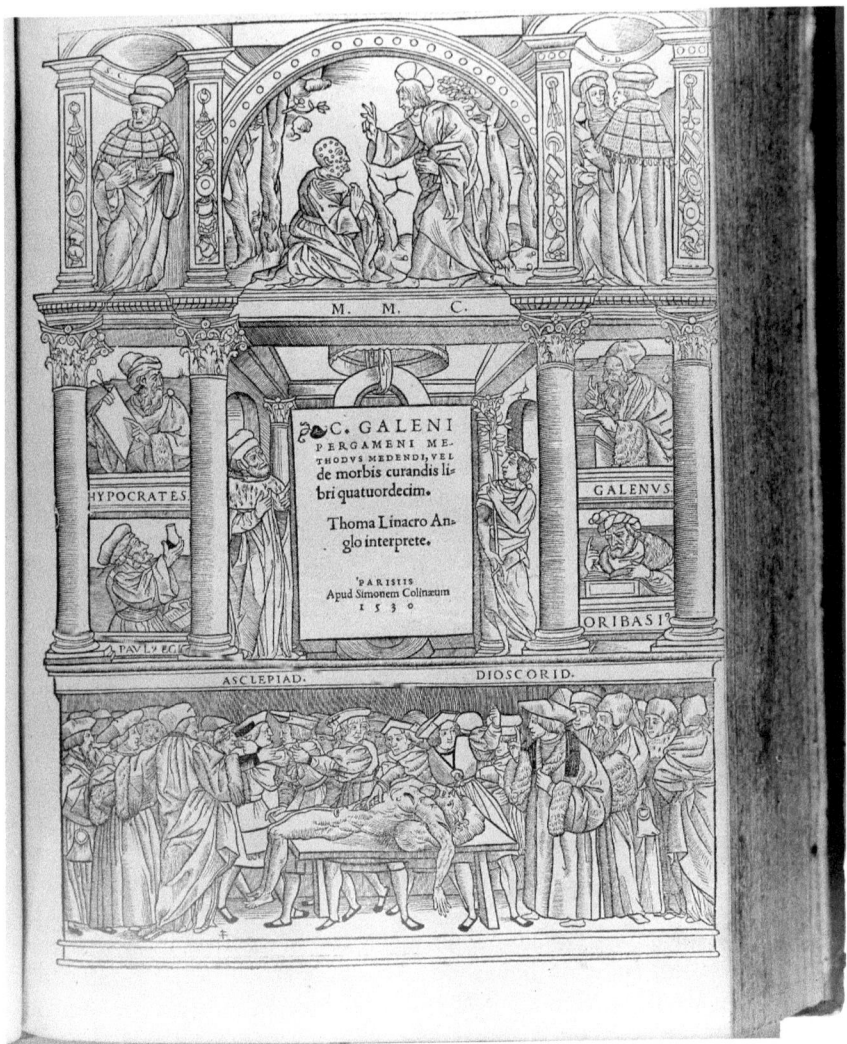

Figure 4.2 The title page of Thomas Linacre's translation of Galen's big *Method of Healing*, Paris, Simon de Colines, 1530. Not only does it depict some of the great ancient Greek physicians, but it shows Galen performing a dissection. Although this book contains little on anatomy, the same block was used for the following year's publication of Guinter's extremely influential version of *Anatomical Procedures*.

Barbaro, one of Leoniceno's critics, produced his own translation and commentary, although it was not published until 1516. There were four Greek editions between 1499 and 1529, but the later ones of 1549 and 1598 appeared alongside a Latin translation. The earliest translators and commentators concentrated upon philological questions, but a greater interest in

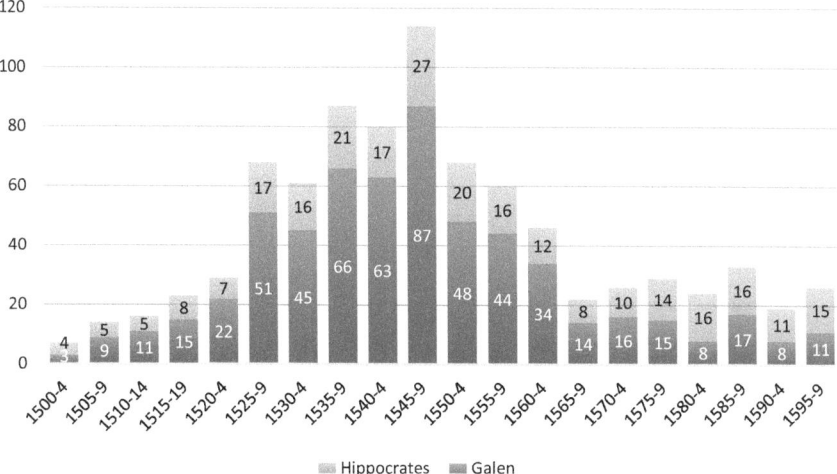

Figure 4.3 Editions and translations of Galen and Hippocrates in the sixteenth century.

the medical value of Dioscorides's listings came to the fore in the 1530s and was developed further by others with more botanical or pharmacological interests. Some, like the obscure Hollander Cornelius Petrus in 1533, made a deliberate effort to tailor his information about plants, their names and their properties for a local readership, and the later editors and commentators, as we have seen, sought to integrate Dioscorides's descriptions into the ever-widening world of botany and natural history. Particularly striking is the extent to which the *Materia medica* was translated into languages other than Latin. Mattioli's commentary, first written in Italian and constantly revised, was available also in two different French versions, another in German and yet another in Czech as well as a posthumous enlarged and corrected Italian edition. There were independent vernacular versions of Dioscorides in Dutch (1520), German (1546), French (1553) and two in Italian (1542, 1547). No other ancient medical writer, apart from Hippocrates, reached such a wide non-Latinate audience, but, as has already been noted earlier (p. 16), an interest in plants and their usages was not confined to the medical profession.[65]

For much of the sixteenth century versions of Hippocrates took very much second place to Galen. Calvo's 1525 translation and the Aldine Greek edition of the following year largely put an end to the older medieval versions, although the old standbys of the *Aphorisms*, *Prognostic* and *Epidemics* continued to attract far more attention than the treatises that were made available for the first time.[66] The pattern of publication resembles that of Galen, but in much smaller numbers and with a decade's delay,

with one major exception. Although there is some falling off in Hippocratic printings after 1555, those of Hippocrates show a smaller fall and
maintain a roughly similar average of annual printings to those of Galen
until the end of the century.[67] The second half of the century also saw the
gradual supersession of Galen by his master. Not only were sumptuous
editions of Hippocrates put out in 1588 by the Giuntine Press and in 1595
by that of Wechel, but the so-called Paris Hippocratics produced large
commentaries on texts like *Coan Prognoses* which had been neglected for
centuries. Anutius Foesius of Metz, the Wechel editor, also brought out
in 1588 his *Oeconomia Hippocratis alphabeti serie distincta, Hippocrates
Alphabetised*, a work that is at one and the same time a Hippocratic lexicon
and a detailed study of the words and concepts found in the Hippocratic
Corpus.[68] A change in the statutes of the German university of Ingolstadt
around 1563 neatly shows the increasing authority of Hippocrates over
that of Galen. From now on, only the genuine works of Hippocrates and
Galen were to be the subject of lectures in the medical Faculty. Anatomy
teaching was to begin with the Hippocratic *Nature of Bones, Anatomy,
Glands* and *Fleshes*, while the pathological texts now included *Places in
Man* and *Breaths*.[69]

The doctors or teachers who translated these classical texts, whether they
were concerned with Galen, Hippocrates, the Byzantine encyclopaedist Oribasius, or the minor writers most accessible in a collected volume largely
translated by the Paduan teacher Junius Paulus Crassus, all subscribed to
the humanist creed that the recovery of the works of Antiquity was a mark
of progress.[70] It was not just a question of style and accuracy, although
these factors figured prominently in prefaces bemoaning their predecessors'
lack of eloquence, their paucity of appropriate Latin words, and their tire-
some and virtually unintelligible adherence to a word-for-word translation
technique. Rather, there was a universal conviction, following Leoniceno's
unanswerable demonstrations, that "medicine in the Middle Ages had
been buried and overwhelmed in a great gloom", "utterly corrupt" and
"shrouded in darkness perpetual and silent night". Now medicine had been
raised from the dead to speak again with its true voice.[71]

There was a great deal of truth in this rhetoric. To a student of the Latin
of Cicero and Celsus the minor works of Galen that had been translated
by Niccolò da Reggio with pedantic word-for-word accuracy would have
been forbidding in their ugliness, as well as hard to understand because
of their mixture of Latin and Greek. Only the deeply committed medical
scholar or collector owned a 'complete' Galen, and few bothered to read
more than a handful of the treatises it contained. The story recounted by
Hartmann Schedel (1440–1514) of finding a codex containing many Latin
works of Galen rotting away on the top of a monastic cupboard rings true.[72]
But much of this ancient Greek heritage was never translated, or at best
piecemeal and inaccurately. The minor authors and medical compendia and
encyclopaedias of Late Greek Antiquity, as well as much of Hippocrates

and Galen, remained unknown, and Dioscorides had been read, if at all, only through a very inaccurate Latin version dating from the 11th or 12th century. Above all, the new Greek material provided a very different view of Galen, and one much closer to what he himself had attempted to create, that of Galen the polymath, the thinker and the experimentalist.[73]

Reassessing the Past

As well as developing, and at times rejecting, their classical heritage in anatomy, pharmacology and therapeutics the medical men of the sixteenth century had to work out afresh their relationship with a medical past that was now both more Greek and more extensive. They were aided in this by Galen, who had been concerned to buttress his own authority by invoking that of Hippocrates and had had to find ways of explaining away what he considered to be errors in the writings ascribed to the Father of Medicine.[74] His favoured method was to place individual treatises, or parts of treatises, along a spectrum of authenticity. Though all were in some way Hippocratic, some tracts were more closely linked to him than others. Some came directly from his pen, others from what he had told his family or taught his pupils, still others were Hippocratic only in spirit. This was a methodology that, in their turn, doctors in the sixteenth century applied when they discovered errors or inconsistencies in treatises that circulated under the names of Galen, Hippocrates or Dioscorides, thus reinforcing the authority of those tracts that, in their view, were demonstrably genuine.

This process was most clearly visible in the two great Latin editions of Galen that were published in the 1540s by the firms of Giunta and Froben in what John Caius called "honourable competition" with a third edition curated by Agostino Ricci and Vettore Trincavelli. All three aimed to improve on existing printed versions by going beyond the Aldine and Basle editions of the Greek to consult other manuscripts and to emend the text before translating it.[75] The Giuntine editions in particular, organised by Agostino Gadaldini (1515–75) between 1541 and 1565, became for many physicians the simplest way of consulting Galen. From 1550, this task was assisted by a massive index compiled by Antonio Musa Brasavola which until the age of the computer remained the only way in which one could discover quickly what Galen had said on any given theme.[76]

This attempt to use Galen's own methods to separate his genuine writings from those that had simply acquired an association with him over time was necessary, for the 1490 edition of Galen's collected works had contained many that were not by him, and the first translators from the Greek lacked discrimination.[77] Four of the Galenic tracts published by Giorgio Valla in 1498 were later shown to be inauthentic, as were two of the three published in 1536 by Struthius, the genuine *Antidotes*, an *Astrologia* (the simple title of a work otherwise known as *Prognostics from Taking to One's Bed*) and a short tract on urines.[78] Struthius's enthusiasm outran his scholarship.

The treatise on astrology was quickly shown to have no connection at all with Galen, and that on urines, although incorporating some of Galen's ideas, was soon identified as a summary dating from Late Antiquity. Giovanni Battista da Monte (1489–1551), the editor of the 1541 Giuntine edition, explained why he had placed the *Prognostics* in the separate volume of spurious writings but not the tract on urines. This he had included alongside other therapeutic works, merely marking it as "ascribed to Galen", because it was still a valuable contribution to medicine, whereas *Prognostics* was neither genuine nor useful.[79] This distinction between genuine and supposititious material, which was also followed in the Froben edition, condemned it and the ancient writings that were likewise exiled to the volume of *Spuria* to centuries of neglect, despite their valuable evidence for alternative points of view in the Greek world of Galen's day.[80]

But most physicians of the sixteenth century were interested in new information that might be useful in their practice, and not so much in history of medicine. Nonetheless, even here, the new Greek material added considerably to their knowledge of Galen's life and his struggles with his competitors in Rome. Until the recent discovery of Galen's *Avoiding Distress* in 2005, all his biographers depended heavily on his own accounts in three different treatises. Two of them, *My own Books* and *The Order of My Own Books*, had been unknown before the Aldine edition, while the third, *Prognosis, for Epigenes*, had been little read in the Latin version of Niccolò da Reggio. Gian Giacomo Bartolotti (c. 1470–c. 1530), who wrote a tract on *The Antiquity of Medicine, De antiquitate medicinae*, in 1498, would appear to have been the first to make use of the last treatise, almost certainly reading it in the 1490 edition of the Latin Galen.[81] The new data allowed doctors to challenge in their prefaces to Galenic translations and in individual pamphlets some of the legends that had been transmitted in the Arabic tradition. They disputed at length where and when Galen died. Was it at the age of 70, 87, 95, 105 or even 140? (This last was the hypothesis of the humanist Caelius Rhodiginus (1454–1525) in his *Lectiones antiquae, Readings from Antiquity*, a popular reference book.) Had he died at Pergamum or on a pilgrimage to the Holy Land, the origin of a strange debate as to whether he was a Protestant or Catholic *avant la lettre*? Whatever his precise religious views, all were agreed that he was undoubtedly a man of upstanding moral purpose, although today's historians will be surprised to find him held up by Antonio Fumanello (fl. 1536) as "thinking nothing of insults" and "not seeking glory", or by Conrad Gessner as "liberal, humane, truthful, and unwilling to do harm".[82]

Those who preferred to study Hippocrates faced yet greater difficulties, for they knew from Galen that not every tract published in 1525 and 1526 came unmediated from the pen of the Father of Medicine. In one sense this did not matter, for they saw Hippocrates through the eyes of Galen and equated the medicine of Hippocrates with that of his disciple. One of the first tracts of medicine to bear the name of Hippocrates alone, Johann

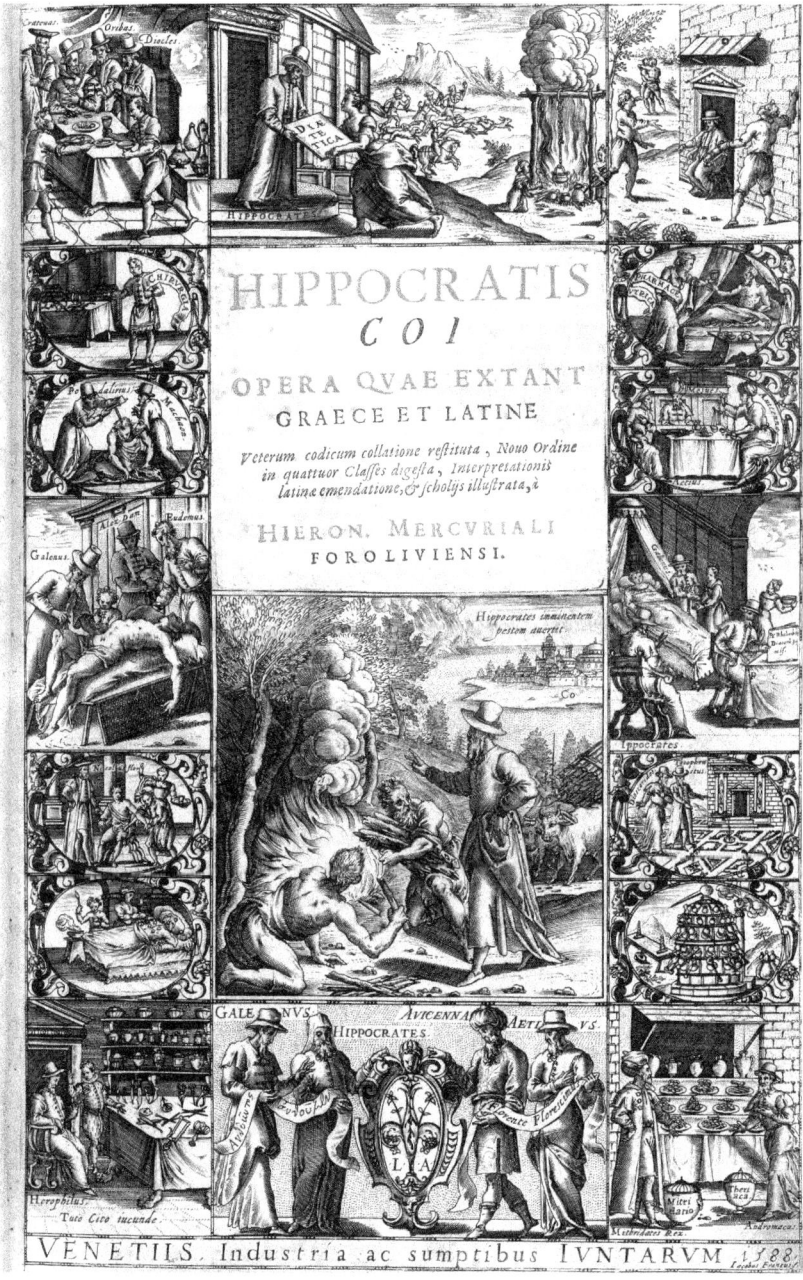

Figure 4.4 The title page of Girolamo Mercuriale's edition of Hippocrates, Venice: Giunta, 1588. The incidents depicted are generic or based on the pseudo-Hippocratic *Letters*.

Schroeter's *Sketch of Hippocratic Doctrine, Idea doctrinae Hippocraticae*, published at Vienna in 1550, was no more than a summary of Da Monte's opening lectures on the *Aphorisms* and was intended to show the complete unity between Hippocrates and Galen.[83] Indeed, Janus Cornarius went so far as to claim that it was only through Galen's championship of his ideas that Hippocrates attained the honoured place that he now held.[84]

But, compared with those of Galen, biographers of Hippocrates had little new to offer their readers. True, they could now read in the pseudo-Hippocratic letters of his dealings with the King of Persia, the King of Macedon and the philosopher Democritus, but their gist was already known to them through Galen.[85] When Pierre Vernay (fl. 1540) wished to write a life of Hippocrates to accompany a version of the *Oath* and *Prognostic*, he had little choice but to rely upon the highly imaginative traditions of the Arabs.[86] The contrast between the two biographies can be seen clearly in the illustrations that fill the huge frontispieces to the Giuntine editions of the two authors. Incidents from the life of Galen fill the entire page in the editions from 1541 onwards, whereas Hippocrates features personally in only five of the 17 scenes in the similarly large historiated frontispiece to the 1588 printing of his complete works.

This edition, curated by Girolamo Mercuriale (Figure 4.4), exemplifies the methods and the ambitions of those who believed in the importance of their classical sources. A large folio edition, it presented in elegant fonts both Greek text and Latin translation in facing columns. Although Mercuriale had been frustrated in his hopes of seeing an ancient Greek manuscript that was rumoured to exist on Crete, he was the first to make use of one of the oldest of all surviving manuscripts, Vatican, Graecus 276, and improved the text and translation by his own suggestions.[87] He prefaced his edition with a detailed investigation into the authenticity of the Hippocratic writings, participating in a controversy that had been reignited by the rediscovery of Galen's commentaries and had divided scholars for 50 years.[88] It had acquired added significance through the decision of universities such as Ingolstadt (see earlier, p. 112) to base their curriculum on the genuine works of Hippocrates and Galen. To solve what is today termed the 'Hippocratic question' was no easy task. Mercuriale's solution in 1588 was his third attempt to build on Galen's four-fold classification as he revised his judgement on the style and 'weight', *gravitas*, of these miscellaneous treatises in the light of others' comments. He now included rather more tracts among those he believed were written by Hippocrates himself, but placed the *Oath*, *Ancient Medicine*, and *Glands* among those where there was no real link with the historical Hippocrates.[89]

Mercuriale's edition of Hippocrates, for all its merits, marks the end of what might be termed the philological approach to medicine. The ancient writers continued to be studied and their ideas discussed, criticised and developed, but few doctors now accepted Leoniceno's credo that medical misconceptions could be best corrected by a search for forgotten ancient writings and improving the meaning of ancient authorities by emending the text or seeking out better manuscripts. In the following century there were still eminent physician-philologists such as René Chartier (1572–1654) in Paris and Jan van der Linden (1609–64) in Leiden, but they were far fewer in number, and none could compare in the intensity and scale of their philological activity with sixteenth-century predecessors such as John Caius or Janus Cornarius.[90] Cornarius (1500–58) who interspersed periods of teaching at the universities of Basle, Marburg and Jena with serving as a civic physician at Nordhausen, Frankfurt and Zwickau, had a Europe-wide reputation as an editor and translator of classical texts, and the emendations he made in the margins of his editions of Hippocrates and Galen are still highly regarded by modern editors (Figure 5.1). But his vigorous conservatism did not always endear him even to like-minded colleagues, and his passion for past medicine created problems in the present.[91] By 1553 the town council of Zwickau, his home town, which had appointed him as town physician in 1546 with an unusual ten-year contract at 100 guilders a year (equal to the pay of the Burgomaster), had received so many complaints about him for neglecting his medical practice in favour of his translations that they sought permission from the Elector of Saxony to pay a deputy for the last three years of the contract. Their wish was granted. The son-in-law of a former town physician was appointed his deputy, and Cornarius was left to his translations.[92] He was not reappointed, and he moved to a professorial chair at Jena in 1555. John Caius was more successful than Cornarius as a physician. He made enough money from his medical practice in Tudor London to allow him to re-found his old Cambridge College, while still devoting much of his time to editing and translating Galen. He covered his copy of the 1538 Basle edition of Galen with thousands of notes, many taken from manuscripts or collections of notes by others that he had seen in Italy in the 1540s or later in England. He was nine times elected President of the London College of Physicians, where he joined other like-minded doctors, such as John Clement and Edward Wotton, in stressing a detailed knowledge of Galen and Hippocrates as the sole criterion for admission.[93]

Such reverence for the Classics, and certainly the belief in philology as the key to an improved medicine, diminished noticeably in the last quarter of the sixteenth century. But earlier, in the first half of the century, and particularly after 1525, it had stimulated new ideas in medicine as the rediscovery of ancient authors, especially Galen, revealed a rich heritage that had been unknown to the Western Middle Ages. This renaissance resonated with wider ideas about the importance of Antiquity as a model for culture and morality that long continued. But medicine itself moved on rapidly, and classically orientated professors were literally left behind. Van der Linden in his old age lectured to near-empty classrooms, as the young deserted him to hear the new chemical philosophy of De le Boë Sylvius (1614–72). It was a sad end to a distinguished career and to a movement that a century earlier had promised so much.

Notes

1 Machiavelli 1979: 124.
2 Nutton 2020a. For Galen's anatomical studies, see later, pp. 246–7.
3 The history of Galenism from 200 to 1490 is covered in detail in Bouras-Vallianatos and Zipser 2019, sections 1–3; Nutton 2020a: 133–8.
4 Overwien 2019.
5 Harig 1974; Ventura 2019.
6 The history of Galenic translations in the rest of this section depends on the various contributions in Bouras-Vallianatos and Zipser 2019, sections 2 and 3. For translations of Arabic medical writings, see also Siraisi 1987: 19–75, 1990; Burnett 2011.
7 Bloch 1986: I, 98–110, 127–34; Green 2019 adds much new material.
8 Agrimi and Crisciani 1988.
9 Nutton 2020a: 132–3.
10 Jacquart 1980; Agrimi and Crisciani 1994.
11 Reeve 1983 summarises briefly the over-abundance of information given by Marx 1915: XXX–LXIII; Nutton 2020c.
12 Nauert 1979, 1980.
13 Mugnai Carrara 1979 is fundamental; Lonigo 2019. For the Ferrara background, Nutton 1997b.
14 Mugnai Carrara 1979: 188.
15 Mugnai Carrara 1989 presents a late treatise long thought lost.
16 Wilson 1992; Giacomelli 2021.
17 Mugnai Carrara 1991: 35: of the items inventoried in his library, in both print and manuscript, at his death, 247 out of 340 concerned medicine, philosophy or mathematics.
18 Leoniceno 1492: sigg. a.3v, 4r, 4v; for Arabs and modern druggists, sigg. C.3v–4r.
19 Details of this controversy are easiest found in Reeds 1991: 19–21; Godman 1998: 96–108; Grafton 2001: 3–9; Ogilvie 2006.
20 Several are collected in Leoniceno 1509.
21 Leoniceno 1508; Mugnai Carrara 1983.
22 Leoniceno 1506; Hirai 2007, 2011: 19–45.
23 Leoniceno 1497; Arrizabalaga *et al.* 1997: 70–87.
24 Valla 1529, but first published as part of a larger work in 1501, see Landucci Ruffo 1981; Raschieri 2012. For the development of ideas on skin disease at the end of the century, Murphy 2020.
25 Maddison *et al.* 1977.
26 Nutton 1987a: 39–40; for Bessarion, Lowry 1974–5; Labowsky 1979; Giacomelli 2021.
27 De Vecchi 1932; for Alessandro Benedetti (later, p. 250), Giacomelli 2021.
28 Manardi, *Ep. Med.* XIX, 5: 1556: 192, of December 1535.
29 Sicherl 1976: 42–50.
30 Legrand 1885: I, 75; II, 312–3.
31 The absence of a large enough readership for such an expensive author may explain Wilson's surprise (1992: 161) at the long gap between the rediscovery of Galen in Greek and real efforts to read his many works.
32 Arbenz 1891: 248.
33 Nutton 1987a: 29, 37.
34 Valla 1498.
35 Sonderkamp 1987: 1–6. The author was a tenth-century author, Theophanes Chrysobalantes. The Nuremberg 1496 edition of Hippocrates's *Aphorisms* involved a substantial selection, reworking and reorganisation of an older Latin version.

36 Nutton 1997a: 166–9.
37 Clemen 1907a edits three medical letters of Sturtz.
38 Nutton 1997a: 166–9.
39 The papal privilege of the 1526 Hippocrates promises these authors, and one of the Aldine editors, Georg Agricola, certainly collated codices of Aetius and Oribasius, Nutton 1993: 23.
40 Jurina 1985: 7; cf. also Nutton 1987a: 48.
41 Rabelais 1532; on Rabelais's knowledge of Galen, Nutton 1988b.
42 Orozco 1540: sigg., Aa 6–7.
43 Labowsky 1961: 125; Giacomelli 2021.
44 Wenkebach 1925; Fortuna 2019a: 443–5.
45 Nutton 1987a: 39–40.
46 Nutton 1987a: 38–9.
47 Wenkebach 1925; Reed 1925–6; Nutton 1987a: 58–9; Pietrobelli 2008: CCX-CIV–VII; McDonald 2013; Beta 2019.
48 Nutton 1987a: 59; Pietrobelli forthcoming.
49 Gundert 2006.
50 Pratensis 1527: sig. A.5v–r.
51 Cardano 1663: 6, 7. Alciati (1492–1550), the leading jurist of the day; Erasmus, later; Guillaume Budé (1467–1540), the great French humanist; Caelius Rhodiginus (1469–1525), Professor of Greek in Venice.
52 Caius 1570c: f. 18r; Nutton 2018a: 70.
53 Perilli 2012.
54 Flood and Shaw 1997: 70.
55 Burckhardt 1917: 34, 133–4.
56 Manardi *Ep.* XIX, 5: 1556, 192.
57 Flood and Shaw 1997: 70; Hieronymus 2005: 68–9.
58 Tarchagnota 1549 (one of three different Italian versions of this tract).
59 Lowe 1597; Geyer-Kordesch and MacDonald 1999: 41–78.
60 Erasmus 1526, 1969.
61 Mugnai Carrara 1979: 200.
62 Berengario 1529: fols. 2v–3v; for the date, Nutton 1987a: 36, note 72.
63 Durling 1961.
64 Durling 1961: 238, n. 42; Savino 2019, 2020.
65 Riddle 1980: esp. 8–11, and 58–9 (Petrus). For Mattioli and the development of medical botany, see earlier p. 16–7.
66 Hippocrates 1525, 1526.
67 The comparable survey to that of Durling, Maloney and Savoie 1985, is far less reliable because of the doublets and omissions, particularly of pre-1560 Hippocratic printings. I have excluded commentaries without texts. Rütten 2008 compares the patterns.
68 Hippocrates 1588 (edited by Mercuriale); Hippocrates 1595 (edited by Foesius); Lonie 1985; Foesius 1588.
69 Nauck 1956, arguing for 1555, but in the form he presents them, the Statutes refer to books published in 1557 and 1562. This curriculum was also adopted at Freiburg.
70 Crassus 1581; for Oribasius, Savino 2020: 29–46.
71 Durling 1961: 239, gives typical examples.
72 Stauber 1908: 58. He later acquired the manuscript, now Munich, Staatsbibliothek, CLM 2.
73 Nutton 2020a.
74 Smith 1979.
75 Caius 1570c: sig., 6v; Nutton 2018a: 58.

76 Garofalo 2004. The index to the standard bilingual edition of Galen by K. G. Kühn is a much abbreviated version of Brasavola's.
77 Fortuna 2020.
78 Struthius at Galen 1536: pref., 112v–13v, showing how much at this date astrology was highly respected within medicine and studied even by bishops; 136r–v.
79 Galen 1549: 10; 1565: 10, 12r–v; 1549: 4, 473–4; 1565: 4, 123v–5v.
80 Fortuna 2019a: 449; Savino 2020; Petit *et al.* 2021.
81 Schullian and Belloni 1954: 58–60.
82 Nutton 2009.
83 Schroeter 1550.
84 Cornarius 1536, fol. 81r.
85 For an early humanist life of Hippocrates, of c. 1506, by Cuspinianus, Siraisi 2007: 220–1, 329.
86 aa.vv. 1552: 495–6. For the legends, Rubin Pinault 1992.
87 Jouanna 2008: 291–9.
88 Sylvius 1539.
89 Jouanna 2008: 269–90.
90 Boudon-Millot *et al.* 2012.
91 Clemen 1912; Mondrain 1997; Montfort 2018.
92 Uhlig 1938: 305–6. Contrast the enthusiastic praise of him in 1548 by Melanchthon 1977: no. 5073.
93 Nutton 1987a, 2018a.

People

5 The Kaleidoscope of Healing I
Physicians

When illness struck, an individual in the sixteenth century was faced with an at times bewildering variety of people offering cures of one sort of another.[1] It was a choice constrained by geography, for those who lived in the countryside, even in well-populated regions such as Northern Italy or the Southern Netherlands, had less access to graduate physicians or sworn surgeons who preferred the companionship and wider opportunities available in a town or city. Economics mattered. Despite frequent injunctions to care for God's poor, the services of the elite practitioners were likely to be more expensive, although not always more effective, than those of a local healer, a literate cleric or a well-educated lady of the manor with a wide range of remedies of proven efficacy. Besides, a hamlet or small town could not provide the range of profitable patients that every physician expected and needed if he was to maintain himself and his family in an appropriate station in life. But although local circumstances might differ, the general picture of the providers of healing is roughly the same across Europe from Portugal to Poland. One hears the same complaints or success stories, and the leading practitioners worked within similar structures of universities and local guilds. Career patterns are also similar and were facilitated by the development in the sixteenth century of better methods of communication which allowed both more frequent and lengthier periods of travel and a swifter access to new information, whether passed on in books, letters or personal contact. This chapter concentrates on physicians, their education and their possible career paths. It does not deal except in passing with what they were taught or how they practised, which are considered elsewhere.[2] Instead, it looks at the various stages in their medical life, from becoming a student to obtaining a permanent position as a local doctor or something more prestigious, culminating in an appointment as personal physician to a nobleman or even a monarch.

The Medical Student

Medicine prided itself on being a learned profession, one based on texts, usually in Latin, and requiring a long period of study before obtaining an

DOI: 10.4324/9781003223184-8

acceptable qualification. As well as attendance at a school that taught Latin until the age of 16 or so, a prospective physician needed to have studied at a university for several years, rarely fewer than five and often more, before obtaining a medical degree. Surgery was taught in some Italian universities, but elsewhere it usually involved a form of apprenticeship that might include some lectures as well as examination by a local college or guild of surgeons. A medical education was expensive, although the rewards for success were universally accepted as likely to be huge.[3] But even if, as we shall see, there were ways in which these expenses might be reduced, it required a high initial investment that was available only to a few. Consequently, most of those who studied medicine, if not from medical families themselves, came from the mercantile bourgeoisie or, like William Harvey, from solid yeomen or minor country gentry, reasonably well off, although not as wealthy as many of the students who flocked to study law in Germany or Italy.[4] It was this ambiguous status that so exercised the French lawyer André Tiraqueau (1488–1568) that he devoted over 250 pages to pondering whether being a physician derogated from any nobility of birth that he might have possessed. His arguments for and against this proposition ranged from the presence of physicians in the ranks of saints, angels and poets to their involvement with faeces and urine and finally to the generally low opinion of them held by their patients from Ancient Greece onwards.[5] In the end he accepted the argument that medicine was the noblest of the arts, but he remained doubtful that it was a profession fit for a nobleman, warning that nobility once lost in this way could never be regained.[6] But that, of course, did not deter those who were not noble, and who saw in medicine a way of enhancing the wealth, and indeed the status, of their family.

In Northern Europe the medical course was often begun after one had already obtained a degree in Arts, sometimes after a lapse of several years, but in Italian universities one usually gained a degree in both subjects at the same time.[7] This preliminary training in arts explains why, at the end of the sixteenth century, the London College of Physicians contained two Fellows who had been headmasters and another the Provost of Oriel College, Oxford, before turning to medicine, while, earlier, John Clement and Edward Wotton had both previously taught Greek in Oxford.[8] The Saxon Georg Agricola had similarly obtained a degree in Arts at Leipzig and served as headmaster of the town school at Zwickau in Saxony before returning to Leipzig to study medicine.[9] At least one doctor managed to follow both careers simultaneously. The Dutch humanist Gisbert Longolius (1507–43), after taking his MD degree in Italy, combined the posts of civic physician and headmaster of the town school at Deventer before moving to Cologne as Professor of Greek and personal physician to its Archbishop.[10]

Although the MD was the summit of medical qualifications, it was also possible in some universities, such as Oxford or Cambridge, to take a lesser medical qualification, either a medical licence or an MB, which allowed one to practise within a restricted geographical area, but this does not seem to

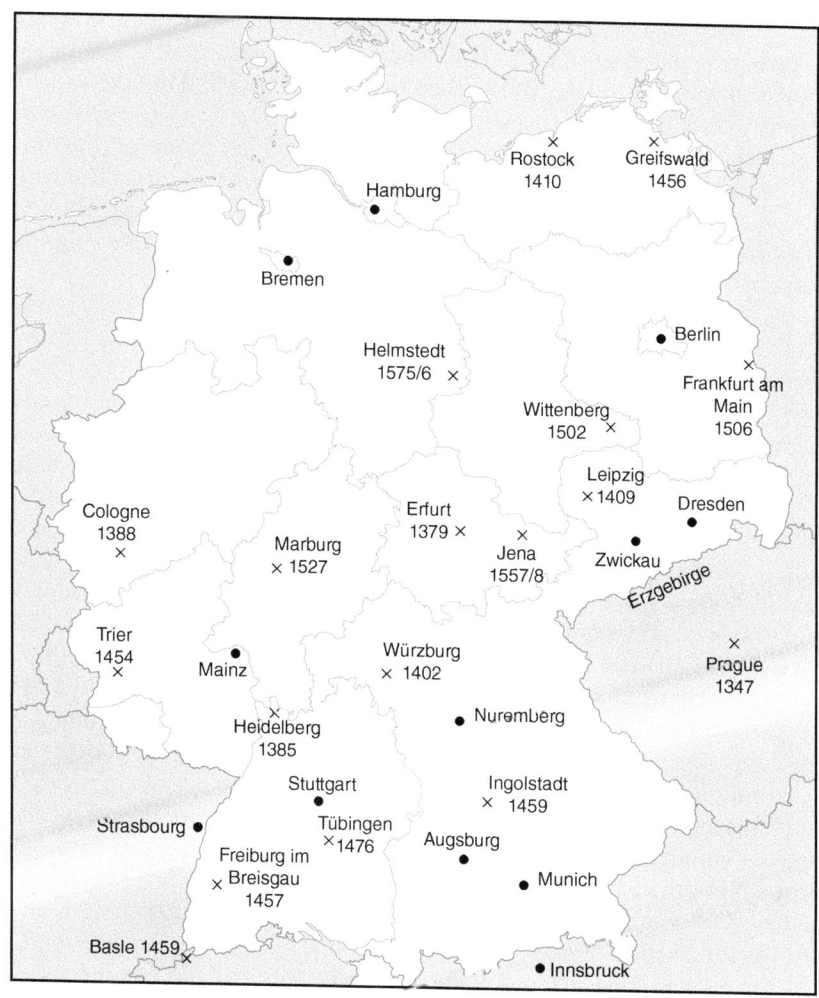

Map 5.1 Towns in Germany with universities before 1600.

have been the case in Italy. Roughly a third of Cambridge's 95 medical licentiates in the sixteenth century went on to complete a further medical degree, but one-third of those who had previously graduated in Arts did not, while only one-third of those who took the intermediate MB went on to take an MD.[11] Very often a student who had begun at one university went on to take his degree at another, particularly if it was the MD. Vesalius, for instance, began his studies at Louvain, moved to Paris, then back to Louvain, where he took an MB, leaving almost at once for Padua, where he graduated MD less than a year later in December 1537.[12] Several students from Padua took an MD degree from the *Studio* of Venice, almost certainly because this was cheaper than that of Padua itself.[13] By contrast, because medical graduates of Paris enjoyed a monopoly over medical practice there and in much of France, any non-graduate who wished to practise there had to take a further degree, unless granted a special royal permission or willing to run the risk of prosecution for unlicensed practice.[14] This Parisian privilege was hotly contested throughout the century by the University of Montpellier, which was almost as old and equally distinguished and which in the sixteenth century produced such famous names as Guillaume Rondelet (1507–66) and Laurent Joubert (1529–82).

Not all universities, particularly in France, had a medical Faculty, and most of those that did had only a handful of medical students. Ferrara's total of five or six medical graduates a year in the early 1540s compares poorly with Bologna and Padua, with three times that number, although it was still far more than in most universities that taught medicine, including Oxford or Cambridge, which produced only a handful of MDs over a decade.[15] Universities had often been set up primarily with a local focus to provide the ruler with a cadre of professionals, lawyers, doctors, administrators and, in Northern Europe, clerics. Particularly in the sixteenth century, universities were founded to ensure that the young studied in an appropriate religious environment, whether Protestant, like Marburg (founded in 1527) and Jena (founded in 1558) or Catholic, as at Würzburg (reopened 1582) or Fermo in Italy (founded by Pope Sixtus V, a native of the region, in 1585). A reputation for promoting learning added to the fame of its founder, and there was a general expectation that the arrival of rich young students and their retinues would boost the local economy. When Nuremberg set up its own high school in 1578, it was precisely to tap into the market of wealthy students coming from further east in the Holy Roman Empire, although the town council, wary of what students might get up to in the city itself, decided to build it in a small town, Altdorf, some 25 kilometres away towards the border with Bohemia.[16]

Those responsible for running the university, especially in Northern Italy, were keen to retain its reputation as a place where students could reliably expect to hear and consort with the best medical minds of the day. A collaborator praised Antonio Musa Brasavola for attracting large numbers of students to Ferrara from outside the local area during his first years of teaching there from 1536 to 1540, a claim not entirely confirmed by the matriculation and degree figures.[17] The success of Padua was closely watched by Venetian officials who oversaw the university. In 1517, concerned about a decline in student numbers, they instituted reforms that were to prove the foundation of the university's success over the next century. The introduction of a ban on chairs being held by native Venetians opened up the faculties to talent from all over Europe, while, in the second half of the century, the relative laxity of the Venetian Inquisition allowed Protestants to study there who would have been in grave danger from the Inquisitions in Rome

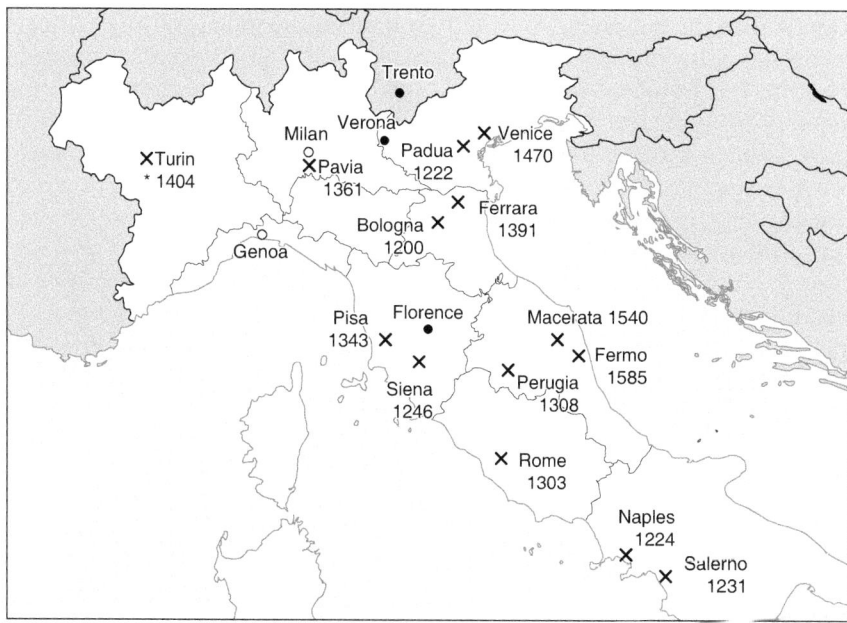

Map 5.2 Towns in Northern and Central Italy with universities before 1600.

or papal Bologna. Venice also granted students certain privileges: they were allowed, for instance, to bring their own property in and out without being subject to onerous border tolls.[18]

Although residence at a local university was always an option, if one did decide to travel, one could save money by making private arrangements to stay with friends. Felix Platter stayed while at Montpellier with an apothecary friend of his father whose son in return stayed with the Platter family during his education in Basle.[19] Often older students found jobs in the town or region. The editors of the Aldine editions of the Greek medical classics were all studying, or had just finished studying, medicine at Padua and elsewhere.[20] Others turned to teaching in public or in private. John Caius augmented his stipend as a Fellow of Gonville Hall by lecturing publicly at Padua on Aristotle's Greek texts, a very junior and poorly paid position, and also repeated some of his lectures for the benefit of wealthy English aristocrats.[21] Others made their way to university thanks to loans and grants. Christopher Langton (1521–78), a Yorkshireman, was supported during his time at Eton and in Cambridge by a local magnate, Sir Arthur Darcy (c. 1495–1561), to whom he dedicated his first book.[22] John Clement was granted £10 a year by Henry VIII to travel overseas, taking his medical degree at the much cheaper University of Siena.[23] A frequent source of such grants in Germany was the Fugger family of Augsburg who expected in return that the beneficiaries would report back to them on any business opportunity for the firm and keep them up to date on the political situation elsewhere in Europe.[24] In Germany a town might subsidise a citizen in the hope of his return to practise among them. The town council at Zwickau gave Clement's colleague at the Aldine press, the Saxon Georg Agricola, leave of absence in 1523 from his post as headmaster of the local school and a grant to go to Leipzig to study medicine.[25] He soon moved on to Bologna and Padua before returning very briefly to Zwickau in 1527 and then settling as a town physician at Joachimsthal and later Chemnitz. Zwickau had already in 1520 given a seven-year grant to one of its citizens, Janus Cornarius, to study arts and medicine at Wittenberg, and then to go on a long tour of Europe after his graduation.[26]

The indefatigable historian of Zwickau, Otto Clemen (1871–1946), also traced the variety of support given to another local medical student of modest means and considerable ambition, Georg Pylander (c. 1513–44). The son of a clothier who had died when he was a small child, he was educated in part at a school in Annaberg, where a Zwickau relative was headmaster. In 1531 he obtained his first grant from the Zwickau town council to go to Wittenberg, and three years later Melanchthon arranged for the Elector Johann Friedrich to transfer to him for three years part of the stipend of a recently deceased cleric at Altenburg, several kilometres away. In 1537 the city council agreed to give him a further three-year grant to study abroad, which he rejected as soon as he discovered that they wished him to study in Protestant Denmark, not Italy. He was saved once again by the Elector, who gave him a grant to go to Italy for two years, on condition that on his return he put his skills at the Elector's disposal. In 1539 Pylander appealed to the Elector again, explaining that he had already spent six months in Paris and a whole year in Montpellier, and now, finally, was planning to begin a one or two year stay in Italy. Zwickau had given him a grant of 40 guilders over the previous two years, but a stay in Italy would cost between 100 and 150 guilders a year at least. He now wished the Elector to persuade Zwickau to continue their support and himself to add a further 30 guilders. He did not reach Italy on his wanderings until 1540, when he wrote to his Zwickau friend, the town clerk, excusing his slow progress on the grounds that the slow detour via Paris and Montpellier had reduced the danger to his health from any sudden change of climate. But the cost of living in Italy was frighteningly high, commensurate with the learning of its teachers. Whether the Zwickau council continued their support is not clear, and Pylander implies that the town clerk himself gave him money out of his own pocket for further study. He was in Rome in 1541, before going on to take his degree in Naples, and he moved slowly around Italy, presumably supplementing any grant by treating patients. He is last heard of in Northern Italy in 1544 when he wrote the preface to a small book on cosmology, but he must have died soon after, for he talks in it of his weakness of both body and mind. Neither the Elector nor Zwickau ever profited from their investment in Pylander.[27]

Travels in Search of Knowledge

It is not hard to discover why such students should choose to spend many years away from home gaining a medical degree and sometimes journeying for yet more years around Western Europe before they settled into a permanent position.[28] Pylander put it succinctly. One was likely to benefit greatly by associating with the most learned and acute physicians, hearing what they had to say and learning from their lifetime of experience.[29] The Zwickau town clerk, Stephan Roth, was already familiar with this argument, for he had been the dedicatee in 1531 of a short oration in praise of travel from Janus Cornarius. In this essay, which had been originally delivered at Wittenberg as a lecture on Hippocrates's *Airs, Waters and Places*, the well-travelled Cornarius provided a variety of reasons for a medical tour. It broadened the mind and introduced one to new people, new diseases, new drugs and new ideas; it confirmed the truths of Hippocrates's meteorological medicine; it furthered international friendship and understanding; and it also gave one the reputation of a world traveller. The delightful prospect of being able to test what others had said about far-flung lands was doubtless enhanced when it was being subsidised by others. Cornarius took full advantage of his good fortune, visiting Courland, Lithuania, the Baltic coast, the Netherlands and even distant England, where he spent a few days by the Thames in London watching drugs being imported from exotic lands.[30] To support himself he also lectured, published and occasionally treated the sick on his travels.

Cornarius noted that increasing numbers of young students were now visiting the distant lands of the North, including Britain. One who did so was a young man from Landshut, Lorenz Gryll (1524–60), helped by a travel grant from the Fuggers, but it was not an enjoyable experience.[31] It was his misfortune to arrive in London in 1553 as the young Edward VI lay dying and the supporters of the Protestant Lady Jane Grey as Queen were struggling for supremacy with those of the Catholic Mary Tudor. No one would talk to him as he wandered bemusedly around London for a fortnight, suspected of being a foreign spy, until he was forced to retreat hurriedly to Flanders, still uncertain of what was going on.[32] He recounted this experience, and many others, during his inaugural lecture at Ingolstadt in 1558. It was a memorable occasion, not least because it had to be delivered from a camp bed, as Gryll had recently broken his leg. He described a remarkable journey, undertaken, he averred, to gain knowledge of the latest ideas, the best practices and the most effective drugs, both plant and mineral (especially from mines in Goslar, Eisleben, Mansfeld and the Erzgebirge). He had visited almost everywhere of note, from Venice, Ferrara, Tuscany, Rome and Naples, to Montpellier, Toulouse, Lyons and Paris, crossing the

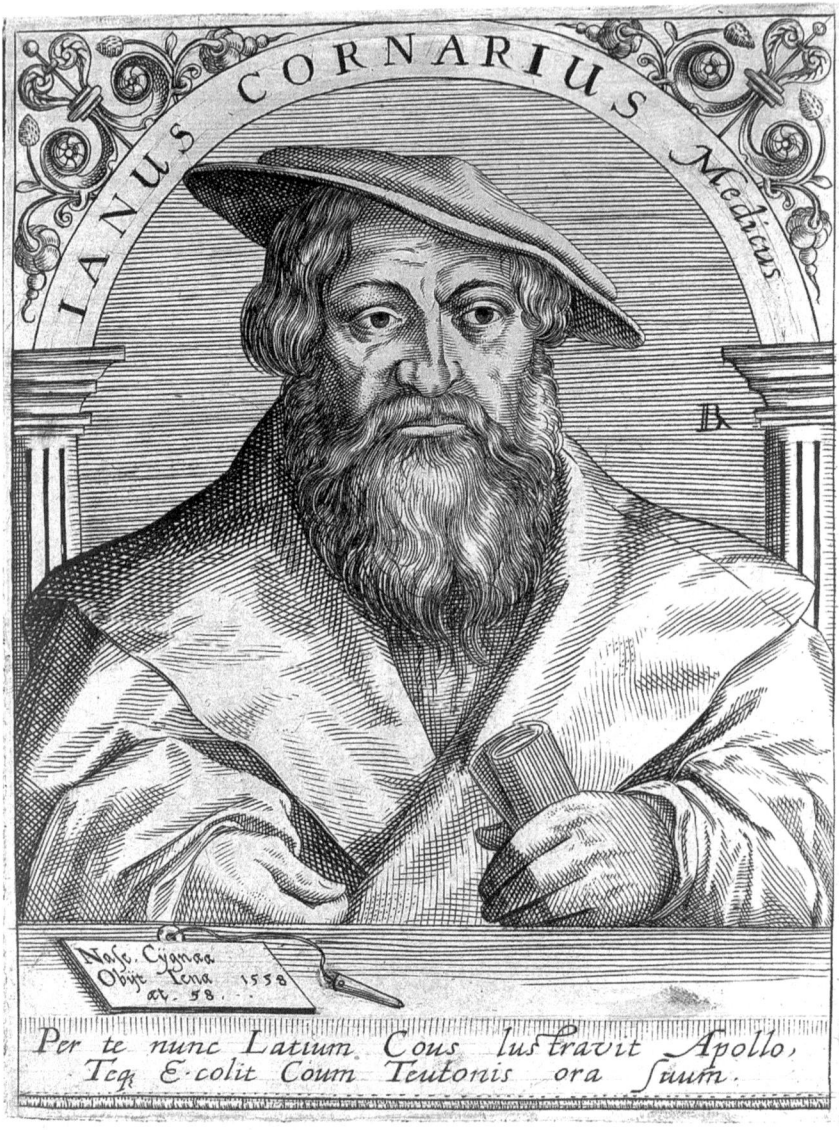

Figure 5.1 Janus Cornarius (1500–58), translator and professor of medicine at Marburg and Jena. Engraving by T. De Bry. The accompanying poem reads: Through you the Coan Apollo [Hippocrates] has illuminated the Latin world, and the German shore admires you as its own Coan [a reference to his 1546 Latin translation of the works of Hippocrates].

Channel to England and back to Belgium and Louvain before he made his final return to Germany. Even the final stages of his journey home were not without incident, for fighting forced him to take a very roundabout route, by ship from Amsterdam to Hamburg, and then slowly overland via Braunschweig and the Harz to Leipzig, Dresden and across the Erzgebirge back to Augsburg. He records that he had met and even studied with all the great names in medicine of the period – Da Monte and Brasavola in Italy, Rondelet at Montpellier, Valleriola in Arles, Julius Caesar Scaliger at Agen, Fernel and Sylvius in Paris, Drivère in Belgium, Cornarius and Agricola in Germany and many more. In Zurich in 1555 he met with Gessner, who dedicated a tract on rare plants to him along with a hint to recommend him to his patron, and hoped-for sponsor, Ulrich Fugger.[33] He visited botanic gardens and pharmacists' shops, attended anatomical dissections by Falloppia and others, both in private and as part of a normal medical course, and talked with Vesalius in Brussels. At Padua he was particularly struck by Fracanzano's habit of taking his students every day to the hospital and discoursing to them about diseases at the bedside.[34]

To achieve a better understanding of practical medicine was one of his great aims. While on his travels he worked in hospitals in Padua and Florence, whose Great Hospital, S. Maria Nuova, he found particularly welcoming, and in Rome, where, like other northerners, he toured the wards with Gisbert van der Horst, a Fleming, and a long-time resident and superintendent of one of the Roman hospitals.[35] In Marseilles he talked with knowledgeable monks and travellers from Africa and Greece about the plants of their region, and he helped to dissect corpses in Paris and elsewhere in order to learn the technique of post-mortem investigation. This was a very full and protracted journey, lasting roughly seven years and allowing also for some sightseeing in Campania, where Vesuvius was in eruption, and visits to the baths at Abano, Aachen and Karlovy Vary. It was all the more surprising for a man, who, as he explained at the beginning of his lecture, was always in weak health and had decided to take up medicine for that very reason. Sadly, the expertise he had acquired did not avail him much, for he died only a few years later, in 1560.

Eight years later, in the somewhat unlikely setting of a preface to the translation of a Byzantine medical manual, one of his pupils, Hieremias Martius (d. 1585) gave a long account of his own education and travels.[36] Like Gryll, he had been supported as an Augsburg native by a member of the Fugger family, who had encouraged him to study at Ingolstadt and then to embark on a long peregrination to improve his medical knowledge. He spent three years at Montpellier before returning home briefly and receiving another grant and further encouragement to study in Italy, beginning with six months in Padua. A letter from his patrons then sent him on to Florence, where they had gained permission from Cosmo de' Medici for him to work for a year in the Great Hospital, where he discovered just how different medical practice was from listening to lectures. He left with a glowing testimonial from the head of the hospital and at least one other leading physician. He obtained permission from his sponsors to visit Rome (for its sights as well as for its physicians), but he did not wish to incur any further expenses after that and decided to return home. Unwilling to face the hardships of overland travel, he took a ship from Pesaro to Venice, surviving a frightening storm on the way across the Venetian lagoon from Ravenna. An unfortunate surprise greeted him once back in Augsburg. He could find no job immediately, and it was only the support of his old teacher who encouraged him to speak once more with the Fuggers and, with their help, to approach the Augsburg city council that gained him the post of doctor to the hospital for syphilitics. His anxieties, hinted at in the several references to the costs of his education from his earliest years and the problems he faced at home and abroad before finding a middle-range position back home, are likely to be a truer reflection of the problems of coping with life abroad than the cheerful lion-hunting of Gryll.[37] As another doctor who had made a similar tour remarked, travellers were always beset by problems, and a friend of a friend might well be prevailed upon in a crisis to provide a subsidy or a loan.[38] But every medical traveller expected that after such a long period of study at home and abroad he would find suitable employment immediately on his return, even without much experience as an independent practitioner.[39] Great learning and some guided experience mattered above all, and friendly contact with teachers and doctors with a European reputation opened many doors.

Physicians' accounts and reminiscences of their student travels (surgeons are less informative) often emphasise how what they studied or discovered in the wanderings determined or deepened their medical interests. Gryll's focus on his encounters with different types of drugs or his visits to mining areas explains why his executor thought it worth publishing his travel account as an appendix to a much more academic discussion of the sense of taste, while Martius's emphasis on his hospital experiences foreshadows his work in the syphilis hospital. For Jordanus in Moravia it was discussions and friendships in Vienna far more than his visit to Paris, Montpellier, Bologna, Padua, Pisa and Rome that determined the shape of his future career as a specialist in epidemic diseases – and gave him an entry into Crato's circle around the Emperor.[40] Similar reminiscences of his time with Gisbert Horst in his Roman hospital, as well as his experiences in the Bolognese hospitals with Benedetto Vittori (c. 1481–1561) and Elideo Padoani (fl. 1540–76) established the Dutchman Pieter van Foreest's credentials as an expert in practical therapy.[41] John Caius, who overlapped with him in Padua, concentrated instead on his two passions, anatomy and ancient Greek manuscripts. His *Autobibliography, De libris suis*, describes his visits to libraries and collections of manuscripts in Northern and Central Italy, and his meetings and discussions with leading anatomists in Padua, Venice, Ferrara, Rome, Pisa and Bologna, as well as in Louvain on his way home.[42]

It was not unusual for such students to take private patients or even accept a public appointment while on their travels. Van Foreest was recommended by the distinguished Parisian teacher Jacobus Sylvius for the job of a public doctor in the small French town of Pithiviers, south-east of Paris, but although he records a few cases from there, he does not appear to have stayed there for long and he was back home in Alkmaar only a few months later, in mid-1546 after ten years of study.[43] On one occasion, two such travellers clashed in Nantes. When around 1534 Pietro Baptista of Cremona, who had already spent time in Pavia and Paris, arrived there as part of his European tour to learn medicine, he found that another Italian, Giovanni Agostino Capalla, had preceded him, and was creating a stir by his lectures and by his treatments of the sick. Baptista was not impressed, claiming that he had mixed up drugs, preferred hellebore to the gentler rhubarb as a purgative, failed to cure a simple case of paralysis and recommended a clyster fit only for Gargantua and Pantagruel (the earliest recorded reference to Rabelais's masterpiece). In his first letter to Capalla, he complained that his compatriot was letting down the reputation of Italy by his misspelled Greek words, confusion of terms and simple mistakes in grammar, as well as his ignorance of what Dioscorides and Aetius had written. No proper Italian would be so stupid, or so neglectful of the niceties of humanist learning. Two further letters continued this assault on his competitor.[44] Whether they had any effect, how they were distributed and the ultimate fates of both men are alike unknown.[45] But Baptista's short pamphlet was aimed less at correcting Capalla than at establishing his own superior credentials as an up-to-date and well-trained physician in a competition for patients.

Finding a Position: The Importance of Collegiality

Acquiring a post may not have been as easy for a newly qualified physician as might appear from the accounts of those who were successful, and Martius may not have been the only one who found it hard to step onto the first rung of the professional ladder. Physicians regularly complained about the sick who preferred the services of wise women, clerics, travelling salesmen, astrologers, uroscopists, charlatans and a wide range of purveyors of dubious remedies, "idle old trots, coblers and costardmongers" or, in the florid words of the surgeon William Clowes, "Mountebanks, Landlopers, Fugitives and other masterless makeshifts".[46] But competition from these healers was perhaps less severe in a metropolis like London or Rome where there were many wealthy patients than in a smaller town, like Mantua or Strasbourg, where in addition there might already be several physicians and surgeons.[47] New graduates who came from local medical families had an easier entry to the profession (and cheaper, since some fees were reduced), but others, like Martius and Pylander, had to seek the support of a local bigwig or of someone like Melanchthon well attuned to the arts of patronage on behalf of his students. Positions as a hospital physician or a civic physician were not well paid, but they at least offered the possibility of making contacts with rich members of the community and occasionally beyond its boundaries. But in smaller towns and in the countryside the population could not always satisfy the expectations of a physician or even a learned surgeon. Mattioli's enforced move from his high-status post as personal physician to the powerful Cardinal Archbishop of Trento to become a civic physician at the frontier town of Gorizia was a comedown, despite the opportunities it gave him to continue his botanical researches. The town itself might want to hold on to him, but he had his mind set on higher and more lucrative things.[48]

Doctors and surgeons were also adept at excluding those whom they did not want to practise in their communities by imposing local barriers through some form of guild membership involving an examination. In Spain, parts of Italy and occasionally elsewhere a 'chief physician' appointed by the government or ruler had the task of overseeing all medical activities, including setting standards and examinations for permission to practise. Often this was delegated to a local guild or college who decided who should be allowed to practise in their community. Such institutions had long been found on the Continent. In some places, as in Padua, and Rome, its membership overlapped, and was occasionally co-terminous, with that of the medical Faculty of the university. More often than not, as in Verona or Mantua, it was confined to graduate physicians, but in some places admission to practice was lightly controlled: the Guild at Florence, which brought together medics and *speziali*, spicers and apothecaries, was notorious for accepting a wide range of healers, including even a bonesetter.[49] Elsewhere, particularly where there was no local university, as in Lyons and London, the requirements for membership were tougher than those for a medical degree.[50] Like other guilds, both inside and outside Italy, medical colleges and surgical guilds expanded in numbers and authority throughout the century as part of a growing trend to professionalisation.[51] But in the eyes of those who might have to pay for their services, the formation of such a supervisory college of physicians was not always a good thing. When it was proposed to create a Medical College at Nuremberg in 1571 to oversee all the medical practitioners in the city, the city councillors at first demurred, requesting only that each academically trained physician should give their opinion on foreign immigrants who were thought to be leprous, a task that suited their civic priorities better. Not until 1592, and several proposals later, was a civic medical ordnance agreed and a *Collegium medicum* with supervisory powers created.[52]

Although in many ways anomalous, the history of the London College of Physicians neatly illustrates the role of such colleges, as well as the problems that might be encountered in exercising its authority.[53] Medieval Britain, as in so much else, lagged behind the Continent in developing institutions that might supervise healing practices. London had had very briefly around 1423 a joint college of physicians and surgeons, and a company of barbers, including some surgeons, had been chartered as a company as long ago as

1387. In 1435, the surgeons properly split from the barbers to form their own Fellowship, although the latter had their rights to practise surgery confirmed in 1451. Elsewhere, as in Norwich, numbers of healers were too small to constitute an effective guild, and they joined other occupational groups in a wider association. In the early sixteenth century, however, the population of the city of London began to grow enormously, thus providing a ready market for those offering healing services, while Henry VII and Henry VIII, following the upheavals of the Wars of the Roses, set about creating a new monarchy along modern lines (i.e. adopting ideas from France and Italy).[54] But although the superiority of physicians to surgeons in matters medical was widely recognised at home and abroad, and at least one physician, John Smyth, served as examiner for the Company of Barber and Surgeons in 1497, there was no organisation or official oversight of physicians themselves until 1511.[55] Then Parliament enacted that no person was to be allowed to practise as a physician or surgeon in the City of London and seven miles around without being first examined and admitted by the Bishop of London or the Dean of St Paul's, assisted by four doctors of physic and an appropriate number of surgeons, and subsequently by four of those who had been approved under the new procedure. Elsewhere, a similar responsibility was handed to the bishop of each diocese with appropriate assistance. (Given that the church had an administrative structure that covered the whole country, this was a sensible move.) Nothing was to prejudice the privileges of the two universities of Oxford and Cambridge, which could grant licences to practise throughout England. Little is known of the workings of this Act, save that in 1514 72 surgeons were examined and admitted.[56]

Physicians, however, sought an authority commensurate with their learning and status. In September 1518, a few months after the first English plague orders on a continental model had been issued, Henry VIII granted permission for the establishment of a College or Commonalty of the Faculty of Medicine of London. Its leading spirits were royal physicians, not least the Galenist translator Thomas Linacre, backed by the Lord Chancellor, Thomas Wolsey, who had been his patient.[57] Its writ, like its predecessors', ran only in London and its environs, and it had the duty to examine all those who wished to practise medicine and the right to punish those who failed to obtain a licence with a fine and even imprisonment. Exactly what constituted the examination at this date is not known, but the statutes of 1541–2 emphasised five subjects, medical theory, semiotics, methods of treatment, materia medica, and the use and practice of medicine. No books are prescribed for the last section, but for the rest, the candidate had to display a remarkably detailed knowledge of at least 17 treatises of Galen (in Latin translation). This was a deliberately severe test, both to reduce the number of frivolous applications and to ensure a high standard of learning among its members. Graduates of Oxford and Cambridge were excused the first three sections of the examination, but foreigners wishing to practise took the full examination, and, if successful, were charged £4, double the fee of native Englishmen.[58] Such examinations, as well as a discriminatory level of fees, were typical of Continental colleges, which, like universities, adopted more and more works by Galen and Hippocrates into their systems. The division between Fellows, candidates and mere licentiates, which became more prominent as the century wore on, is also found in some Continental colleges, as is the emphasis on collegiate solidarity both intellectual and moral.[59] John Howell, a licentiate, was expelled in 1553 for failing to take his doctorate within the prescribed time and for ethical breaches of the oath of membership. He was reinstated in 1556, penitently promising not to damage another's reputation, show off or cause divisions or factions within the College: he had also to pay a fine and give a dinner to the President and Fellows. Two years later, after three warnings, Christopher Langton was expelled for annoying his colleagues by his constant arguments with them in front of patients, and for his boastfulness, stupidity and incontinence – behaviour which seems to have continued long after, since in 1563 he was paraded through the streets in ridiculous attire as a punishment.[60]

Typical too was the right of the College to oversee other medical groups and to inspect the wares of the apothecaries who provided them with their drugs. Antonio Musa Brasavola's books on remedies were specifically designed to help future physicians of Ferrara in any inspection of the apothecaries' stores they might undertake, and the series was organised according to the types of preparations they would encounter, linctuses, powders, waters and oils, for example.[61] The distinguished Lyons physician Jacques Daléchamps (1513–88) wrote an angry letter in 1557/8 to Jacques Fernel in Paris complaining about the misdemeanours of his city's apothecaries and comparing the success of the Parisian College in enforcing their writ over their miscreants, thanks to royal backing, with the difficulties of his own College in the face of conflicting local authorities.[62] The London College's relationship with the surgeons was more harmonious, and in 1540 the physicians were instrumental in helping them to secure an Act creating a new Company of Barbers and Surgeons with similar provisions for the control of surgery, and the physician John Caius took charge of its annual anatomies for more than 20 years.[63]

But what seems to have worked well in an Italian or a French town ran into problems almost immediately in London, for two reasons.[64] The first was a conflict of authority. The two universities resented any infringement of their rights, and both Parliament and the city of London raised objections from time to time, especially as several of those whom the College refused to admit or pursued through the courts were physicians to leading citizens and members of the court. It is no coincidence that what the historian of the College, Sir George Clark, termed "the resolute action" of the College in attempting to enforce its authority with some success occurred between 1555 and 1564 under the almost uninterrupted presidency of John Caius. Both he and many other Fellows then enjoyed the favour of both Queen

Mary and Queen Elizabeth before the College's not unjustified reputation for Catholic sympathies collided with an increasingly Protestant court, city and Parliament. After that, despite the presence of many royal physicians in its ranks, the College struggled to maintain its privileges. Far more damaging to its pretensions was the growth in the population of London. A tiny group of Fellows, rarely more than 16 in number until the end of the century, could not hope to examine, still less control, all those who flocked to offer their healing services in London, with a population running into hundreds of thousands, let alone throughout the whole country, as was specified in the Parliamentary Act of 1523 that confirmed the Charter of Henry VIII.[65] It may have been a recognition of this major difference between London and towns elsewhere that led Parliament in 1542–3 to pass what became known as the Quacks' Charter, an Act mainly directed against the surgeons but including the physicians almost incidentally in its consequences. It allowed "any subject of the monarch with knowledge and experience of herbs, roots and waters legally to treat any outward sore, wound, or outwards swelling or disease with them". Such unlicensed practitioners were not to make use of cauteries or incisions, the province of the surgeons, or prescribe internal medicines, which was reserved for physicians. The vagueness of the wording of the Act did not entirely settle the issue, and the College continued to be involved in such territorial disputes for centuries to come.

What membership of a college like that of London or Lyons ensured was permission to practise within a town or region and an acknowledged status with access to the wealthiest of patients. It provided an arena where one might discuss new ideas and, at least in London, Fellows were required to play a full part in giving lectures and in supervising the annual dissections. Throughout Europe colleges brought together learned men who might express their learning either in books, antiquarian research or poetry. John Caius, for instance, was closely involved with a distinguished group of London historians around Archbishop Matthew Parker.[66] Mercuriale was a member of the antiquarian circle around the Cardinal Farnese, and the first book of his *De arte gymnastica* constitutes a remarkable reconstruction of the institutions and buildings involved in ancient athletics, many of their ruins still visible in Renaissance Rome.[67] His description of the Last Supper and the accompanying illustration in his book were praised by none other than Anthony Blunt for being the first historically accurate representation of Christ and the apostles at the Last Supper reclining at table rather than, as Leonardo and all previous artists had shown them, sitting upright.[68] Other physicians, from Cuspinianus to Girolamo Rossi (1539–1607), the historian of Ravenna, whose treatise on good and bad physicians, *De probitate et improbitate, Scientia et ignorantia. Felicitate et infelicitate medicorum*, seems lost or never to have been printed, wrote accounts of their towns and regions.[69] Still others, as well as composing liminary odes in Latin or even Greek to adorn the early pages of their own or their friends' publications, turned texts of Hippocrates and Galen into verse or wrote medical poetry, of whom Eobanus Hessus and Fracastoro are the most famous examples.[70] Alas, all trace appears to have disappeared of a Latin poem by Luca Valenziano of Tortona (d. before 1538) on the construction and functions of the body, praised by a contemporary for making a respectable job out of such an unpromising subject.[71] Medical information also fed into prose. One of the most famous of all Renaissance writers, François Rabelais, a distinguished physician in his own right, revised his acquaintance with Galen's embryological treatises before finishing the relevant sections of his satire on gynaecology in his *Tiers Livre* around 1545.[72] All these intellectual activities, within and without the collegiate community of physicians, helped to define what a doctor was or should do, as well as how he should be regarded by his fellow practitioners.[73] The stress in many collegiate statutes on moral values both in dealing with patients and, perhaps more important, in maintaining a collaborative and respectful attitude towards fellow-members also proclaimed a certain behavioural stance to prospective patients who shared these values. Even after death, tombstone inscriptions and printed funeral sermons continued to promote the virtues, academic, familiar and collegiate, of the physician as he and his relations saw them.[74]

Aiming Higher: University Professors

Two groups of physicians, each in its own way, enjoyed a superior status to the average practitioner. Modern historians have written much about the first group, university teachers, but far less about the second, the medical attendants of rulers and magnates. The former have been praised for their medical ideas and for the development of anatomy, physiology and materia medica. Many of them are rightly applauded for their insights and for bringing about a renaissance in medicine, contrasted in both their own and in modern rhetoric with the stagnation of the preceding centuries. Many of their ideas will be discussed further in this book, but three caveats are in order. Although there have been some excellent accounts of individual teachers and individual faculties, there is no detailed European-wide survey that collates these varied accounts.[75] Secondly, historians share with the students whose reminiscences have already been discussed, the notion of a hierarchy of universities and consequently direct their attention mainly to the medical schools of Northern Italy, Paris and Montpellier. The Swiss Johannes Ulmer who came in 1563 to study medicine at Oxford for a year was a rare foreign visitor to an English university, as opposed to London, and his stay there may best be explained by his family's relationship with English Evangelical exiles in Switzerland who had returned to England after the death of Mary.[76] The biographies of teachers at these less prestigious or unfamiliar universities such as Siena, Freiburg or Helmstedt are known only to a few regional historians or have yet to be reconstructed from the archives. They may have enjoyed a certain local celebrity and been regarded in their own town as supremely talented, but their unnoticed career and restricted reputation may be more typical than those of a Corti, a Fernel or a Vesalius.

Thirdly, even within a prestigious university such as Padua, Bologna or Montpellier, there are many teachers who remain in the shadow of others more celebrated, and, just as today, students' views of their teachers may not entirely coincide with those of their colleagues. Few today remember Luigi Bellocato, praised at Padua by Martius and Jordanus, or Elideo Padovani at Bologna, mentioned affectionately by both Gryll and Pieter van Foreest.[77] The primary aim of medical teachers was to transmit their knowledge effectively to their students so that they could become good doctors. Novelty, however valuable, was secondary, and it is hard to assess the living impact of a given teacher from a printed page, a passing reference or the near silence of the archives.

Attending the Great: The Dangers of Success

One must not forget that, however attractive a professorial chair at a major university might seem to a modern academic, it was rarely the limit of a doctor's ambitions. At the apex of the medical profession in the sixteenth century were those who served a ruler or a wealthy magnate, whether clerical or lay.[78] Although, as Sebastianus Montuus put it, the proper aim for a doctor was the maintenance of health, not money-making, no one could fail to notice the wealth and honours given to court physicians.[79] Their income was in general far higher than that of academic teachers, let alone those who were in civic service or who attended a merely local clientele. Writing in 1549, the German physician and metallurgist Georg Agricola (1494–1555) gave a list of the average incomes of lawyers and doctors.[80] An academic lawyer could earn 800 gold ducats a year, although the most famous teachers at Pisa or Bologna could get over 1200. The income of a professor of theoretical medicine rarely exceeded 600 a year, and his more lowly academic colleagues received much less than that. When Andreas Vesalius (1514–64) was appointed to lecture on anatomy at Padua in 1537, he received a mere 40 florins, which had increased to 200 by the time he left for Basle in 1542. According to Agricola, only one medical teacher in the whole of Italy had an income equal to that of the lawyers, Matteo Corti (1475–1544), who had been paid 800 ducats a year while teaching at Padua from 1524 to 1532 and 1200 in Bologna in 1538 and later in his second spell at Pisa.[81] His stipend can be compared with that of his contemporary Giambattista da Monte (1498–1552), the most influential of all medical teachers at Padua, who was paid 1000 florins in 1546.[82] But Corti and Da Monte were stars with a European reputation, and Corti's increased salary in his last years may also reflect his simultaneous position as doctor to Lorenzo di Medici, the grandson of Lorenzo il Magnifico, as well as the 1000 ducats a year he had been paid during his three years' service in Rome between 1531 and 1534 with Pope Clement VII.[83] More typical was Agostino Ricci (1512–64), who received 200 gold scudi on his appointment as a papal physician in 1550, roughly double his salary as a university teacher. Andrea Cesalpino (1524–1603), who was paid only 400 scudi a year at the end of 36 years of teaching at Pisa, resigned to become doctor to Pope Clement VIII for 1000 a year.[84] Vesalius likewise increased his income substantially on his appointment as a physician to Charles V on June 3, 1544. He was appointed at the same salary as his friend Cornelis Baersdorp, another imperial doctor, of 30 shillings a day, or 1,825 gold Flemish crowns a year. This was three times more than his brother-in-law Nicolaus Bonart received as an assistant barber, and he would have received further emoluments while attending the Emperor on campaign as well as the possibility of having his own patients.[85]

Cynics also noted that those summoned in an emergency to advise on a cure for the Pope could expect to be paid even more than his usual attendants.[86] When Girolamo Cardano (1536–1606) was called from Italy to Scotland in 1551 to treat John Hamilton, Archbishop of St Andrew's, he first of all received 300 gold crowns, some of which he used for his expenses on the journey, and agreed a payment of 20 gold crowns a day for his attendance, and yet more if he effected a cure. He stayed for 75 days, receiving in addition a further 1800 crowns, a gold chain worth 125 crowns, and a good-tempered horse for his return journey. He also treated a variety of patients on his journey to Scotland and during his stay, charging on one day 19 gold crowns. When he left in September 1552, he and his servants were provided with a cavalry escort as far as London to prevent his boxes, containing some 5,000 crowns, from being stolen. No wonder that he took the advice of Sir John Cheke in London to avoid France, a country overrun with bandits, and follow the longer and safer route via the Netherlands, Cologne and Basle.[87] With such a profitable practice, it is not surprising that he should turn down the offer of the French Marshal Brissac to join him as a mathematician and designer of war machinery for a 1,000 crowns a year. He dealt similarly with an offer from King Christian of Denmark to become his personal physician at an annual stipend of 800 crowns (twice his salary at the University of Pavia), free maintenance for his household and three horses, along with the assurance that he would make the same amount or more from attending nobles at the Danish court. This offer did not tempt a man who thought the Danes little more than barbarians and their damp, cold climate "an entrance to death's caverns".[88] Family ties and a desire for independence, as well as his teaching, will also have played a part in his refusal, even if the details he gives of his practice suggest that his major activity as a therapist had ended by 1560.[89]

This offer to Cardano is a reminder that a royal physician could also expect to have his income increased in a variety of ways, and not only by attending wealthy nobles and their families. In many of the smaller German courts, doctors attached to the palace household had also the job of civic physician in the surrounding locality, and even in larger ones only the

Leibarzt, the ruler's body physician, was kept fully occupied in the palace.[90] Physicians who were ordained, and many who were not, could expect to receive significant funds from grants of ecclesiastical benefices. John Chambre (1470–1549), physician to Henry VII and Henry VIII and one of the founders of the London College of Physicians in 1518, was unusual only in the number of such offices he held. He was a prebendary of Lincoln and Salisbury, a Canon of Windsor, Archdeacon of Bedford, treasurer of the Cathedral of Bath and Wells, as well as enjoyed preferments in one Irish and three English dioceses. Warden of his old Oxford College, Merton, from 1524 until 1544, he became also Dean of the Collegiate Chapel of St Stephen's, Westminster, on whose behalf he paid for the construction at enormous cost of new cloisters that were almost immediately torn down in the Henrician Reformation.[91] Another Mertonian, George Owen (1499–1548), profited from the Reformation by receiving a variety of manors and abbey sites from Henry VIII and his successor Edward VI in and around Oxford, including Godstow Abbey, where he resided, and the buildings and grounds of Durham College, which he then sold.[92] Clerical physicians at the papal court could expect to receive similar preferments. Gian Francesco Manfredi, doctor to Pius IV, received a variety of benefices in the dioceses of Brescia, Teramo and Sessa, and he was appointed in 1561 Corrector and Revisor of the Vatican Library for life with an additional salary. Four years later, he lost his papal appointments, and was imprisoned in the Castel Sant Angelo, following an accusation of treason.[93]

Not all those who attended a ruler are counted today among the most significant practitioners of the period. Most of those who were on the royal payroll in England during the sixteenth century are familiar today only with specialist historians of the court and the London College of Physicians.[94] Elisa Andretta's long list of papal physicians contains a few names, like that of Mercuriale, with a wider reputation, but most are scarcely remembered today.[95] Many of them had studied at a leading university – Perugia seems to have had a favoured school of surgery – and some also lectured at the papal university of Rome, but they made little impression outside the city. A chance encounter could catapult a physician to wealth and social eminence. Simone Castelvetro, who treated Cardinal Sfrondrato when he fell ill in Modena in 1590 on his way to the papal conclave, was immediately summoned to Rome when his patient emerged from the conclave as Gregory XIV.[96] Service in some distant lands or at minor courts appears to have attracted medical adventurers rather than real experts. When Stephen, ruler of Moldavia, was troubled with an old wound in 1502, he was treated by a Venetian doctor, Mattheus Murianus. When he too fell ill, Alexander of Verona was summoned and paid the substantial sum in advance of 300 gold pieces. Alexander never arrived, although it is not clear whether he got lost on the way, died or simply kept the money, for he is not heard of again. In 1504, when Stephen died, he was being attended by another Italian, Lionardo da Massari and a German doctor from Nuremberg, Johann

Klingsporn. Although some of these men may have had medical degrees, nothing is otherwise known about them.[97]

Two letters, some 50 years apart, offer an insight into the qualities required of a papal doctor, and their advice would doubtless have applied to many other courts. The first was written around 1545 to a member of the papal entourage by Andrea Turini, a former lecturer at Pisa and Bologna, who had been a personal physician to two Popes, Clement VII and Paul III, before joining the French court of Francis I.[98] In it he recommended three experienced doctors, Pietro Bayro, a long-time professor in Turin, Ludovico Panizza of Modena (although he may no longer have wanted to continue in practice) and a certain Omobono at Cremona. Both Bayro and Panizza were known personally to him, but for Omobono he could only suggest that his correspondent check with Cardinal Salviati, who had experience of some of his excellent work as a physician in Piacenza. Both Bayro and Omobono had sons in the church, which guaranteed their orthodoxy. But what counted most was their ability to conform to the expected behaviour of courtiers. Bayro is "a good courtier, very pleasant and without any traces of boorishness", Panizza is "used to service at court", and Omobono, of whom the writer knew least, is "pleasant and used to dealing with men of importance". Cardinal Aldobrandini seeking similar advice in 1604 had a mere two questions. Was the doctor a person of breeding who could deal with princes? And was he strong enough to cope with the fatigue of office?[99]

Fidelity, gentility and stamina here outrank medical ability in determining the choice of a personal physician for a monarch or a major dignitary such as a cardinal or a duke. Stamina is perhaps unexpected, if one forgets that the physician and surgeon had to be perpetually on call, not only advising on diet but also attending to their master's every ailment.[100] Crato in 1574 apologised to his wife for not being able to see her and complained that his service with Emperor Maximilian II gave him no chance to think about his health or his own life. He could not decide whether it would be better to die and be spared mortal concerns or find himself worn out in what he described as "splendid misery".[101] Some of the Popes, and not a few of the monarchs, were frail or sickly, and it was the duty of their medical attendants to keep them alive or at least to assure them that they would do so. Cardano's prophecy that the medical horoscope of Edward VI, "the young Solomon", showed that he would have a long and prosperous reign proved notoriously wrong, and not everyone believed Cardano's defence that it would have been politically disastrous to have revealed the truth about the sickly monarch.[102] He was not alone in being asked to exercise his expertise in astrology in royal service, for many royal physicians from Lewis of Caerleon at the court of Henry VII of England at the beginning of the sixteenth century to Thaddeus Hagecius and others in Rudolfine Prague at the end utilised their medical expertise in astronomy to explain the future.[103]

The medical attendant was constrained in what he could or could not do. Vesalius hesitated for some months in 1543–4 whether to become an imperial physician or accept the lucrative offer from the Medici Duke of a chair at Pisa.[104] Intervals of activity were matched by periods of boredom, when, according to Aretino, one could not cough or blow one's nose for fear of annoying one's master.[105] One had to go wherever one was ordered. Vesalius had to move to Spain when Philip II left his Brussels capital for Madrid, which deprived him of opportunities to perform or observe dissections. His skill as a physician and surgeon also meant that he could be lent to other rulers as a diplomatic gesture. Along with his colleague Daza Chacon he attended the French King Henri II in 1559, when he was fatally injured in a joust, and twice treated members of Italian ducal families allied to Spain. He treated Francesco d'Este when they were together at Ratisbon in 1546, and first treated and later performed an autopsy in Brussels on Ferrante Gonzaga in 1557.[106] His voyage to the Holy Land, which ended with his death in 1546 on Zakynthos on his return journey, also involved diplomacy, for he was chosen to accompany the annual gift of 500 gold ducats by the Spanish King for the support of Christian churches in the Holy Land.[107] The rewards were high but so were the demands, and it was an advantage to both parties if, like Vesalius, the son of a royal apothecary, the doctor or surgeon came from a family with links to a court.[108]

The intimacy between doctor and royal or noble patient also imposed choices on the patient, particularly if he or she might be new to the country or estates over which they ruled. Should one continue with one's predecessor's household or choose instead someone like Mercuriale or Johannes Lange at the Palatine court with whom one shared many intellectual interests in literature, art or Classical Antiquity?[109] Spanish cardinals and Popes preferred to bring in medical attendants from home who might prove more trustworthy and purvey less gossip than local ones. Not surprisingly, few papal physicians came from Rome itself, and many hailed from same native region of Italy as their employers. In England, which produced only a handful of learned physicians a year from its less medically advanced universities, future royal physicians had either to be sent to study in Italy, or were themselves immigrants from Portugal, Spain or Italy.[110] But this in turn presented different problems, simply because of their proximity to the monarch and the influence this might give them. Sometimes their non-medical activities are evident. Sir Thomas Wendy (1499–1560), royal physician to English monarchs for almost 20 years, served as a member of Parliament and acted as a conduit of information concerning his University of Cambridge. In 1559 he served on the committee that inspected the university to ensure that it had eliminated papists from its midst after the Protestant Elizabeth had succeeded the Catholic Mary the previous year. At other times, the influence of royal physicians remains no more than supposition, however plausible. Historians are divided over the extent to which an earlier royal physician, Sir William Butts (1486–1545), promoted the Evangelical cause under Henry VIII and assisted his relative Anne Boleyn in her support for the new Evangelical religion in the 1530s.[111]

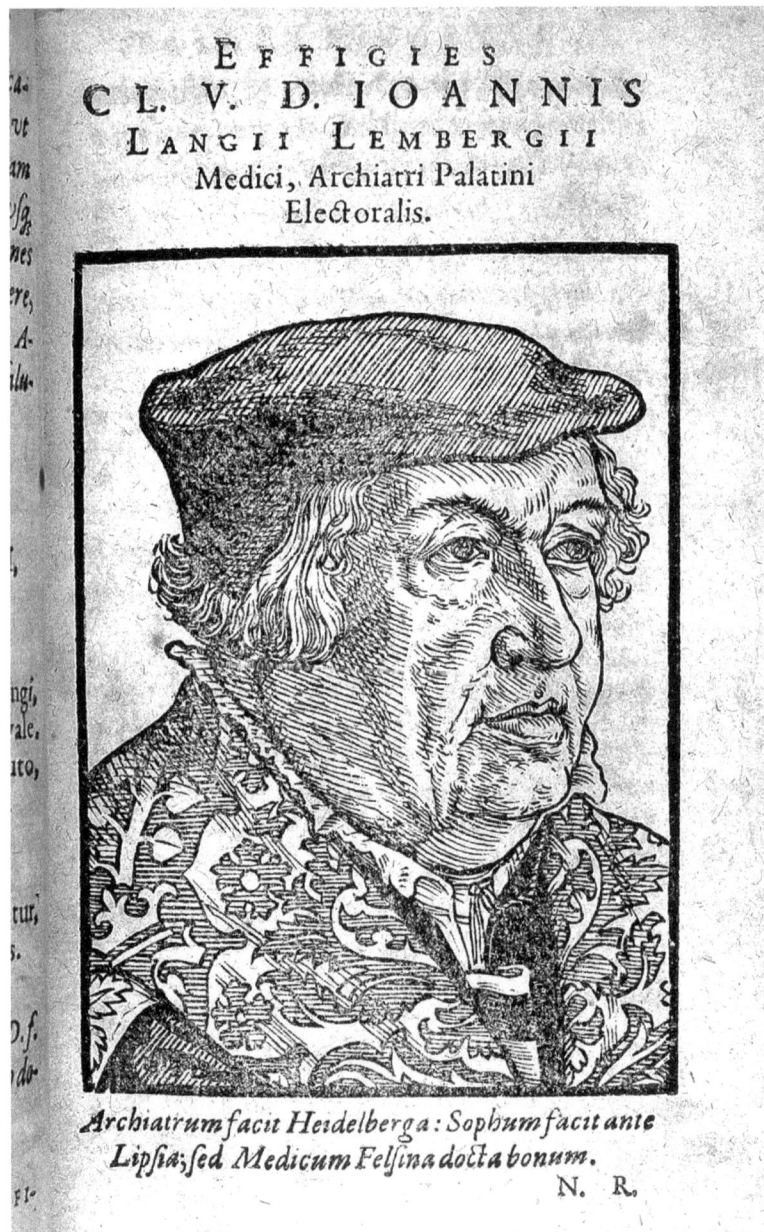

EFFIGIES
CL. V. D. IOANNIS
LANGII LEMBERGII
Medici, Archiatri Palatini
Electoralis.

Archiatrum facit Heidelberga : Sophum facit ante
Lipsia; sed Medicum Felsina docta bonum.

N. R.

Figure 5.2 Johannes Lange (1485–1565), professor of medicine at Heidelberg and doctor to the Elector Palatine. The frontispiece to the 1589 edition of his *Medical Letters*. Frankfurt, heirs of A. Wechel, C. Marnius and J. Aubrius. The poem beneath gives his biography: Heidelberg made me a royal physician; before that Leipzig made me an intellectual but learned Bologna a good doctor.

This perception of backstairs influence on the part of highly placed medical attendants did not always work in the doctor or surgeon's favour. The untrue rumour, circulating within months of his death, that Vesalius's fatal visit to the Holy Land was the result of a decision on the part of Philip II to make him do penance and avoid serious punishment for performing a human vivisection, was spread widely around Europe within a few years.[112] Others were, rightly or wrongly, suspected of spying or worse. Simone Simoni (1532–1602), who fled from Italy to Calvinist Geneva, moved on to become doctor at the courts of the Palatinate, Saxony and Poland and Prague before ending his career as physician to the Catholic Bishop of Olomouc (Olmutz, Moravia). He was widely believed to have acted as a spy, although no one was entirely sure for whom.[113] Agostino de Agostinis, doctor to Henry VIII and Cardinal Wolsey, was also paid for his advice as a spy, and acted as a go-between between England and the Continent.[114] Another Italian exile who treated members of the English court, Giulio Borgarucci (c. 1525–80), was accused of being a secret Catholic, and was involved in a whole series of lawsuits before he could clear his name.[115] The saga of his wife's adultery, and his suing for divorce, which sorely exercised the saintly Archbishop Grindal (1519–83), provided ample cause for gossip, and his precipitate flight to Catholic France was, in the opinion of a diarist far away in Cornwall, only to be expected of a foreigner.[116] Hector Nuñez (1521–91), a Portuguese Jew who had moved to London in 1550 and became in 1554 a Fellow of both the College of Physicians and of that of Surgeons, had a better reputation despite his heavy involvement in secret diplomacy between England, the Porte and Spain.[117] His Jewish compatriot, Rodrigo Lopez (c. 1517–94), was less fortunate. Having arrived in London in 1557, he was long used by two of Elizabeth I's chief ministers, Cecil and Walsingham, as a conduit for communicating with Spanish spies. A royal physician since 1581, he was convicted in 1594 of plotting to poison the Queen and was hung, drawn and quartered as a traitor. To what extent he was guilty of more than receiving money from Philip II is unclear, and his conviction reveals more of the murky world of Elizabethan espionage and court politics than the truth of his involvement.[118] The perils of life at the top, especially for foreign physicians and surgeons, should not be underestimated.

But such positions were accessible only to a few, whether talented, ambitious or lucky. Most practitioners were content with relatively high wealth and status in their own urban communities, roughly on the same level as lawyers, wealthy tradesmen and civic councillors, whose interests they often shared. Many of them will have come from medical families or similar social backgrounds, able at least to pay for an education up to the level of a local medical school, if one existed, and even for a period of travel to one more prestigious. But for those who did not have these advantages, it was difficult to break into the medical profession. There might be grants available for early schooling, and both Germany and Tudor England saw an increase in such scholarships and local schools, but to go further demanded wealthy sponsors and patrons. Study at a major university might be expected to lead to success at home, for, as Cornarius and others insisted, one had been exposed to the very latest of ideas and trained by the best masters of practical medicine. This would guarantee the intellectual calibre and medical experience of the aspiring physician, but to go further he needed one further attribute, gentility, the knowledge of how to behave in polite society, and that was not something that could be easily attained by those who were not brought up in the right circles. Prospective clients, however, were not always swayed by the displays of coats of arms in physicians' portraits.[119] Tiraqueau's lengthy discussion of the arguments for and against a high status for the physician, and *a fortiori* of lesser healers, in sixteenth-century France reveals that, coats of arms notwithstanding, medicine was not for the nobility. It still retained the taint of trade, a social barrier that many medical families acknowledged covertly and tried to circumvent by sending their sons off to study law, not medicine.[120]

Only a few practitioners could reach the heights of a university chair or a palace preferment, or even attain the status of a local grandee, and most were content with posts as town physicians or at a hospital or simply to build up a local practice, happy in the company of their colleagues. The rewards of even a local practice were not inconsiderable, particularly in the eyes of those who did not come from wealthy families and needed help with the considerable investment of time and money required to gain a medical degree, and still more if they wished to embark on a long peregrination in search of experience and contacts. It is no wonder that, once they had established themselves, they saw themselves as superior to other healers and wrote vigorously against those who challenged their authority.[121] But, as we shall see in the next chapter, they were only one group among many offering healing, and their fees and their pretensions may have often induced patients to look elsewhere for assistance.

Notes

1 Stolberg 2021b gives an overview of the doctor-patient relationship.
2 Later, pp. 236–41.
3 Stolberg 2021a: 31–3.
4 De Ridder-Symoens 1996: 416–48, 2010. Possibly over half of medical students came from medical families.
5 Tiraqueau 1561: 234–489, the longest chapter in the book by far; the same question in Montuus 1537: 178–9.
6 Tiraqueau 1561: 520. Contrast Brunetto 1548: 96–100.
7 Grendler 2002: 314–52; Maclean 2002: 32, notes the different lengths of courses.
8 Clark 1964: 127.
9 Karant-Nunn 1987: 193.
10 Finger and Benger 1987: 58–67; Finger 1990.
11 Jones P. M. 1995: 198. The remaining third of the licentiates had a looser connection with the university.
12 O'Malley 1964: 33–73.
13 Palmer 1983.

14 Brockliss and Jones 1997: 10.
15 Nutton 1990c: 235–9. In the first 60 years of the century there were between two and three medical graduates a year in Germany as a whole. Numbers increased later, and were double that at Heidelberg in the 1560s. Matriculation figures are higher in Italy and some other universities than those for graduation because of students moving around.
16 Kunstmann 1963: 14–17. Founded as a *Hochschule* on the model of Strasbourg, it had four faculties, of which medicine was the weakest, and was granted full university privileges in 1622; badly affected by the Thirty Years War and later competition from newer foundations, it closed in 1809.
17 Nutton 1990c: 235–9.
18 Roberts 1912: 55.
19 Tröhler 1991: 17. He was also expected to gain an up-to-date knowledge of drugs thereby.
20 Earlier, pp. 106–7.
21 Caius 1573: 14v; Nutton 2018a: 66.
22 Langton undated, sig. iii r–v.
23 London, British Library, MS Egerton 2604, fol. 6v.
24 Gryllus 1566b: 3.
25 Karant-Nunn 1987: 193.
26 Clemen 1912: 38–42. He served for the first time as *Stadtarzt* at Wittenberg in 1531–2. For other German grants, Stolberg 2021a: 33–4.
27 Clemen 1909.
28 Maclean 2002: 33; De Ridder-Symoens 1996: 416–48, although concentrating on Flemish students, gives useful details of numbers; 2010: 79–83; Enenkel and De Jong 2019.
29 Clemen 1909: 347. Cf. the programmatic Zwinger 1577: 120–2.
30 Cornarius 1531: 55–76.
31 Cunningham 2010; Haye 2019.
32 Gryllus 1566b: 3r, with supplementary funding from a local professor of law; 8r.
33 Gryllus 1566a: 43v; Serrai 1990: 336, 361; Blair 2017: 181–2.
34 Later, pp. 222–4; Stolberg 2014.
35 Stolberg 2021a: 58–63 gives other examples. For Horst's role in Roman medicine, Andretta and Pardo-Tomás 2019: 22–3; Margócsy *et al.* 2018: 309; as international correspondent, Egmond 2018c: 84–5.
36 Martius 1568: sigg. 5r–1r; Maclean 2017.
37 Martius 1568: sig. 3v. The implication throughout is that he was a 'scholarship boy' from a relatively humble background.
38 Purkircher 1988: 161. For medical problems caused by travel, Hrubetius 1610 (with Hieronymus 2005: 3, 1984–6, who prints the theses defended).
39 John James (1550–1601) spent some 17 years in higher education before returning to England as doctor to the Earl of Leicester, Pelling and Webster 1979: 190.
40 Jordanus 1580: sigg. A2v–3v.
41 Bosman-Jelgersma 1989: 14–17; Santing 2010. For Padovani, Pomata 2010: 229, n. 89.
42 Caius 1573; Roberts 1912; Nutton 2018a.
43 Bosman-Jelgersma 1989: 17–18; Santing 2010. For Sylvius's reputation as a teacher, see the poems in his honour collected by Badali 2013: vol. 2, 1906, VI–XXIV.
44 Baptista (1534?); Screech 1976.
45 Baptista may be the same man as Pietro Manna, d. 1560, a doctor from a wealthy family of Cremona, whose portrait in old age by Lucia Anguissola (1536–65) is in the Prado Museum, Madrid.

46 Nutton 1996, quoting from the abridged version in Hart 1623: sig. a.iv; Gentilcore 1998, 2006. For Clowes, Poynter 1948: 80.

47 Cipolla 1976.

48 Fausti 2004.

49 Park 1985: 24–34; Conforti 2008: 329–33.

50 For French cities with medical colleges but no university, Brockliss and Jones 1997: 179.

51 Mocarelli 2008, 2018. For the consequent downgrading of female healers, see later, p.

52 Dross 2010; Murphy 2019: 150–65.

53 Pelling and Webster 1979 compare the situation in London with that in Norwich.

54 The most immediately relevant to medicine was the planning for the Savoy Hospital, earlier, p. 60.

55 For the complex relationship between barbers and surgeons, extending to actual terms used to describe them, Decamp 2016: 7–19.

56 Clark 1964: 9–36; Decamp 2016: 8–9.

57 Clark 1964: 54–80; Webster 1977.

58 Clark 1964: 98–101; for future Fellows and licentiates failing the examination, including an MD from Padua, *ibid.*, 165–6.

59 Clark 1964: 95–7, 108–9.

60 Roberts 1912: 46.

61 Brasavola 1561.

62 Schmitt and Bono 1979; Schmitt 1989: IV, 100–27.

63 Clark 1964: 85, 122; for comparable squabbles between physicians, surgeons and apothecaries in Paris, Brockliss and Jones 1997: 205–23.

64 Pelling and Webster 1979: 179–85; Pelling 2003.

65 Clark 1964: 132. Numbers were fixed at 20, raised to 30 in 1590; in 1597 there were 31, in no way keeping pace with the mushroom growth of London.

66 Grafton 2017; Nutton 2017a.

67 Agasse 2006; Mercuriale 2008; Kavvadia 2021; later, pp. 234–6.

68 Blunt 1938–9.

69 Siraisi 2007, esp.: 193–206; Cuspinianus 1553; Rossi 1572. Rossi's lost book is cited several times in Carrarius 1581. For Crato's (lost) history of Wrocław/Breslau/Vratislavia, Lambrecht 2002: 253, note 41, and for the prolific Sigismund Schorckel of Naumburg, Grafton 2012: 144.

70 Eobanus Hessus 1524 (and often reprinted), with Krause 1879: 388–95; Fracastoro, earlier, pp. 25–6. Some random examples of odes by medical men, Johannes Agricola preceding Gryllus 1566b; Johannes Lange: Clemen 1898: 110–12; Johannes Albert Cygnensis: Clemen 1943–4: 14–17; Purkircher 1988: 145; poems in honour of Jacobus Sylvius, Badali 2013: vol. 2, 1906, VI–XXIV; Achilles Pirmin Gasser, preceding Martius 1568: sig. (..)r.; plague poems, Rädle 1982: 325–8; Dutch medical poets, Heesakkers 1996: 119–28; for the *Aphorisms* in verse, Roseler 1554, Fryer 1567; for Galen's *De usu partium* versified, Lygaeus 1555; for a doctor poet writing on medicine in French, Bretonnayau 1583; cf. also the poems and plays of Jacques Grévin, later, p. 277; and for an expert versifier in both Latin and Hungarian, Ferenc Hunyadi, Huniadinus 1586 with Evans 1984b: 18, cf. 19–20.

71 Sacchi 2020.

72 Rabelais 1532; Antonioli 1976; for his annotations Nutton 1988b.

73 Biow 2002; Stolberg 2020, 2021a: 93–113 discusses all aspects of the doctor's *Habitus*.

74 Lenz 1984; Zahn 2009/10.

75 Valuable information is scattered throughout De Ridder-Symoens 1996.

76 Robinson 1846–7: II, 418–20.
77 Gryllus 1566b: 4r; Martius 1568: sig. (..) 8r; Jordanus 1580: sig. A 2v; van Foreest, earlier, p. 43–5, 59.
78 For the problematisation of court medicine, Lammel 2018. For the role of a *protomedico* in Spain and Spanish Italy, earlier, p. 47.
79 Montuus 1537: 178–9, 183. In general, Nutton 1990a; Stolberg 2021a: 397–401, 410–22.
80 Agricola 1550: 324. A ducat, a florin and a scudo were roughly equivalent and originally a gold piece, but their value could fluctuate substantially. An equivalent in today's money is hard to determine: on present UK salaries, a ducat would be worth some £130.
81 O'Malley 1964: 77; for Pisa, Davies 2009.
82 Padua, University Archives Reg. 662, f. 25r (information from Richard Palmer), up from 700 in 1543.
83 De Ferrari 1983; Nutton 1987b: 176; Palmer 1990a: 68–9.
84 Schmitt 1974: 6, 1989: IX, 6.
85 Martinez Millan 2000: 244, a reference I owe to Maurits Biesbrouck. Anne Vesalius, probably his wife rather than daughter, was appointed a washer of the body in 1551, *ibid.*, 247.
86 Andretta 2011: 275–6.
87 Cardano 1663: 1, 23–4, 92–3 and 9, 123–52; Wykes 1969: 123–37; Fierz 1983: 16–21.
88 Cardano 1663: 1, 23–4 (giving details of other offers made to him by rulers and magnates), 92–3; Wykes 1969: 121–2.
89 Siraisi 1997: 29–40.
90 Schlegelmilch U 2021; Walter forthcoming.
91 Moore and Bakewell 2004.
92 Furdell 2001: 31; Lee and Wallis 2004.
93 Andretta 2011: 277–8.
94 Furdell 2001: 16–97, although her list is overly wide.
95 Palmer 1990a; Andretta 2011: 232–84, 572–5. Both Mercuriale and his Padua colleague, Francesco Frigimelica (1491–1559) turned down permanent appointments, *ibid.*, 262–3, 269–73.
96 Palmer 1990a: 60.
97 Florescu and McNally 1973: 200.
98 Andretta 2011: 258–60.
99 Palmer 1990a: 60.
100 Siraisi 2013: 48–9, noting some of Lange's reminiscences of court life in his *Medical Letters*.
101 Gillet 1860–61: II, 6–10; Fichtner 2001: 84.
102 Wykes 1969: 133–5; Siraisi 1997: 38.
103 Carey 1992; Evans 1984a: 203–4. Azzolini 2010 adds many examples of political astrology from Italy.
104 Soulier 2020a: 43–6 describes his hesitations in 1543–4 about taking a post or returning to lecture at Pisa, because of the indifference of his colleagues to his dissections. Venice expected his period in imperial service to be relatively short.
105 Palmer 1990a: 59.
106 O'Malley 1964: 283–8, 295; Chambers 1990: 96.
107 Dirix 2014: 112–13.
108 Although he was annoyed at being passed over in 1544 as personal physician to the Emperor on grounds of age, Soulier 2020a: 40–7.
109 Siraisi 25–6, 133, 2007: 168–224, 2012: 39–60.
110 Andretta 2011: 265–7.

111 Furdell 2001: 26–7 (Butts), 31 (Wendy); Nutton 2018a: 120–1. For the influ-ence of Crato von Crafftheim on the religious policy of Emperor Rudolf II, see earlier, p. 86; for Spanish physicians offering political advice, Sumillera 2020.
112 O'Malley 1964: 304–5: Soulier 2020a: 580–2, 1098–1107.
113 Verdigi 1997; Celati 2018a.
114 Hammond 1975; MacCulloch 2018: 586.
115 Firpo 1971.
116 Collinson 1983: 378–9; Rowse 1953: 130.
117 Katz 1994: 54–8.
118 Clark 128 "almost certainly guilty"; Guy 1988: 444, doubtful of any plot; Katz 1994: 49–106, guilty.
119 Two examples, John Caius, Nutton 2018a: fig. 1; Van Foreest, Bosman-Jelgersma 1996a: 11.
120 Tiraqueau 1561: earlier, p. 124.
121 For doctors' views of the qualifications demanded by civic employers, Schlegelm-ilch S 2020.

6 The Kaleidoscope of Healing II
Surgeons, Apothecaries and Outsiders

For most of the population of sixteenth-century Europe recourse to a physician was a last and usually an expensive resort. They had to rely on a variety of healers, if they, or their family, could not provide appropriate treatment for themselves. Those who lived in a town in a well-populated and well-traversed region could consult surgeons and apothecaries, while in smaller and more remote settlements they might encounter an occasional travelling healer, a so-called charlatan, to supplement the therapies offered by a local cleric or the lady of the manor.[1] Few communities were so small that they did not include a woman with some expertise in herbs who also acted as a midwife. All these healers fell at times under the critical eye of the physicians and of those who considered themselves superior enough in learning and expertise to appeal to a ruler or local authorities to take action against those whom they considered a danger to the health of patients. Their requests were sometimes answered, but more often they remained unfulfilled, paper dreams that official reluctance and indifference or the lack of any effective enforcement mechanism, to say nothing of opposition from those whose livelihoods would be affected, prevented from being realised. The variety of healers as well as the economic and geographical circumstances and the administrative organisations of their communities together make any overall historical description illusory or at best partial. The situation revealed in the archives of a typical Northern Italian town of 3,000 or 4,000 inhabitants differs vastly from that in an upland village in Bohemia or England, to say nothing of a megalopolis like London, Paris or Rome, where both civic, religious and medical authorities were faced with a constantly changing and growing population and with a multitude of competing or at least overlapping healers.

Surgeons

One generalisation remains valid: surgeons far outnumbered physicians. Even in Italy, the great majority of employment contracts for civic positions in Italy relate to surgeons rather than physicians, particularly in rural areas where their ability to deal with common complaints such as sprains, ulcers

DOI: 10.4324/9781003223184-9

and the results of accidents (and potentially at a lower fee than a physician) made them a useful investment for a small town.[2] They had learned their craft in an apprenticeship that might last longer than the university training of a physician and that ended in a formal examination of competence before the relevant authorities, the Masters of the surgical guild, often assisted by a physician or someone appointed by the *protomedico*.[3] The quality of this training varied from place to place and from individual to individual. Many surgical apprentices were literate, and some knew Latin, but few would have had the training given to Alois Carséna (1517–1611) by his father, who was barber-surgeon to the Duke of Savoy.[4] By the time he was 15, he had acquired sufficient skill in purging by enemas and laxatives, bleeding and administering emetics for his father to begin teaching him the science of surgery, beginning with anatomy, for which his father obtained parts of hanged criminals for him to dissect.

In some Italian universities there were courses aimed at surgeons, often conducted by a teacher of anatomy, with the possibility of a university degree if a candidate had also attended some medical courses. At Bologna, the list of teachers included such important figures as Bartolomeo Maggi (1487–1552), who lectured there between 1541 and 1552, his nephew, Giulio Cesare Aranzi (1530–89) who taught both surgery and anatomy from 1556 to 1587, Cesare Varolio (1543–75), who taught surgery and anatomy before lecturing on practical medicine, and Gaspare Tagliacozzi (1548–99), who held a lectureship in surgery between 1570 and 1590, and later the chair of anatomy. Tagliacozzi is famous for his advocacy of rhinoplasty, repairing noses by a skin graft, in his book of 1597, although he was not the first to perform such an operation, for his teacher Aranzi seems to have preceded him in the late 1560s, and there are stories of local families of healers in Sicily and Calabria also doing this.[5] At Montpellier, physicians and surgeons mingled together and surgeons gave well-attended lectures, although probably not within the university itself. Lorenz Gryll, on his peregrination, was delighted to find there "as frequent a practice of surgery as of the rest of medicine", something he rarely mentions elsewhere.[6] In Paris in the 1520s, Jean Tagault's lectures on surgery within the Faculty attracted the interest from a few medical students, and would have been attended also by barber-surgeons, whose guild had come to an agreement for such lectures in 1506. The Faculty had a pricklier relationship with the learned surgeons of the community of St Côme, who fought hard to establish their claim to be the equal of the physicians, obtaining letters from the King in their support. Both sides appealed to civil authorities for backing which, even when given, did not always prove effective. A decree of the Parlement of Paris in 1552 that no one could join the community of surgeons without the approval of the physicians quickly became a dead letter. Conversely, in 1576, the request from the surgeons to be recognised as members of the Faculty and give lectures was blessed by Henri III and further enhanced in 1579 when the Pope gave approval for a quasi-Faculty of surgery. But this also long remained on paper, as the physicians, now allied with the guild of barber-surgeons and aided by the Parlement, battled against the implementation of the papal bull.[7] Elsewhere in some Italian towns, such as Florence and Padua, surgeons and physicians were members of the same professional college, although in both cities differences of status and competition for clients also tended gradually to push them apart.[8] In Northern Europe, the division between the two was somewhat greater, although not always expressed with the same animosity as in Paris. Both groups might attend difficult cases together, but it is clear from Van Foreest's surgical observations that, although some individuals might enjoy a good working relationship, this was not universal, and both physicians and surgeons viewed each other with a certain mutual suspicion. Van Foreest's plea for physicians to learn about surgery did not extend to performing manual operations himself and may be interpreted as both an assertion of his own superiority and an acknowledgement of the gulf that often separated them.[9] Likewise Georg Handsch, although interested in the techniques of surgeons around him, seems to have performed only very minor operations, such as using a clyster, and then relatively rarely. His use of a white ointment described to him by a barber was unsuccessful, because he applied it to an open wound, contrary to the instruction of the barber.[10]

The treatments that surgeons provided all involved some form of direct intervention – the term often used to describe them, 'mechanics', indicates the use of instruments. They included dealing with wounds, fractures, dislocations, abscesses, ulcers and fistulae, bladder stones and internal obstructions as well as bleeding, couching for cataract, and cautery.[11] Surgeons might also be called on to destroy a foetus in an obstructed delivery, but a Caesarean operation almost always followed the death of the mother.[12] While there was a general agreement that external conditions were the province of the surgeon, and internal of the doctor, there was a substantial overlap. Tumours, for example, could be treated by medications and diet as a systemic affection or by the knife as a localised excrescence. Skin conditions, including syphilis, fell within the competence of both groups, and sufferers might prefer to describe their condition to a friendly barber than to a more expensive physician or surgeon. One thing was clear to patients: surgical intervention always involved pain, whether it was setting a bone, scraping around the edges of a raw ulcer, or removing a tooth. When a dangerous surgical operation was called for, it was usually because the patient was in such pain that even death might seem preferable. The solution as far as possible was to operate swiftly on a patient sedated with alcohol or opiate drugs and tied or held down by strong assistants, and to have ready a wide choice of instruments (Figure 6.2). Even though instruments in illustrations and museums might appear similar, before mass production in the nineteenth century there was no standardisation, and a local smith would make them to fit the requirements of the individual surgeon, who in turn would be influenced by the type of operation he expected to carry out. The representation of instruments in surgical treatises is often so crude that the subtleties that the author wished to emphasise are not always easy to discern. The surgical chest of a military or naval surgeon would similarly have been different from that of a practitioner who expected to pass his time in civilian life (Figure 6.5). As William Clowes pointed out, such a surgeon would often be forced to rely on his own resources for a considerable time on a voyage or campaign and treat illnesses such as scurvy as well as the results of accidents and warfare.[13]

Evidence for co-operation between physician and surgeon is easier to find than many historical accounts suggest, not least because 'elite' surgeons had far more in common with physicians than with their lesser brethren. So, for example, when the London College of Surgeons and Barbers was established by Henry VIII in 1540, leading members of the College of Physicians joined leading surgeons in the petition to the king and were active in supporting the new group in its first years.[14] Soon after his return from his medical studies at Padua, Henry VIII put John Caius in charge of the annual dissection, a task that he continued to perform for more than 20 years. Henry VIII also approved of the production of Geminus's anatomy book based on the *Tabulae Sex* of Vesalius to serve as a basic manual for surgeons.[15] It may be no coincidence that the largest 'academic' account of medicine in English was written around the same time by an aspiring MD, Christopher Langton (1521–78), and published in 1545. It opened with a long chapter on the organisation of the human body that was replaced in the revision of 1547 with an injunction simply to read Galen and Vesalius.[16] It was also leading London surgeons like Thomas Gale and George Baker who encouraged translations of some of Galen's surgical books into English, basing them on earlier French versions.

Surgical Developments

In France the centre for vernacular translations of classical surgery was not Paris, but Lyons, a city without a university but where there seems to have been good co-operation between physicians and surgeons. Both Jean Canappe (fl. 1538–52), a Paris MD, and Jacques Daléchamps (1513–88), better known as a botanist, gave lectures on surgery there. Pierre Tolet (c. 1502–80), like Jacques Daléchamps, a Montpellier pupil of Rondelet and later Dean of the Lyons College of Physicians, drew up a programme in 1574 for the proper academic study of surgery. Both Canappe and Tolet were concerned that surgeons had no Greek or Latin, and hence could not access the riches of ancient surgery. As another translator, Guillaume Chrestien put it, although they were highly intelligent, they lacked only one thing, a good education, but, he mused, if they had had that, they might have chosen to become doctors rather than surgeons.[17] In his preface to his re-edition of the works of the most famous of all medieval surgeons, Guy de Chauliac (fl. 1363), Canappe hoped that, aided by the new learning and sustained by

Galen, the surgeon would both offer sound advice to his patients and kindness and charity to his confreres, unlike physicians, who were always arguing, offering confusing advice and fighting among themselves like gryphons, horses and dogs.[18] Daléchamps in his *Chirurgie Françoise*, first published in 1569, was more charitable towards physicians, arguing that their reluctance to engage with surgery left a gap that learned surgeons could fill, not least by recovering many forgotten operations that had been described in classical texts such as Galen, Paul and Aetius. Classical techniques, especially as interpreted in Daléchamps's learned commentary (prepared with the assistance of Ambroise Paré), would supplement the best of modern surgery and persuade "weak and delicate" souls to submit to the surgeon's knife.[19]

Similar claims for the importance of Classical Greek surgery were also made by Guido Guidi (Vidus Vidius, 1509–69), whose collection of translations of ancient surgery contained beautiful reproductions of images from a Byzantine compendium of surgery owned by the Florentine Cardinal Ridolfi, his early patron.[20] When Vidius came to Paris in 1542, he brought a copy of the manuscript, along with his translation, as a gift for Francis I. His reward was swift: "Vidus venit, Vidius vidit, Vidius vicit".[21] He was appointed a lecturer in medicine at the Collège de France, where he demonstrated anatomy to large audiences, and a royal physician. On the King's death, he returned to Florence as doctor to Cosimo I of Tuscany and a chair at the newly reformed university of Pisa. In the German world the equivalent of his compendium was provided by Conrad Gessner, who chose to publish a huge volume of 408 folios in Latin, which, he claimed, would sell better and be more carefully looked after by students than individual texts. Based on what he could find in Zurich after he had weeded out books that were written in a "filthy and scarcely Latin" style, it was a curious mixture of ancient and modern.[22] Vidius and two writers on gunshot wounds, Bartolomeo Maggi of Bologna and Alfonso Ferri of Naples (1515–95), rub shoulders with medieval authors such as Jacopo dei Dondi (fl. 1350), and the volume ends with a short text designed to help the layman choose doctors and surgeons. Books like this were intended to appeal to the learned and Latinate surgeon, like the 'sworn surgeons' who occupied official positions in German towns and in Paris and who had the responsibility for carrying out inquests and, at times, cutting off the fingers or hands of criminals as punishment.[23]

Many of these surgeons served for shorter or longer periods of time in the armies, and occasionally navies, of their respective lords, some, like Hans von Gersdorff (1455–1520), writing up their experiences in manuals of military surgery.[24] The most important task of a royal physician or surgeon was to accompany his master on campaign, and be on hand to deal with any emergency. Both Vesalius and the distinguished Spanish surgeon Daza Chacon were in the entourage of Charles V at the siege of St Dizier in 1545, and Vesalius may have been present eight years later at the siege of Hesdin, if he is the imperial physician who carried out an autopsy there

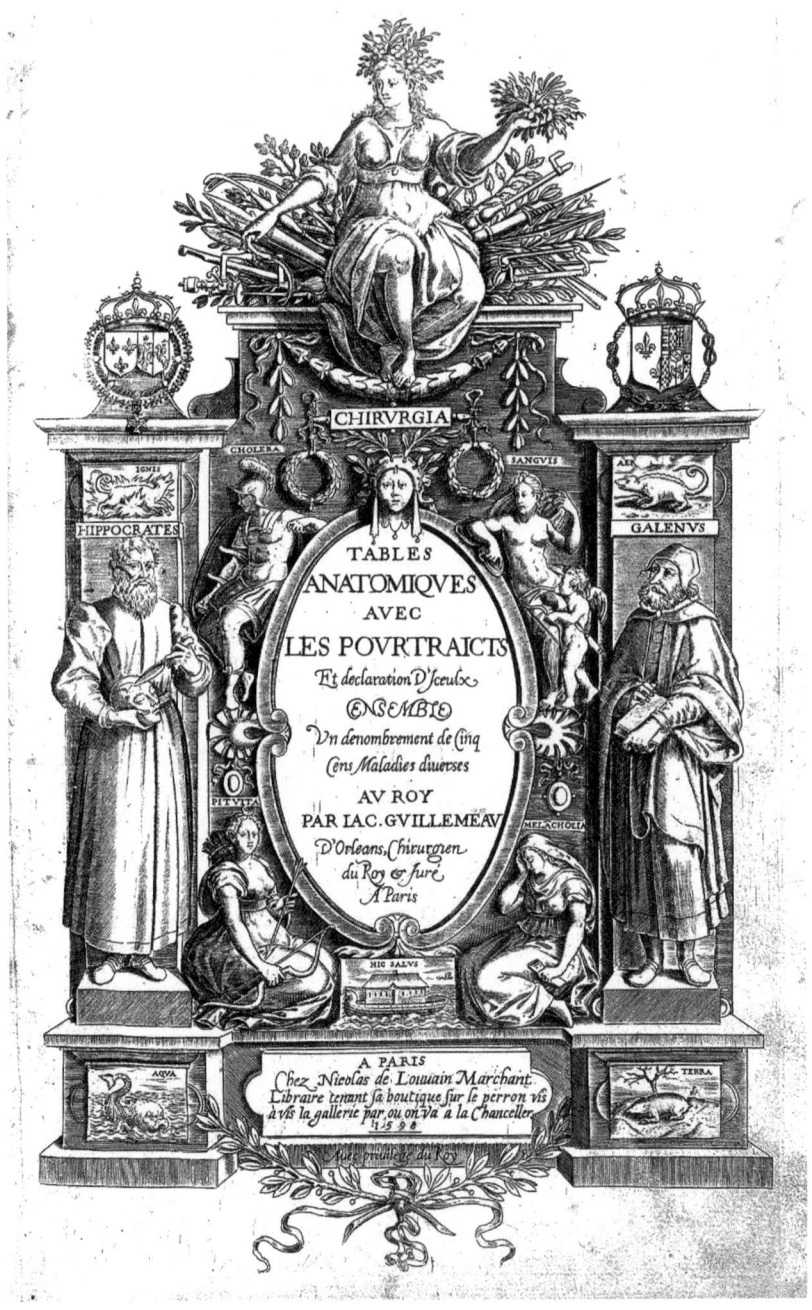

Figure 6.1 Jacques Guillemeau (1550–1613), *Les Oeuvres de Chirurgie*, Paris, N. de Louvain, 1598, frontispiece. Hippocrates and Galen stand within representatives of the four elements.

with Ambroise Paré (1510–90).[25] Paré's career is by far the best known of all Renaissance surgeons, largely thanks to his *Apologie et Traité*, *Apology and Treatise*, first published in 1585, which includes a long account of his work as a military surgeon on campaigns with his noble employers.[26] In it he tells of his rise from a small town barber-surgeon in the French provinces to become, briefly, an employee of the Paris Hôtel-Dieu, a military surgeon (although not officially admitted to the Paris barber-surgeons guild until 1541) and then in 1552–3 one of the royal surgeons of Henri II and, finally, in 1554 a member of the company of St Côme. Such a career, as Paré knew, was extremely unusual. So also is the range of his writings, which treat topics as varied as gunshot wounds and monstrous births.[27]

He made his most famous discovery in 1537 at the siege of the castle of Villane in Savoy, when, like others, he at first treated those who had been wounded by gunfire by using boiling oil. But when his supply of oil ran out, he decided instead to apply a 'digestive' and soothing mixture of egg whites, oil of roses and turpentine, as well as an onion plaster for burns. Finding to his surprise that his new patients fared better than his first ones, he decided to abandon for good his earlier method, thereby earning the thanks of his patients and the plaudits of subsequent historians.[28] He may have found this out for himself, but others had preceded him in treating such wounds similarly. Indeed, applying boiling oil was a relatively new remedy, strongly backed by a leading Italian surgeon, Giovanni de Vigo (1460–1525) in his widely published *Practica of Surgery*.[29] Vigo had concluded from observing dark marks around wounds and the speed with which those who had been shot died that the bullets themselves in some way poisoned the body: heat was the standard remedy for poisoning, which was classed as a cold disorder. Paré in his writings attacked the notion of poisoning, reverting to an earlier opinion that the darkness around the wound was some form of contusion or burn for which a gentler cooling therapy was required. He himself visited a distinguished surgeon in Turin who was independently advocating a similar treatment, and the Bolognese surgeon and teacher Bartolomeo Maggi had reached the same conclusion in his posthumously published treatise on the treatment of gunshot wounds.[30] Maggi may have been the Italian Master Bartolomeo who introduced Vesalius and Daza Chacon to these new methods at the siege of St Dizier, and Vigo also had earlier recommended an onion paste for treating burns.[31] But one should be careful about overestimating Paré's influence. The participants in a debate at Montpellier in 1580 on how to treat gunshot wounds did not mention him by name but argued over the superiority of Paracelsian remedies over those of Hippocrates, Galen and Guy de Chauliac.[32]

A second innovation has also been credited to Paré, the use of ligatures to tie off blood vessels before an amputation. This method he had used as early as 1552, although he did not make it public until 1564 as a safer and less painful alternative to cautery for staunching blood flow, and he never claimed credit for it, even spending the first section of his *Apology* in providing a list of examples from books and from others' experiences.[33] An earlier variant of his method was adopted by the German surgeon Hieronymus Brunschwig (c. 1460–1512) who had recommended in his *Surgery* sewing and tightening a thread under the skin of the thigh after an amputation.[34] Nonetheless, surgeons continued to use cauteries as the main means of stemming the flow of blood, and, at the end of the century, the German Fabry von Hilden (1560–1634) suggested that it might be worth first heating the saw or cleaver so that the heat would cauterise the blood vessels during the actual cutting process.[35]

Like physicians, surgeons often collaborated with one another in difficult cases or where the patient was a person of high status. Both Paré and Vesalius were among those summoned to the bedside of Henri II after he had been fatally injured in a tournament in June 1559, while Daza Chacon was also present, although apparently not called upon to advise or treat. Daza Chacon and Vesalius were also among the physicians and surgeons called in 1562 to treat Don Carlos, the eldest son of Philip II, who had injured his head when falling down some steps.[36] This time dissension between the medical attendants seems to have been greater. Vesalius's contention that the prince was suffering from an internal lesion of the head was strongly contested, and not everyone approved of his decision to make an incision just above the eyelids into the cranium to relieve pressure by removing pus from inside the skull. His earlier demand for trepanation, the making of a hole in the skull, had also been rejected.[37] Collegiate loyalty was important in avoiding public disagreements but was not always present. William Clowes was criticised in 1576 for abusing most of his fellow-surgeons with scoffing words and jests, and the following year his row with another senior surgeon George Baker ended with a fight in the fields outside the walls of London, although they later seem to have become friends and collaborators again.[38]

Paré was almost equally combative in his argument with François Rousset (c. 1535–98), who had argued in 1581 that it was possible to perform a Caesarean section without losing either mother or child. He had not performed the operation himself, but he reported seeing a successful operation at Easter 1556, although some of the evidence he cited was unreliable, as his opponents gleefully pointed out. However, both he and another surgeon Scipione Mercurio had talked with women who had been delivered in this way and who showed them their scars. Nonetheless, all were agreed in emphasising that this was a very dangerous procedure, only to be performed in extreme cases. (Removing a dead foetus was usually carried out with specially designed instruments and did not necessarily involve cutting into the abdomen.) Others, like Paré and Jacques Marchant, doubted the value of such an operation, which they believed would lead inevitably to the death of the mother.[39]

Rousset stirred up further controversy for his views on the correct way to extract a bladder-stone. This had long been the province of lithotomists, specialists (like operators for hernia) who travelled around and who were

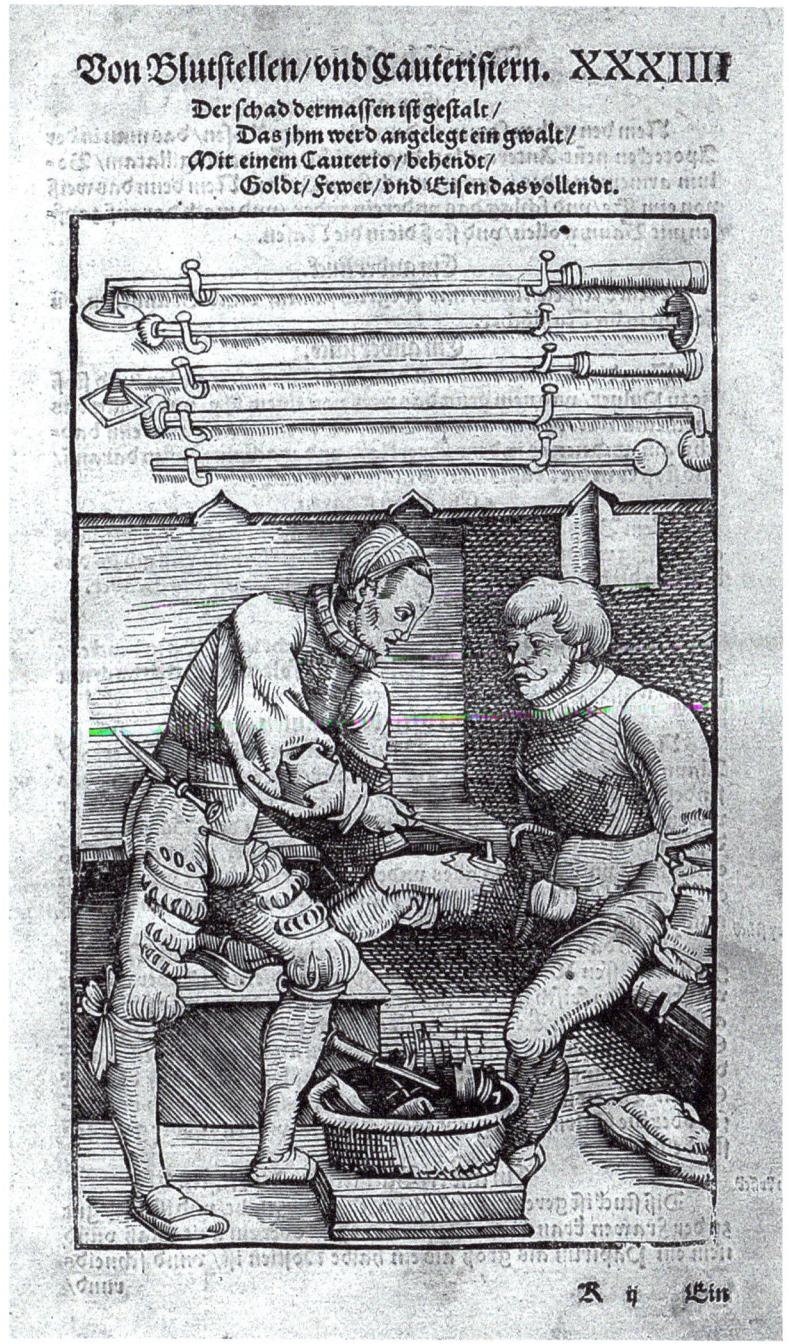

Figure 6.2 A military surgeon saws off the leg of a soporific patient, from the *Feldt-buch der Wundartzney* of Hans von Gersdorff (d. 1529), Frankfurt, H. Gülferichen, 1551.

largely illiterate, although far from unskilled. The standard procedure, familiar from Roman times, was for the lithotomist to grasp the stone with two fingers inserted into the rectum, make a small incision in the perineum and then drag the stone down and out with a hook. The wound was then left open to drain. In 1556 Pierre Franco (c. 1500–c. 1565) described two other methods. In the first, the so-called small method, he passed a probe via the urethra into the bladder to locate the stone and used its tip to bring it down to the site for the perineal incision. He also suggested the less complicated but much more hazardous way of cutting into the body above the pubis, but he recognised its potential dangers, and preferred the small method.[40] It was Rousset in 1581 who most strongly advocated the suprapubic incision, although he may never have performed it himself. However, he noted that if the bladder was filled with fluid and the penis tied, a suprapubic incision need not open the peritoneum, the inner covering of the abdomen, which Franco had warned against in his book.[41] A further method, the so-called grand apparatus, was advocated by the Italian surgeon Mariano Sanzi in 1535. The discovery of his teacher, this involved the insertion of scoops and forceps rather than the fingers to bring down the bladder stone through the perineal incision. Although this method continued to be practised for a long while, its superiority over the others is doubtful, and it still left the patient with potentially dripping urine and often a fistula.[42]

Debates and developments such as this, as well as the growing number of books in vernacular languages, encouraged surgeons to portray themselves as progressive and working at a higher level than many others who performed similar tasks such as lithotomy. The long list of successful cures described in books, often illustrated with pictures of instruments they had specially devised, emphasised their learning and expertise.[43] But unlike the boundary between physician and surgeon characterised by a university degree, that between surgeons and other so-called mechanics was far more fluid. Very few towns had enough practitioners of surgery to form their own guild, and, as in London, they often joined with other practitioners, especially with barbers, some of whom, the so-called barber-surgeons, carried out minor operations such as bloodletting (regularly sought each spring by many people as a simple way of avoiding what they believed was an otherwise inevitable harmful increase of blood at this season) in addition to their shaving and cosmetic work. They might also be involved in treating patients with syphilis, a practice that put them at odds with physicians. Their use of instruments above all equated at least some of them in popular opinion with surgeons, the subject of the same jokes and pretensions. Surgeons, however, made their superiority clear by insisting on primacy within their joint guilds, and certainly wished to differentiate themselves from those who merely practised barbering. In Amsterdam in 1597 the Guild of Surgeons took the decision to exclude barbers who were capable only of shaving and bleeding.[44] In London, despite their amalgamation, barbers and surgeons took their seats in the Common Hall on opposite sides of the room.[45]

Apothecaries

One further group of organised practitioners also had medical interests that overlapped with those of physicians and surgeons. Apothecaries, whose name derives from the storehouses where they kept their wares, were originally involved in bringing in and selling spices as members of the trade guilds of spicers or grocers (Figure 6.3). But over time, some spicers became more and more specialised in dealing with medicinal substances, and some, as in Florence, operated large establishments selling medicinal drugs.[46] By the sixteenth century, if not earlier, they had obtained a monopoly of the local supply of drugs throughout Europe. A Swiss town physician in 1551 was allowed to plant medicinal herbs in his own garden but forbidden to interfere with the rights of the apothecary to supply and sell drugs to the community.[47] Physicians, and particularly surgeons, prescribed medicines, creams and the like, but these had to be prepared by apothecaries according to the instructions of the medical man, who was often repeating remedies that had been handed down for centuries. In this division of labour the physicians claimed, and were usually granted, the right to inspect apothecaries' shops to see that they held an appropriate stock in good condition. The Ferrarese professor Brasavola's series of little tracts on medicines enjoyed great success because they were organised in such a way that the inspecting physician could easily discover and check whatever was available in the shop, whether an ointment, a pastille or a syrup and so on.[48] It was also physicians who were behind the printing of collections of recipes and drug-lists that over the century came to have an authoritative status and had to be followed by apothecaries. Some, like the Florentine *Nuovo Recettario* of 1499 or the 1546 Nuremberg *Dispensatorium* of Euricius Cordus, were private reform initiatives that were backed by local authorities, but they quickly became used as a means whereby the town and the physicians could exercise control of the apothecaries and any others who sold drugs.[49]

Like the other professional groupings, the apothecaries often sought to join a trade guild that would protect them both from rivals and from intervention by the authorities. In St Albans and Ipswich for example, they were included in the Guild of Mercers along with physicians, and in Shrewsbury around 1560 some apothecaries were members of the Glaziers Guild, while others joined the Merchant Adventurers.[50] In London, the apothecaries had undoubtedly benefitted from the 1543 Act that allowed non-surgeons to minister "outward medicines without payment", an acknowledgement of the competence of some apothecaries. But their attempts to separate themselves from the grocers were at first unsuccessful, and their separation was not authorised by the monarch until 1617, and formal acknowledgement of their right to practise medicine was the subject of bitter argument throughout the next century. Elsewhere in the provinces the lack of competition from other medical practitioners gave the apothecaries greater opportunities for offering medical assistance regularly. At Exeter in 1580 the apothecary

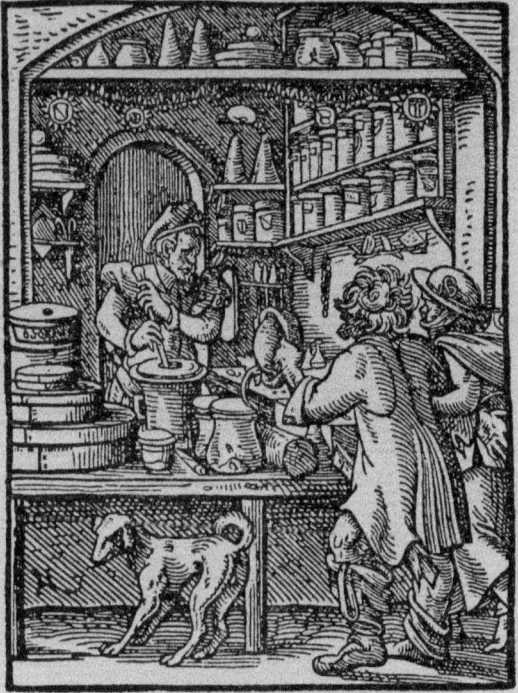

Der Apotecker.

Ich hab in meiner Apoteckn
Viel Matery die lieblich schmeckn/
Zucker mit Würtzen ich confieier
Mach auch Purgatzen vnd Clistier/
Auch zu stercken den krancken schwachn
Kan ich mancherley Labung machn/
Das alles nach der Artzte raht
Der seinen Brunn gesehen hat.

Der

Figure 6.3 The apothecary, from Jost Amman's *Stände und Handwerker*, Frankfurt, S. Feyerabend, 1560. The translation of the poem by Hans Sachs (1494–1576) reads: I have in my pharmacy / many tasty things. / I mix sugar and spices / and make up purges and enemas. To strengthen a weak patient / I can sometimes provide a cordial, all according to the advice of the doctor who has examined his urine.

William Dove was licensed to practise medicine and surgery, an acceptance by the authorities of what will have been the *status quo* rather than an innovation. The local population may well have found it more convenient to entrust themselves to a man whom they knew rather than to an unknown surgeon or newly arrived physician.[51]

By the end of the sixteenth century almost all physicians, surgeons, barbers and apothecaries had come together in some form of association, a college or a guild, whether it was a largely religious confraternity or, increasingly, an occupational body concerned to protect the interests of its members. Medieval in origin, the numbers of specialised medical guilds increased as temporary rules became permanent, groups split from one another, and civic and state authorities found them useful for their own purposes as a means of control, gaining political support or, like Henry VIII, simply waving the flag of their own modernity.[52] The proposal of Peter Lowe, who had been a member of the College of St Côme in Paris, for the creation of a College of Physicians and Surgeons in Glasgow in 1599 not only responded to perceptions of the evils brought about by "ignorant, unskilled and unlearned persons who under colour of Surgeons abuse the people to their pleasure" but also had the backing of the town council eager to show its superiority to its rival Edinburgh, where there was only a College of Surgeons, founded almost a century earlier in 1505.[53] In Flanders in the sixteenth century, surgeons became more and more involved in advising the magistrates in reporting on cases of wounding and in autopsies, a task that the magistrates had earlier carried out by themselves.[54]

Whether long established or new creations, these groups imposed conditions for membership that usually involved some form of examination following a medical degree or a long period of apprenticeship, as well as evidence of competent practice. Guild or college membership provided both an indication of professional quality and proof of a respectable position within civic society, expressed by public processions, dinners and the like. All endeavoured to protect their rights against anyone whom they believed were intent on usurping them, sometimes appealing directly to judicial authorities, at others publishing their complaints in sections of their writings or in entire books. But, as we have seen in the history of the London College of Physicians (see earlier, pp. 136–7), their complaints were not always heard, and their demands for action against the dangerous activities of unlicensed healers often foundered against the habits and expectations of the sick themselves, who preferred to follow their own judgement and consult practitioners from what Brockliss and Jones have called the medical "penumbra".[55]

The Medical Penumbra

This term usefully covers a wide range of healers and healing beyond the officially recognised bodies and can include almost anyone from astrologers and uroscopists to religious healers and even monarchs, who in Britain and France long continued to apply the royal touch to sufferers from scrofula.[56]

Brockliss and Jones's model of a penumbra of overlapping circles also avoids such simple dichotomy as popular and elite medicine, literate and illiterate, and official and unofficial, for boundaries between specialties, competences, availability and acceptability were fluid and often differed from place to place. The Florentine medical Guild, for example, could accommodate bonesetters, oculists, hernia doctors as well as a blacksmith-cum-dentist, Dominic the Teeth, although that did not stop more academically qualified members from demanding their exclusion and attending their funerals, an obligation for Guild officers, only with great reluctance.[57] Civic authorities in the Netherlands took a more pragmatic attitude. They allowed resident lithotomists and hernia doctors who had proved their competence to the relevant bodies to practise freely. Itinerants could not join a surgical guild but could practise at certain limited times, at a weekly or a yearly market, provided that they paid a fee to the surgeons.[58] In England, the licensing of practitioners by bishops, enacted in 1512, was slow to start, and very sporadic in application, while the so-called Quacks' Charter of 1543 effectively left large parts of the country dependent on unlicensed healers.

This does not mean that such healers were unskilled. Many of the so-called itinerants were widely recognised in their locality for their expertise in a particular operation. The administrator of the hospital at Troyes in Central France in 1569 did not hesitant to call in an itinerant surgeon to deal with two young children with hernias, although the treatment of hernias, including strangulated hernia, was widely described in books of surgery.[59] Cataract operations and cutting for the stone were frequently the province of itinerants, attacked by Pierre Franco for their eagerness to rush into operations they should have avoided and for their willingness to accept payment in kind for their cures – a blanket for a hernia, a tablecloth for a kidney stone, a couple of serviettes or headscarves for a cataract, and beer money on top.[60] Learned surgeons, like Felix Platter, constantly warned patients against trusting in operators whom they did not know, but, as Conrad Gessner explained when writing to a fellow doctor about his own eye problems, he was in a dilemma: on the one hand, he had poor sight and various eye problems, but, on the other, he did not wish to entrust himself to just any eye doctor and empiric. His own doctor, Peter Hafner, was very experienced, and he hesitated to employ another practitioner in the town, Jacob Baumann of Nuremberg (1521–86) (Figure 6.4), whom he described as an empiric with far more boldness than experience.[61] No wonder that Geneva introduced a regulation in 1569 forbidding any cutter for the stone, hernia, cataract or resolver of fractures and dislocations to act without the presence of a physician and surgeon of the patient's choice, or to perform any operation beyond his specialty, and without express permission.[62]

Some of these oculists, like Peter Hafner, gained a considerable reputation for their specialty, and settled down in a city to enjoy life as a respected surgeon and member of society. Jacob Baumann returned from Zurich to Nuremberg, where he became a member of the surgeons' Guild and

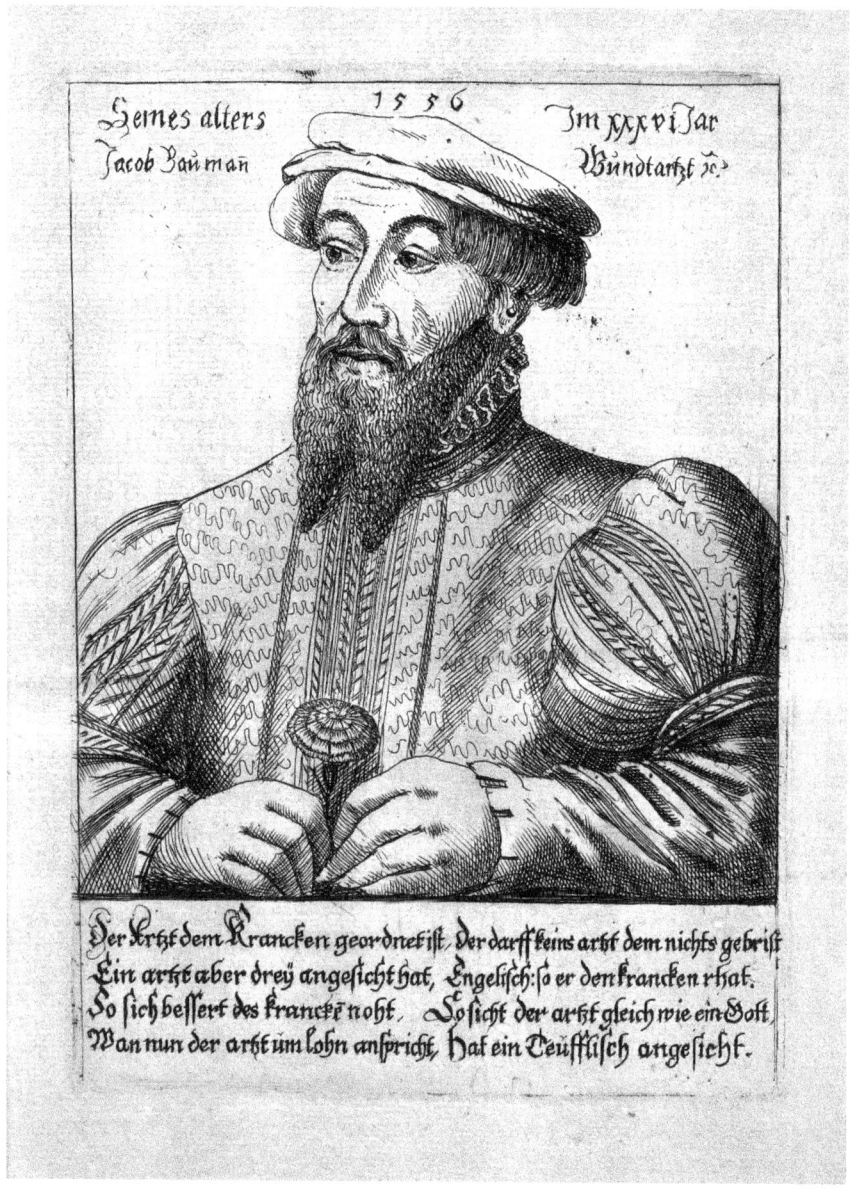

Figure 6.4 Jacob Baumann (1521–86), oculist and surgeon. Etching attributed to a follower of Hans Lautensack, 1556. The poem below may be translated thus: The doctor is instructed by the patient, who should not for that reason despise the doctor. / The doctor has three personae: of an angel when he advises the patient, / and of God when he relieves his need. / But when he talks about a fee, he takes on the appearance of the very devil.

co-operated in a German summary of Vesalius's *Fabrica* "for the use of surgeons of the German Nation". His portrait depicts him as a wealthy citizen holding a flower.[63] A similar practitioner, Georg Bartisch (1535–1607), was apprenticed to a barber at the age of 13 and ended his career as court oculist to the rulers of Saxony. For 30 years or more he travelled around Saxony and Bohemia as a specialist in cutting for the stone, wound surgery and eye diseases, on which he wrote the first major treatise, illustrated with 92 woodcuts.[64] It opens with 25 pages of testimonia from individuals and from municipal officials praising his abilities as an eye surgeon and lithotomist, and emphasising his successes in a variety of eye conditions in both old and young. Others had their techniques copied by others of greater standing: Tagliocozzi, for example, may have owed his understanding of rhinoplasty from his acquaintance, at first or second hand, with a Sicilian family of surgeons called Branca.[65] Others, however, preferred to keep their methods a secret. A secret technique of lithotomy in adults was used by eight generations of the Colot family from Laurence Colot (c. 1520–90) until 1727 when it was published by François Colot. The similarity of their operation to the grand apparatus procedure advocated by the Italian Mariano Sanzi was explained away as the invention of an even earlier (and implausible) Germain Collot (*sic*), who had practised with his instruments on corpses and whose successes had allegedly inspired Sanzi and his teacher.[66]

Unless they settled down in a major city, like Baumann later in Nuremberg or Colot in Paris, with a sufficiently large and well-heeled body of patients or, like Bartisch, found employment as a specialist at a wealthy court, specialists in only one or two operations were compelled to travel in search of patients simply to make a living. In this they resembled the typical object of complaints from all types of urban healer – the so-called charlatan, also known in English from his sales methods as a mountebank or quacksalver. A widely used multi-lingual Latin dictionary of the period translated the phrase '*medicus circumforaneus*' as 'a seller of theriac', 'an itinerant', 'a quack', thereby combining three different aspects of his activity, his location, his wares and methods, and his reputation.[67]

This description emphasises that he travelled around, like the oculist or the lithotomist, going from market to market, the literal meaning of '*circumforaneus*', sometimes from a home base, even if he was not a citizen there. There are many examples, from Antiquity onwards, of such healers who followed a circuit, probably living in one town or village and travelling out from there to service outlying communities or, more often, attending markets where potential patients from the wider district would regularly congregate either weekly or at certain times of the year.[68] As such, they were subject to market regulations, and hence some form of public scrutiny, but not always that of other medical professionals. The licences given to them by many towns around Europe show how they were often integrated into the medical world, supplementing what others could offer. In areas where there was no resident doctor or surgeon, as in parts of Southern Italy, they

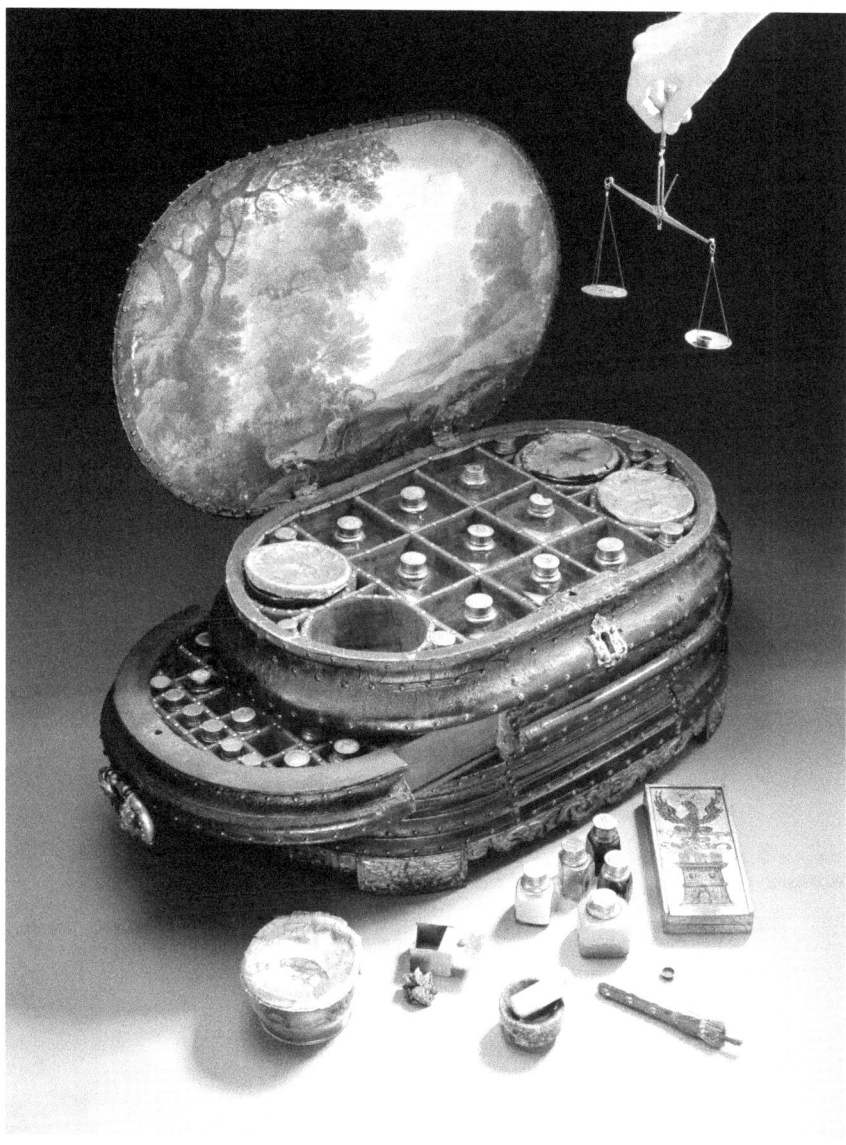

Figure 6.5 A Genoese medical chest for use on board ship. Made between 1562 and 1566.

provided a vital service to those who fell ill.[69] Any successful cures would only add to their reputation and continue to provide them with an income. They need not have been trained by another healer, but many were, and a servant who accompanied such a man on his rounds might well be also learning the trade.[70]

Another characteristic emphasised by the lexicographer in his description of the travelling doctor is the way in which he advertised himself. He might arrange to have the walls of an inn strategically located by the town gate plastered with adverts for his arrival. Once there, he would have a market stall, sometimes with a banner advertising his wares, and often a stool or bench on which he would stand to shout out to attract customers (hence 'mountebank'). Other words to describe him stress his patter (Italian '*ciarlare*', from which comes 'charlatan') and the way in which he hawked his drugs (Dutch '*kwakzalver*', 'ointment boaster', hence 'quack') like any good salesman. Above all, descriptions in both art and writing mention his extravagant clothing, often with fantastic headgear, which can form part of a deliberately theatrical display, in contrast to the sober clothing and austere image of the learned doctor or surgeon.[71] Rabelais had Gargantua class sellers of theriac among the spectacles worth seeing on a rainy afternoon, along with acrobats and card-sharpers, whose deceitful tricks were no different from hawking theriac.[72] But not every mountebank was a showman as well as a salesman, and one may wonder how far the theatrical performances and clothing associated with the quack doctor developed in this period to fit the image expected of him. At least one early image, in a French manuscript of around 1470, now in Dresden, shows him in normal clothing, and the change from the flashy outfit of the military surgeon or a wealthy townsman to the colourful jacket and hat of the quack in an Italian *commedia* is not large.[73] Significantly, when in 1545 Jacopo Coppa, faced with complaints from the surgeons of Florence, was allowed to make a public trial of his wares in the main square, he appeared from a sort of theatrical tent "in sublime majesty", wearing a black velvet tunic and skirt, a black cap and a golden chain given him by the Duchess herself, precisely the sort of clothing that appears in portraits of leading physicians. His dress was a sign to his enthusiastic audience that he was the equal of any physician.[74]

The third element In Junius's translation is his specific reference to theriac, an association that goes back to Classical Antiquity and is the occasion for the depiction of the mountebank in the Dresden manuscript just mentioned. A mixture of many different substances, both vegetable and animal, it appears to have been devised in the second century BC, and one variant became associated with King Mithridates of Pontus, who was believed to have used it successfully as an antidote against poison, hence the alternative name Mithridatium. Several famous doctors produced their own versions, whose ingredients grew in number and complexity. The Emperor Marcus Aurelius used it as a tonic, employing Galen among others to prepare it for him, and its usage became common again in imperial circles in the first decades of the third century. Two treatises on theriac from this period survive under the name of Galen, thus adding to the reputation of the drug when they were rediscovered in the late fifteenth century. It was favoured by medical writers in Arabic as a panacea, and as such passed into the Latin West, which obtained many of their supplies of it from the Eastern Mediterranean via Venice, hence the common English name, 'Venice treacle'. Other towns like Montpellier also prepared their own theriacs using a very similar formula and even arranging for it to be made in public to demonstrate its purity.[75]

It was a drug with many advantages for the travelling salesman. Once made, or obtained from another dealer, it was easy to transport, and, even if it was not the genuine article (and who could tell?), the method of making such a complex confection was one of the trade secrets of the seller. The name alone and its long and apparently successfully history were guarantee enough of its efficacy. It was famous as an antidote to poison, something attested in literature, archives and medical writings, as poisoning was widely feared by all classes. Above all, it was a panacea, a *catholicon*, touted as a remedy against an enormous range of conditions, which obviated the need for the itinerant to travel with a broad range of specifics, whether against a particular disease or to fit the humoral balance of the individual.[76] It could work as a purgative – and many believed that their diseases were the result of something nasty in the body that was required to be removed – or as an analgesic, for it included substantial amount of opium and similar substances. The use in it of viper's flesh can be regarded as a sort of sympathetic magic, here working against a potentially harmful substance, poison, that may have come from the viper itself. Learned physicians had their doubts about panaceas of all kinds, particularly when prepared without their supervision, but those who bought a small jar of theriac believed that they were buying something that could not only cure the present condition but also protect against, and even successfully treat, something similar in the future. A mid-sixteenth-century customer in a market in Milan or Heilbronn would have been acting little differently from one who four centuries later bought from a stallholder in a Bradford market a tin of Sercuro, a zinc and wax based ointment that claimed to resolve most types of boils, styes and skin ailments – and indeed did.[77]

But very often accusations of charlatanry were levelled at outsiders simply because they were outsiders who offered types of healing that seemed to challenge the status quo. This was particularly the case in the second half of the century when Paracelsian and similar remedies began to become familiar. Valentin Rasworme, the object of vitriolic attack from William Clowes and others, had been a well-respected lithotomist in Cologne before moving to London, and his success with Paracelsian remedies among the London elite and members of the court was a direct threat to the pocket of leading surgeons.[78] Clowes had a much more ambiguous relationship with John Hester, who faced strong opposition in the 1570s when he attempted to set up a business selling large quantities of Paracelsian remedies at his shop at St Paul's wharf. Hester had been a strong defender of Rasworme, describing him as a "wise Alchemist", and duly came under attack from Clowes. But once the College of Physicians took up the cudgels against Paracelsians, Clowes and fellow-surgeons like George Baker changed tack, supporting

Paracelsian remedies and translating Paracelsian treatises. Baker even recommended a visit to Hester's shop, calling him a painstaking and well-travelled expert. But once Hester in turn began to encroach upon the surgeon's claims to treat syphilis, Clowes and his friends reverted to their former position. They denounced Hester and his associates as mere empirics and retold the saga of Rasworme in splendidly rhetorical English (Figure 6.6) that distinguished between their own proper understanding of Paracelsus, Hippocrates and Galen and the counterfeit Paracelsian quacksalver.[79]

Rasworme's career as a man with a respectable reputation and distinguished backers who found himself in the wrong place and advocating the wrong type of medicine finds a parallel in the experiences of Leonardo Fioravanti (1517–88), a much more significant figure as both healer and publicist.[80] Fioravanti may have picked up some medicine while a young man in Bologna, his home city, but he claims to have learned far more from travelling around the Mediterranean and learning from the experiences, experiments and secrets of healers of all kinds, from physicians and surgeons to shepherds and country women, precisely those whom the learned practitioners frequently denounced. He learned the art of distillation to make his secret balsam, and in 1549, instructed by an elderly surgeon from Naples who had performed similar operations before, removed an enlarged spleen from the wife of an army captain. He did not hesitate to trumpet his results and was almost immediately appointed as a surgeon at the hospital for syphilitics in Palermo and then as a surgeon at

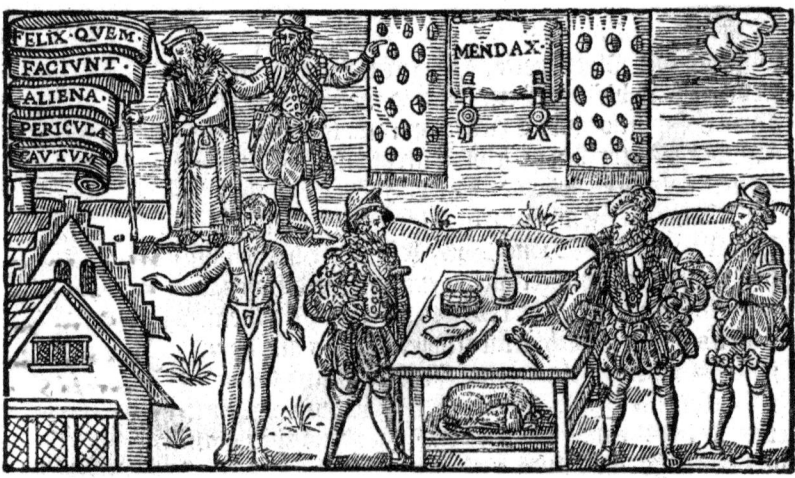

Figure 6.6 An Elizabethan quack, as portrayed in William Clowes, *A briefe Treatise*, London, T. East for T. Cadman, 1585. The Latin words advise prospective patients to take care: "Happy the person whom others' dangers make cautious"; and: "Liar".

the court of the Spanish Viceroy of Sicily in Messina before returning to Naples as *protomedico* of the Viceroy and his son there. A further spectacular cure, replacing a nose of a Spanish gentleman by rhinoplasty, a technique he had learned from a family of surgeons in Calabria, increased his ambition.[81] In 1555 he moved to Rome, gaining a licence to practice, but his competitors, including Realdo Colombo, accused him of purveying secret remedies and he was forced to leave the city for Venice. Once there, he began a lucrative new career as a publicist and writer of books of secrets as well as continuing with his surgery and pharmacy. These books, dealing with medicine, surgery, plague and domestic medicine, were published by well-known publishers such as Valgrisi, explaining in vigorous language for an eager literate audience his 'secrets' and denouncing the evils of more orthodox practitioners.[82] He made enough money from his writings and his drugs to turn down an offer in 1564 from the Emperor to join him as a doctor on campaign. He was again threatened with a ban for practising medicine without a medical degree, which he avoided by being granted a doctorate in medicine from Bologna at a reduced fee as a native of the city. This did not stop attempts in Venice to prosecute him as an itinerant charlatan – though patients provided him with testimonies of his miraculous cures – and he was jailed for eight days in Milan at the insistence of the physicians there. He was still in Venice during the plague of 1575–6, attempting to cure what in an earlier tract he had stressed had been sent as a punishment from God for the sins of its citizens, a typical comment by healers of all types, although expressed with particular force by Fioravanti. In 1576 he moved to Spain, where he was welcomed by Philip II, to the annoyance of orthodox physicians at the court, who accused him of ignorance of Latin, giving patients drugs of his own invention, and using unorthodox and unapproved remedies, almost certainly deriving from Paracelsian tracts as well as the medieval alchemical tradition of Ramon Lull.[83] He remained at court for about a year, experimenting on tobacco and other New World plants he had read about in Monardes, gaining the friendship of at least one court doctor and leaving behind a disciple, an empiric and alchemist from Bologna. He returned to Venice and to his writing, including a new edition of his book on surgery, but apart from a few references to him as a charlatan and vendor of secrets, he disappears from the record after 1582, and he may have died back in Bologna in 1588.

Fioravanti is an extreme example of the complications of categorising the practitioners of healing in the sixteenth century. He did not obtain a formal medical qualification until at least 25 years after he had begun to practise, and even then its validity continued to be challenged. His writings show considerable flair and erudition, as well as a talent for publicity. He had learned his surgery by associating with other experienced surgeons, and was aware of the important role of the surgeon in assisting in formal university anatomies (see p. 248, later). His remedies differ little from those available in other books, and even his adoption of alchemical and probably Paracelsian remedies was in no way unusual. His crime in the eyes of his competitors lay in adopting the ways of the outsiders, the itinerants, the empirics and the purveyors of secrets, in emphasising the wonderful cures that he had performed and in relying on information from groups that they regarded as suspect and appealed to the authorities to suppress.[84] There is ample evidence that, like Baumann in Nuremberg, he too would have preferred to settle down, as he did at the end of his life in Venice, and enjoy the privileges of a physician to a magnate or monarch.

In an increasingly corporatist profession, with growing numbers of guilds and universities all with their own regulations as to who should be allowed to practise in their region, any outsider, however experienced, was seen as a threat. Authorship of a book of secrets, even if published by reputable Venetian publishers as Valgrisi and Sessa, still carried a taint of magic and mystery, despite the emphasis that writers like Fioravanti placed in them on their success. Such books, with authors like Alexis of Piedmont, were aimed at prospective patients as well as those who might seek in them for home remedies, but by publicising substances that apothecaries regarded as their own province they also incurred considerable hostility from official guilds.[85] But whatever physicians and apothecaries might think, these books sold well, going through more editions and in more languages even than plague tracts, evidence that in this too the public took a different view from the disciples of Aesculapius.

Fioravanti's career also shows how the rich and powerful could disregard the advice of more orthodox practitioners and employ an outsider with a track record of healing. The Viceroy of Sicily and his counterpart in Naples, as well as Philip II later, were eager to attach him to their suite, and although he did not find the employment he had hoped for at the papal court in Rome, he was allowed to practise by the papal *protomedico*. When Henri II was fatally injured in a tournament in 1559, an itinerant healer was summoned to his bedside alongside Vesalius and Paré.[86] For those who lacked either the money or the physical access to a graduate physician or a learned surgeon, the itinerant healer was both cheaper and, in all likelihood, no worse. He could be seen in action in the marketplace along with his testimonials from grateful patients. His performances to drum up clients were no less effective than the joint consultations of sober physicians, and his condemnations of other healers may have served as a greater warning of medical incompetence than the respectful agreement and judicious silence of the learned, who were forbidden by many College Statutes under pain of a fine to utter abuse or make any show of public dissent when attending a case with a colleague.[87] Besides, as a lawyer put it in 1575 when defending a woman accused of charlatanism, "How many savants in medicine have been outdone by a simple old peasant woman who with a single plant or herb has found a remedy for illness despaired of by physicians?"[88]

Choices and Perceptions

Historians of medicine have long moved away from considering the choices available to the sick as a dichotomy between officially qualified medical personnel, principally physicians and surgeons, and other healers. This division, although useful as a way of organising data, is doubly misleading. It reflects the bias of the sources, principally written by the literate and urban medical community, and it underestimates both the complexity of what was available and the perceptions of all those involved in the healing process, from the sick and their families to royal physicians and university professors. Even the more accurate metaphor of a spectrum of healers, which rightly stresses the way in which one type of healing could easily merge into another, is too static, for it minimises the social interactions that will have determined whether a sick person sought help or not, and whom they chose to provide that assistance. Hence the choice in this and the previous chapter of the metaphor of the kaleidoscope: the pattern of healing and healers can remain both recognisable, like colours and shapes, while being transformed, sometimes substantially, without any change of focus.

One major result of research into European archives and the availability of databases of population and social groups has been to challenge the old idea of the paucity of medical assistance available in the sixteenth century; the choices available to the sick were far wider than literary accounts had appeared to indicate. But, since researchers have used different parameters, statistics are not easy to compare across regions. Carlo Cipolla in 1976 suggested that in 1630 Florence had 33 graduate physicians, a ratio of approximately one physician for every 2,400 of the population, a typical percentage for a large Italian town. Smaller towns like Montepulciano and Poggibonsi had a smaller percentage, but, if surgeons are also included, their inhabitants were looked after by a roughly similar number of officially recognised practitioners.[89] Figures for England are harder to come by, but Roberts suggested that four or five physicians were in practice at Exeter, a regional hub, with a cathedral and a population of around 9,000, at the end of the sixteenth century, and Pelling and Webster give a similar figure for the larger city of Norwich.[90] Figures for France are roughly similar. But the percentages change substantially when other practitioners are included. In Poitiers throughout the century there was on average at least one apothecary per thousand of the population, and a similar proportion in Exeter and Norwich, while at Montpellier, a university town with more physicians and surgeons than normal, 31 apothecaries served a population of 12,500 in mid-century, and 27 in 1600. Surgeons and barber-surgeons also usually outnumbered physicians in all regions – Lyons with a population of around 58,000 in 1545 had 30 surgeons and 45 apothecaries compared with eight physicians (although their numbers had grown to 14 by 1571). Norwich in 1575 had 37 surgeons or barber-surgeons, 12 apothecaries, ten women practitioners, six "practitioners of physic", five university educated physicians and three others for a population that did not exceed 17,000.[91] London was very different in size and social composition from anywhere in England, and arguably in Europe. Pelling and Webster suggest that its population of 200,000 or more in 1600 was served by around 50 Fellows, candidates and licentiates of the College of Physicians, 100 surgeons in the Barber-Surgeons Company, 100 apothecaries in the Grocers' Company, and an almost equal number of other healers, some licensed but many not, to say nothing of midwives and nurses.[92]

Towns, of course, also attracted people from outlying villages who, as at Brno in 1577, might come to market, visit the baths to be bled or tramp across the fields bringing their urine in a flask (or even a sabot) for inspection by an apothecary. These practitioners would have served a much larger number than the town's population as recorded in a census, and many of them would not have spent their time exclusively in treating the sick.[93] But one also needs to consider the work of nurses, midwives, nuns and barbers as well as itinerants (two of whom were ordered in 1562 to be whipped by the Exeter magistrates for claiming to be surgeons and tooth-drawers), and the suggestion that one in 250 of the population, and around one in 400 in London, was in some way involved in healing appears reasonable.[94]

The choice of what to do when illness struck was large and was made first by the patient or their family. It could range from simple resignation to the will of the Almighty to the employment of a variety of practitioners, not all of whom were medical graduates or guild members. Particularly among the wealthy, seeking advice from a number of individuals widened the possibilities for a cure: if one recommendation did not work or find favour, another could be chosen. When in 1574 the Brandenburg court decided that Duke Albrecht of Prussia was mad or an imbecile, they first sent his urine to a celebrated Paracelsian, Leonhard Thurneisser (1531–96), in Berlin, who diagnosed him as melancholic to be cured in both body and mind by a disciplined regime of diet, exercise and chemical drugs. The Galenist court doctors strongly disagreed and his advice was rejected. But at almost the same time court officials decided to consult another healer, not a physician, whose advice was to use different herbal remedies.[95] At the other end of the social spectrum the sick poor may have preferred an itinerant or a wise woman to a surgeon or learned physician precisely because they came from the same milieu and shared the same ideas on treatment.

All parties emphasised their successes and their superior abilities to diagnose and to prescribe appropriate remedies and derided the follies and pretensions of their opponents. The same jokes about doctors and surgeons appear and reappear over the centuries – the incompetent who killed more than he cured, the lecherous practitioner who enjoyed sex with his patients and did not stop at murdering a husband to get his way, or the atheist hiding behind a cloak of respectability. The doctor in Marguerite de Navarre's comedy wants to bleed the patient, even when he has recovered, and to have his fee even if he has done nothing towards the cure.[96] Critics still argue whether Shakespeare put the real John Caius on stage in his comedy the *Merry Wives of Windsor* as a gabbling Frenchman, or how far Molière's doctors who spout egregious platitudes to bewilder their patients represent reality. The blood and gore of surgeons on stage was meant to invoke horror (or at times amusement) in the audience, which might well contribute further to any reluctance to go under the knife.[97] At least two of the literary productions of the Italian writer Ercole Bentivoglio (1507–73) can be connected directly with the medical Faculty at Ferrara, where he spent most of his life. His most popular play, *Il geloso, The Jealous Husband*, features an elderly physician who marries a young wife, a typical theme in comedy, but one with a direct relevance in Ferrara where the marriage in 1535 of the 73-year-old Giovanni Manardi to a young bride (and his death a year later after the birth of a daughter) occasioned not a few ribald jokes.[98] Bentivoglio was a friend and patient of Antonio Musa Brasavola, to whom he dedicated the third of his *Satires*. In it he contrasted Brasavola's kindness and learning with the crowd of semi-learned young doctors riding around in silks with their retinues, who had gained their degree quickly through favouritism or simply paying a fee and who knew no Aristotle or Avicenna and only a couple of recipes from Galen. How much wiser, he concluded, is the peasant who doesn't go hunting for a doctor when he has a fever but drinks cold water or, when he is tired after hard work, forgoes massages and purges like rhubarb that destroy his strength and his appetite further! Nature's ways are best.[99] A Strasbourg patrician Eckart zum Trübel put it more succinctly, baldly warning his Christian readers to beware of all doctors and apothecaries as conspirators against the common people.[100]

One accusation, familiar in a range of media from poems and jokes to paintings, played on the three aspects of a patient's relationship with his or her physician, before, during and after the cure. The physician appears first as an angel, arriving opportunely to offer his assistance; after a successful cure he seems a god; later, when demanding his payment, he is the very devil. A version of this trope even appears at the foot of a copperplate etching of a portrait of Jacob Baumann (Figure 6.4), although its opening line suggests that he himself was far too respected as a surgeon to be characterised in this way.[101] But for every avaricious physician there was always a penny-pinching patient. Doctors frequently complain about bad debts and the unwillingness of patients to pay.[102]

The image of the triple-faced physician also suggests that his services were widely sought after even by those who found difficulty paying, and that, perhaps more significantly, they believed in his ability to cure. How they came to make their selection from an overlapping range of choices can rarely be known, but one cannot assume that modern ideas of a successful cure – and, still more, of failure – are the same as those of the sixteenth century. A society where many children died before reaching the age of 10, famine and plague were constant threats, and it was an achievement to live beyond

50 will have had a very different attitude to death than our modern age. The failure of a doctor to cure his patient was taken as a normal, if sad, occurrence, and a refusal to treat what one considered an incurable condition was a matter for praise, not condemnation. Mercuriale's failure in dealing with the great plague of Venice (see earlier, pp. 54–5) did not handicap his university career or prevent him from being summoned to treat the good and great. Besides, sociological studies have only confirmed the observations of Roy Porter 30 years ago in a pioneering study of patients that a choice of physician and of treatment depended far more on the compatibility of patients' views on the causes of their illnesses with those of their healers than on any simple calculus of medical efficacity.[103] Familiarity, age and status will also have played a part. The ructions at Montelupo and the travails of Euricius Cordus and Theodore Eccombertus as town physicians were more likely to have been caused, or at least exacerbated, by the youth of the medics and administrator involved, and all involved foreigners from some miles away.[104] Had they been more senior, with roots in the community, the outcome might well have been different. It was this shared sense of belonging that meant an itinerant practitioner who made regular visits to a town or market was viewed as more trustworthy than a newly arrived physician or surgeon, who might not be able easily to speak the same language as his clients. Conversely, when Paré stayed for two months in Flanders treating the Marquis d'Auret, patients came to see him from miles around because the marquis had recommended him to them. The chemical cures of Paracelsian physicians and surgeons were favoured by Evangelical magnates and, equally, distrusted by their religious opponents, in part because of their respective world views.[105] The fact that many of the most active Paracelsian proselytisers were alchemists and astrologers was an advantage in communities like that of Hesse whose rulers took a more than passing interest in these intellectual disciplines.

The kaleidoscope of healing in the sixteenth century does not differ markedly from that of the fifteenth: the overlapping groupings remained the same, save for an increase in numbers of healers of all kinds and in the possibilities for study and travel. Until the 1550s learned medicine remained largely what it had been in the 1450s, and developments in war surgery were relatively small. Only from the 1570s onwards did the advent of Paracelsian ideas and chemically based drugs offer a major challenge to Galenism. There was indeed a move towards corporatisation, with the formation of more universities and new guilds, but this was a slow process even in a typical town of 5,000 inhabitants. Physicians, surgeons and apothecaries, however, all appear to have shared a new sense of moving forward from a distant medieval past, expressed most clearly in the rhetoric of prefaces, even if it is to be viewed with a certain scepticism in the relative absence of similar writings from the previous half-century. But there are also gaps in our understanding compared with what follows in the seventeenth century. There is not the abundance of personal, confessional literature and private diaries detailing individual responses to illness that has altered many historians' approaches to medicine in seventeenth-century England, and the voices of ordinary sufferers that do survive from the earlier period come frequently from legal sources within an institutional framework. But institutions change, albeit slowly, and the rehabilitation of the charlatan and the outsider by historians writing over the last 20 years has provided a new way of perceiving these changes as the kaleidoscope of healers has been shaken again.

Notes

1 For clerics, see, for example, De Waardt 1996.
2 Pomata 1998.
3 For surgeons as 'artisans of the body', Cavallo 2007; Kinzelbach 2014a.
4 Lindemann 2010: 131.
5 Adelmann 1966: 51–2. For rhinoplasty, Tagliacozzi 1597; Gnudi and Webster 1950: 109–14; see later, p. 197.
6 Gryllus 1566b: 6v.
7 Brockliss and Jones 1997: 220–1. For attendance at Tagault's lectures, Nutton 2003.
8 Siraisi 1990: 178–80.
9 Nutton 2017c.
10 Stolberg 2021a: 214–20.
11 Siraisi 1990: 155.
12 See later, p. 158.
13 Clowes 1596: 104–10, 140–3, 1948: 143–50; for examples of chests, Müller 1970; Burnett 1982; Endo 2020. For the development of instruments at this period, Kirkup 2006, although not always easy for the non-surgeon to follow.
14 Dobson and Walker 1979: 26–41; Decamp 2016: 8–13. The first dissections may have been supervised by Thomas Vicary (1495 -1561), royal surgeon and sometime Master, Dobson and Walker 1979: 118–20.
15 Nutton 1985b: 83–7; Langton (undated) (1545?): sig. iii r–v, 1547: sig. a ii r. The relationship of this book to Vicary's *Anatomie of Man's Parts*, possibly of 1547–8, but not printed until 1577, needs further investigation, see Thomas 2006.
16 Nutton 2020b.
17 Nutton 1985b: 83.
18 Canappe 1552: 389.
19 Daléchamps 1569: 4v–7r: a briefer expert surgical commentator on a classical text is Aranzi 1579.
20 Vidius 1544.
21 'Vidius came, Vidius saw, Vidius conquered', a joke based on a famous saying of Julius Caesar. For the story of this book, Brockbank 1956; Grmek 1978.
22 Gessner 1555b: sig. +2r.
23 Brockliss and Jones 1997: 221.
24 Von Gersdorff 1517; Panse 2012.
25 O'Malley 1964: 204–6, 261–2.
26 Paré 1585, 1968; Dumaître 1986 updates the classic account by Malgaigne in Paré 1840–1.
27 Paré 1585; English translation 1982.
28 Paré 1545: fol. 52v, 1552: fol. 45r, 1585: 1215, 1968: 23–4, 137–42; Donaldson 2015.
29 Vigo 1514. A French translation appeared in 1525, a Spanish in 1537, an English in 1545 and an Italian in 1549.

30 Maggi 1552: fols. 45r–v. For a possible link with Alexis of Piedmont, Eamon 1994: 143–4.
31 O'Malley 261–2.
32 Veyras *et al.* 1581.
33 The account in the *Apology* opens with list of authorities for ligaturing, going back to Galen: Paré 1585: 1208–12, 1968: 4–16; a further description, Paré 1585: 419–21, 1968: 149–53. For his advocacy of podalic version, see later, p. 186.
34 Wangensteen and Wangensteen 1978: 28–31.
35 Wangensteen and Wangensteen 1978: 21.
36 O'Malley 1964: 285–8, 296–302.
37 Soulier 2020a publishes newly discovered letters by Vesalius to Ottavio Landi, a diplomat in the service of Emperor Maximilian II, describing the case.
38 Clowes 1948: 23; Harkness 2007: 85.
39 Rousset 1581; Mercurio 1601; Marchant 1598; Wangensteen and Wangensteen 1978: 201–4; Blumenfeld-Kosinski 1990: 38–47. Delivering a live child after the death of the mother was known in the Middle Ages and became more common in the sixteenth century, Foscati 2019. For the crucial roles of Paré and Rousset in the medicalisation of the curious story of the Archer of Meudon, Nutton and Nutton 2003.
40 Wangensteen and Wangensteen 1978: 70, 86. Franco's books were republished with a major introduction surveying Renaissance surgery by Édouard Nicaise, Franco 1895.
41 Wangensteen and Wangensteen 1978: 86.
42 Wangensteen and Wangensteen 1978: 70.
43 Decamp 2016: 48–58.
44 De Moulin 1998: 69–70.
45 Matthews 1962: 36.
46 Shaw and Welch 2011; for shops as sites of training, Pugliano 2018; for convent pharmacies in Florence, Strocchia 2019: 130–78.
47 See earlier, p. 47.
48 E.g. Brasavola 1536, 1561. For the importation of new drugs at this period, see earlier, pp. 13–14. For similar rules in Spain and the New World, Grunberg 2006: 151–9.
49 Schmitz 2005: 189–216; Murphy 2019: 34–43.
50 Whittet 1964: 253–4, 261.
51 Wear 2000: 23.
52 Brockliss and Jones 1997: 170–88.
53 Geyer-Kordesch and MacDonald 1999: 3–11.
54 Dekoster 2021.
55 Pelling 2003: 136–88; Brockliss and Jones 1997: 14–15, 230–53.
56 Bloch 1973; Thomas 1973: 227–36; Clowes 1602: *Letter to the Reader*, 48–9, 1948: 47–8, 53–4, records several cures by Elizabeth I.
57 Park 1985.
58 De Moulin 1998: 66–9.
59 Brockliss and Jones 1997: 252; for hernia treatments, Wangensteen and Wangensteen 1978: 111–12.
60 Franco 1895: 5; Koelbing 1967: 149, with n. 377 for identifications.
61 Koelbing 1967: 157, 148–50.
62 Koelbing 1967: 150. A similar regulation is found earlier in German cities, e.g. Ulm, Murphy 2019: 94.
63 Vesalius 1551; Jurina 1985: 204–5, 286–9.
64 Bartisch 1583; ciii r–eiii r.
65 Gnudi and Webster 1950: 115–21; Lindemann 2010: 132.
66 Brockliss and Jones 1997: 106; Nutton and Nutton 2003: 420–3.

67 Junius 1577: 345b.
68 Nutton 2013: 10, 327.
69 Gentilcore 1995, 1998, 2006.
70 Jurina 1985: 93, pl. 100, shows a military surgeon with a young assistant.
71 Brockliss and Jones 1997: 231; Gentilcore 2006: 320–30.
72 Rabelais, *Gargantua*, ch. 24; *Pantagruel*, ch. 16.
73 Dresden, DB 92, f. 195r., now largely destroyed but available in a colour repro-
   duction in Van Leersum and Martin 1910; Jurina 1985: 91–9, and for quacks,
   278–9. For Van Foreest on quackery, Nutton 1996: 243.
74 Gambaccini 2004: 83–5; Gentilcore 2006: 302–6.
75 Boudon-Millot and Michaud 2020.
76 For a French religious print of 1594, punning on the word *catholicon* and
   showing a performing charlatan, Salmon 1979: fig. 20.
77 *Credite experto* – and it remained effective for a good number of years.
78 Harkness 2007: 80–96; see later, p. 299.
79 Harkness 2007: 85–96.
80 Eamon 1994: 168–93.
81 Gnudi and Webster 1950: 115–21.
82 Coppa in Venice also produced many writings, including a book of *Secrets*,
   his own poetry and a tract on courtly behaviour, Gambaccini 2004: 70, n. 23:
   Gentilcore 2006: 360–2.
83 This episode is discussed by Eamon 2005.
84 Nutton 1996; Siraisi 2013: 42–7; Murphy 2019: 147–71.
85 Eamon 1994.
86 O'Malley 1964: 285–8.
87 Clark 1964: 384.
88 Brockliss and Jones 1997: 236.
89 Cipolla 1976: 78–85.
90 Roberts 1962: 371; Pelling and Webster 1979: 225–7.
91 Brockliss and Jones 1997: 201–4; Pelling and Webster 1979: 225–7.
92 Pelling and Webster 1979: 182–8.
93 Earlier, p. 161; Nutton 1996: 246.
94 Roberts 1962: 371; Wear 2000: 24.
95 Lindemann 2010: 276.
96 Marguerite de Navarre 1946: 26, 32.
97 Nutton 1985c, 2018a: 41, n. 3; Gilly 1991; Sawday 1995; Dandrey 2002, with
   Brockliss and Jones 1997: 336–43; Decamp 2016; Schleiner 2014 gives a variety of examples of Renaissance medical humour.
98 Bentivoglio 1719: 145–239; De Blasi 1966 gives his biography.
99 *Ibid.*, 88–92; Bentivoglio 1987: 57–66.
100 Zum Trübel 1528: sig. B iii r. The allegation goes back at least to Piny the Elder.
101 Jurina 1985: 204–5, 286, 288.
102 Stolberg 2021b: 25–6.
103 Porter 1985: 1–22. For the need for compromise in New Spain between the
    medical ideas of the conquerors and those of the natives and slaves, Slater *et al.*
    2014.
104 Earlier, pp. 52, 48.
105 See later, p. 278, 290, 297.

7 On the Margins of Medical History
Women and Patients

Little has been said so far in this book about the one group that arguably made the greatest contribution to the health of the community, women. Their overwhelming lack of literacy has meant that their ideas and opinions have largely disappeared or require to be reconstructed at second hand from the reports of others.[1] The unacknowledged prejudices of older historians also pushed them to the margins by concentrating on the history of medicine either as a history of discoveries, to which women contributed little, or as a history of institutions, the colleges, universities and associations from which women were excluded almost entirely until the late nineteenth century. In their turn writers like Kate Hurd-Mead focussed on a few exceptional names and pioneering ventures by women in peace and war to create a genealogy for their own medical practice.[2] But this told us little about women's medical activities in general, for the few women who published their own accounts such as Louise Bourgeois or Elizabeth Cellier explicitly contrasted their own methods and successes with the great majority of female healers.[3] It was not until the rise in feminist scholarship from the 1970s that historians began to look more widely at the role of women in healing and explore the history of midwifery and nursing, two areas of medicine in which women predominated but whose history had been largely neglected by generations of male physician-historians. But by comparison with the seventeenth and eighteenth centuries, or even the Middle Ages, the sixteenth has proved unfruitful, with a paucity of printed sources and much archival work still to be done, particularly for the period before 1550.[4]

Women's Work

Women in the Late Middle Ages, it is now clear, were not entirely excluded from guilds concerned with healing or neglected by official medical licensing bodies. In the kingdom of Naples in the first half of the fourteenth century 18 women were licensed to practise surgery compared with 3,000 men, almost all of them the daughters or wives of doctors or surgeons except for Cusina di Filippo di Pastino, licensed as a 'magistra chirurgiae' at Cosenza and the daughter of a kettlesmith. Similar licences were issued to female

DOI: 10.4324/9781003223184-10

barber-surgeons in Venice, and four women matriculated as members in the Florence Guild. Two more are mentioned in tax records there from the 1350s, one of them a ringworm doctor (a common disease in children). The same pattern can be found in Paris and London, where the Guild of Barber-Surgeons seems to have admitted women, almost all the wives, daughters and occasionally servants of members, but without granting them the full privileges of the livery.[5] Widows of apothecaries were also allowed to continue making up drugs, but only under the supervision of an appropriately qualified man. The rise of university-trained physicians, as well as a growing focus on textual knowledge as a basis for practice, handicapped women practitioners still further from the later fifteenth century onwards, for few women could read and write, let alone in anything other than their own vernacular. The ignorance of women healers is a constant theme in complaints made against them. Those literate in Latin and even Greek, like Margaret Giggs, the wife of John Clement, a fine Greek scholar in her own right, belonged to gentry families or higher and had no wish to practise a trade.[6]

Official restraints on women who wished to act as physicians can be found across Europe from the late fifteenth century. In 1471 Pope Sixtus IV forbade any unqualified man or woman from practising medicine in Rome or in papal territory, leaving the supervision of his edict to the Rome College of Physicians and, later, to the papal *Protomedico*.[7] A similar ban on women physicians was in force in France, resulting in prosecutions and the jailing of women who were secretly practising medicine that are recorded from Paris in 1507 and Toulouse in 1558. Charles VIII in 1484 had forbidden women from practising as surgeons, although exceptions seem occasionally to have been granted for widows of surgeons. By 1500 their numbers had, however, dwindled to a mere handful. That did not stop some women from attending dissections 50 years later at Montpellier, where the King's writ was not easily enforced.[8] A few female barber-surgeons are known from the Netherlands, but by the 1550s they were only marginally active in cupping and bleeding, confining themselves to cosmetics and acting as midwives.[9] In all these cases, these were women who had learned their trade within the family, and wished to practise it in the wider town community. In a village the transition from looking after one's family to helping neighbours was a small step that could easily produce a growing medical reputation in the surrounding area, particularly in the absence of male healers.

The line between what was permissible and what was not was also based on ideas of morality and appropriate methods of healing. In England the Act of 1511 that insisted on a Bishop's licence to practice was also partly directed against women who "bodily and accustomably take upon themselves great Cures and things of great difficulty, in the which they partly use Sorcery and Witchcraft". But this Act, as we have seen, was not always enforced and the so-called Quacks' Charter of 1542 allowed "honest men and women" to continue to use herbal medicines.[10] Yet only a tiny number of women seem to have received licences to practise medicine or surgery from a Bishop, and many of them had practised for years before the grant. Prosecutions continued in London and sporadically elsewhere, almost always when it was felt that a woman was treating cases that might normally have been treated by a man. But as with prosecutions of unlicensed males, a word from a highly placed magnate could usually suffice to block proceedings. In 1602 the College of Physicians was intent on charging a Mrs Woodhouse until they received a letter from the Lord Treasurer, Lord Sackville, informing them that it was he who had sent for her to deal with his daughter's dislocated limb.[11] The case of Margaret Kennix in 1581, however, shows that the College might be prepared to defy a letter from even a high Secretary of State, if it thought fit. It wished to prosecute this "outlandish, ignorant, sorry woman", but Sir Francis Walsingham argued in his letter that Queen Elizabeth, no less, wished her to continue to practise "quietly" with her simples amongst the poor and use her "small talent" for the benefit of her sick husband and her family. The College, who had already turned down an informal request from Walsingham, instead suggested a meeting to clear the air and avoid a dangerous precedent. Its outcome or indeed whether it ever took place is unknown.[12]

Any estimate of the numbers of women healers is almost impossible, not least because all women were expected to know about herbs and how to prepare simple remedies from them.[13] The surgeon Thomas Gale, complaining in 1562 that the health of patients at St Bartholomew's and St Thomas's hospitals had been damaged by their treatment by witches, women and counterfeit juiviels [rascals], estimated that there were 60 women in London practising medicine and surgery.[14] But there were likely to have been many more, unless Gale was referring only to those who came into the two hospitals, and there was a common belief then, largely confirmed for late-Tudor Essex by modern archival research, that almost every village would have a women with a knowledge of herbs, and sometimes more.[15] As Bishop Latimer put it in 1552, "A great many of us. When we be in trouble, or sickness, or lose anything, we run hither and thither to witches or sorcerers . . . seeking aid and comfort at their hands".[16] Town councils often paid a woman to attend the poor when they suffered injuries, thus saving money on a male practitioner, and London parishes in the sixteenth century regularly paid poor women to nurse the sick and to check on those shut up and suffering from plague, an easy extension of their household tasks.[17] They were also called in to treat poor children: as in medieval Florence (earlier, p. 181); ringworm in children was often dealt with by women as an extension of home nursing.[18] They regularly assisted their husbands in running 'hospitals' for those most in need – the desperately poor and sufferers from plague or the final stages of syphilis. They prepared food, washed the laundry, provided comfort and assisted with the administration of drugs, and possibly much else. Particularly in Catholic regions there were religious orders of nurses who worked in hospitals and the community, but the papal ruling of 1566 that ordered all female orders to observe the rules of enclosure put an end to this in Catholic Europe for half a century.[19] But elsewhere nursing in the home and the hospital, which might involve some medical skills, was overwhelmingly a feminine occupation. Elsheimer's beautiful painting of St Elizabeth of Hungary serving in a hospital (Figure 2.3) is dominated by female attendants. In German towns, the *Meisterin*, the wife of the master of the local hospital, often played an arguably more important role in directly caring for the sick than her husband. The names of women involved in this task figure far more prominently in the archives than those of midwives or male medics, which suggests that their place in the wider economy of healing has been substantially underestimated.[20] But there were also limits. In 1558, Marieta Colochi, the widow of the late superintendent of the plague hospital, applied for a post as a plague doctor on the ground of her experience in epidemics. Her application did not get far, although she continued to be paid for her services in the *lazaretto* and her family continued to serve there until the end of the century.[21]

There can thus be little doubt that the corporatisation of medicine in the sixteenth century led to the exclusion of women from areas where they had been at least fitfully visible before. Even the paid employment of women by London parishes to attend the sick poor is also a sign of the low esteem in which they were held, for this allowed the community to support another disadvantaged group, elderly women and usually widows.[22] Margaret Pelling has argued strongly that professionalisation also represented a way in which the male practitioners could distinguish themselves from the feminine aspects of caring and curing and move away from the subordination of the domestic servant. They, not their wealthy clients, gave orders about health, and, at least in theory, claimed as a result to be of a higher social status than women attendants.[23] Increasingly also, the textualisation of medicine only confirmed their superior knowledge of women's internal health, thus restricting further the role of female healers and limiting their involvement.[24] Male apothecaries equally sought to distinguish their preparation of complex drugs with many ingredients from the simple remedies of the domestic kitchen. The doctor in Marguerite de Navarre's play is shocked when he hears that the wife of the sick man has proposed using herbs and pigeon broth (something forbidden in Languedoc, he claims) for these are general remedies, potentially dangerous if one does not know the particular humoral constitution of the patient.[25] Historians have also pointed to the wider context of the lower status of women in guilds in general, where they were paid less, only very rarely held office and were progressively forbidden to trade on their own behalf. The rhetoric used against them in all societies emphasised their age, lack of attractiveness and association with witches and sorcery, a link that even those who, like Johann Weyer (see later, p. 306), offered different explanations for women's behaviour, still accepted as true. The fact that many female healers were illiterate only strengthened the belief that their knowledge could not have been acquired from books but only through consorting with practitioners of forbidden arts.[26] It was an opinion that, as we shall see, (later, p. 196), involved both a class and a gender bias, and possibly also a religious one as well among those who believed that the role of the woman was firmly within the home and subject to the will of her husband.

There was one partial exception to this exclusion: midwifery, which often included not only looking after the various stages of pregnancy but also caring for young children. The day-to-day management of women's diseases was also almost entirely the province of women. Celestina, the evil go-between in one of the most famous of all Spanish Renaissance plays, was an old woman with a variety of occupations including those of sempstress, perfumer, cosmetician and, to a certain extent, a magician. (Women's multi-tasking goes back a long way.) She was famous for her knowledge of plant and animal recipes, dabbled a little in magic, and was reputed to have destroyed and repaired hundreds of maidenheads. The author, Fernando de Rojas, described at length the contents of her pharmacy and the still room that she used in preparing her love potions.[27] In a novel of 1524, the author, Francisco Delicado, made his heroine Lozana a similarly expert pupil of Celestina: the book's title page shows her attending to sick women and children while on a boat sailing from Rome to Venice (!).[28] But when things went wrong, it was accepted that even an experienced midwife would have to call in a male professional who had the knowledge and in a difficult birth also the strength to bring matters to a conclusion, even if it ended in the death and dismemberment of the child, or worse.[29] Midwifery was also a special case in that in many parts of Europe it was formally regulated by civic and religious authorities.[30] In many German regions and the Netherlands prospective midwives were not allowed to practise before being examined and approved by a board that usually contained one or two senior midwives, sometimes a medical man, but often a representative of the church or the town, usually an 'honourable' woman, the wife of a councillor.[31] The examining panel was usually provided with a set of questions for the would-be town midwife. Had she children of her own? How many births had she attended? What food and drink would help to ease the birth? What advice would she give to the new mother? The doctor would pose medical questions, the cleric and the patrician lady were concerned with her morality – although some ladies in Southern Germany declined the task of interviewing someone of lower standing and practising a trade.[32] It was important for the ecclesiastical authorities, across the confessional divide, to approve the religious and moral comportment of any approved midwife, for it must often have fallen to her to deal with a child *in extremis* at birth and to be able to administer the baptismal rites that would ensure its arrival in heaven. Hence the suspicion of Jewish midwives or, in Iberia, of women who were *conversos*, recent converts from Islam or Judaism, since by ignorance or design they might fail to act and the child would literally be left in limbo. Morisco midwives were forbidden in 1554 in Granada and in 1561 in Valencia to practise on the grounds that "when children are born they usually circumcise them". They were only allowed to attend a delivery in the presence of an (Old-)Christian physician who would prevent the rite of circumcision. Non-Morisco surgeons who failed to do so or who complained were frequently themselves prevented from practising at all.[33] Catholics after the Council of Trent in the mid-century took an even stricter view of the midwife's responsibility for baptism. A 1570 proposal at a Council in Milan that all midwives should ensure that a new-born child was baptised within a week was eagerly taken up by many French dioceses, and it was extended by a suggestion at the Council of Malines in 1607 that the duty of the midwife was to inform the parish priest if a family had failed to bring the child for baptism. Her spiritual orthodoxy was at least as important as her obstetrical competence, for it would ensure the eternal life of the child as well as, it was hoped, its survival on earth.[34]

Far more than England, Continental Europe in the sixteenth century showed an increasing concern for official standards, and, as Flügge notes, also aroused hostility from those experienced women who failed to meet them.[35] As well as the examination for those who wished to be a town midwife, many places laid down appropriate standards that they expected all midwives to follow. Paris in 1560 established a system of apprenticeship under an approved midwife supervised by the royal barber or via training in the Hôtel-Dieu. The final examination was made before the surgeons of the Châtelet, and the successful candidate was allowed to put up a sign and authorised to appear as a witness in cases of rape, pregnancy and impotence.[36] Similar ordinances were issued in German towns, especially taking into account the Evangelical ideals of the community at large. They frequently specified what practical knowledge they expected of the midwife. Did she know how to turn a child before birth? Did she know the stages of labour and thus how to encourage the parturient to "patience and tolerance" and thereby conserve her strength before the final stage of labour, for it was extremely dangerous for her to become exhausted before the cervix was properly dilated? Could she recognise the existence of a dead foetus? These and similar questions were posed in the examination of midwives for the next two centuries, suggesting little change in practice over this period before the arrival of male midwives in the late eighteenth century.[37] While this may be true for most of the sixteenth century, this static picture may also be the result of a bias within the sources. Eucharius Rösslin's *Rosengarten*, the first printed text on midwifery in 1513, was translated from German into Latin, French and English (1540), and was still being sold well into the seventeenth century.[38] Jacob Rueff's Latin treatise on conception was published in both Latin and German in 1554, and soon after that in Dutch, and an English version, titled *The Expert Midwife*, appeared as late as 1657.[39] But Louise Bourgeois (1563–1636), the wife of a respectable Paris barber-surgeon who developed a very large and profitable practice as a midwife from the 1590s, including acting as a royal midwife, would have rejected the idea that she was merely repeating the advice of past centuries. Her book of

1626 contains many observations drawn from her considerable experience as well as a vigorous critique of the ignorant conservatism of contemporary midwives.[40] However, it may also be significant that the two most celebrated novel techniques in this period were both associated with surgeons acting in desperate circumstances. The debate over caesarean section (earlier, p. 18), was carried on between surgeons, while Paré first learned about podalic version, turning a foetus lying transversally in the womb so that its legs can slip easily into the cervix, from two other surgeons, and they may not have been the first to employ the technique. Convincing evidence for its use by midwives is, alas, missing.[41]

On the Continent the midwife, who in the fifteenth century had been left largely to her own devices, was becoming more and more subject to the supervision of men and for purposes that were not always primarily medical. Being able to appear in court as an expert witness gave her a certain status compared with others who could not, but it was only done in a limited range of cases. The Carolina, the law code that from 1532 became mandatory throughout the Holy Roman Empire, placed the testimony of midwives and surgeons on the same level. But as the century wore on, the midwife became more and more viewed simply as a woman and housewife rather than as a medical expert. Indeed, the testimony of midwives in cases involving virginity or the unexpected death of a child could be openly disputed by male surgeons, and the taint of association with witches, poisoners and illiterates downgraded the value of their evidence in the face of contrary testimony from a learned surgeon like Paré.[42] This presumed superiority of men over women was only one of the reasons why Laurent Joubert, professor of medicine and Chancellor of Montpellier, was aggrieved when he and equally learned colleagues were blocked from attending a woman suffering from "suffocation of the womb" by an old midwife who declared that she was in fact pregnant and thus was her responsibility alone.[43]

Medical Notions of Women

But what did a male doctor or surgeon know about women? Or even women about women? Certainly, through their networks within the family and community women could transmit to one another details of their bodies and their workings from their own experiences that were not readily available to males, who would have had less chance of seeing a female body except at an autopsy.[44] Portraits of doctors attending women show them taking the pulse and examining urine, but not performing more than an external examination, and sometimes not even that, if, as often happened, a family member brought details of the case to the doctor by letter.[45] Surviving case notes show that doctors saw male patients far more often than they did female, and touching a female body, although it did occur, required tact, delicacy and the patient's consent, which was not always possible.[46] Women would have been more familiar with female ailments such as mastitis and uterine prolapse, and their understanding of quickening would have been more accurate than the schematic rulings of the church and the no less fanciful conclusions of physicians as to when and how the embryo became ensouled.[47] But learned women's explanations for these phenomena would have differed little from medical speculations, although they might be expressed with less subtlety and fewer citations of earlier authorities. All parties viewed the suppression of menstruation, except for pregnancy, as potentially hazardous, and warned against the dangers of that most female of complaints, hysteria and the suffocation of the womb. They all believed that imagination or the evil eye could have a direct effect on the unborn child, a notion no more fanciful than the argument of the humanist Juan Luis Vives, who claimed the abundance of monstrous births in Flanders resulted from mothers' overindulgence in beer and cabbage.[48] But there is no sense that apart from the normal process of birth (for the rise of the man midwife was a long way in the future), women's ailments were to be treated solely by women. Even if women's ailments were increasingly being discussed as something separate from those of men, they were still subject to the same range of explanations.[49] Obstetrical and gynaecological problems were not the exclusive province of women, and sterility or miscarriages, seen as the result of internal bodily changes, were a prime concern of doctors as well as of apothecaries who provided drugs to promote and in some instances prevent pregnancy. Indeed, Monica Green argues that in the second half of the sixteenth century, male writings with a specific focus on obstetrics and the birth process, and hence intended for both a male and female readership, were replaced by wider discussions about women's diseases or gynaecology that privileged explanations and experiences, as well as texts, which greatly diminished the authority of women to decide upon their own health.[50]

An intellectual investigation into what a woman was and how she might differ from a man required a complex triangulation between three acknowledged authorities, the Bible, Aristotle and Galen.[51] All of them had been studied and commented on for centuries, and all faced new challenges in the sixteenth century. The biblical account in *Genesis* of the creation of Eve from Adam's rib as well as a literal reading of several Pauline injunctions emphasised the subordinate nature of women. Drawing on earlier Greek polarities, Aristotle argued for the manifold inferiority of women, from the number of their teeth and their intellectual deficiencies to their role in the generation of the human species: woman provided merely the material form that was made human through the formative principle contained within the male semen.[52] His arguments from his biological investigations provided strong support for those, like St Thomas Aquinas in the Middle Ages, who considered woman to be an inferior version of man.[53]

Medieval scholastics had adapted their Galen relatively easily to this Aristotelianism. They knew that Galen differed from Aristotle in his view of generation, but they had no easy access to the texts in which Galen set out his opinions, most of which, like his tract on the formation of the foetus or that on semen, were available mainly or only in Greek or via Arabic intermediaries. Another treatise *On Seed* ascribed to Galen and circulating widely in both Latin and Middle English is a curious astrological text that goes back at least in part to the Greek world of Late Antiquity.[54] Leoniceno had published his discussion of Galen's views on the formative principle of the foetus as early as 1506, but editions and translations of the Galenic originals and of the more extensive and varied texts in the Hippocratic Corpus had to wait until after 1525. (The most important of ancient gynaecological writers, Soranus of Ephesus (around 100 CE), was known only indirectly or in fragments and played little part in Renaissance discussions.) The 'new' treatises showed Galen's considerable disagreement with Aristotle. He believed that both men and women produced seed, and that it was the relationship between the two seeds that determined whether a child resembled its mother, father or both. There were obvious differences between the two sexes, both functionally and in their humoral balance. While all agreed that women were colder than men, and that her colder metabolism allowed them to retain some residues that would be necessary for the nutriment of the foetus and the production of milk, it was not clear whether there was a spectrum of heat among the sexes which would explain why some colder men could be dominated by some hotter women. Galenists rejected the Aristotelian notion of women as an imperfect man, let alone, as some joked, a monstrous birth. Nonetheless, their functional explanations and the strong link they saw between humoral balance (usually better in men) and mental capacity easily led to the same overall view of the role of women. Woman is as perfect in her sex as the male is in his, but at the same time inferior to him for physiological reasons.[55]

Most diseases affecting women could thus be easily treated on the same schema of opposites as those of men. But female physiology did not always fit neatly onto this template. While menstruation was seen as something healthy, the body excreting material it did not need, it was not only medics who debated whether the menses themselves were always harmful. Biblical injunctions, reinforced by church regulations, related them strongly to ritual uncleanness and even to the production of diseases, notably smallpox and sexually transmitted diseases. Fernel declared that they were always malignant, but Mercuriale and others argued that they became so only when the whole female body was unwell – still retaining at least some of the ancient prejudices about female blood.[56] A similarly long-standing prejudice related to the role of the uterus, and not least to the belief, found in the Hippocratics and Plato, that the wandering movements of the womb up and down the female body were responsible for a range of hysterical illness (although exactly what these were continued to be debated) and to engender both garrulity and an excessive desire for coitus. It was, said Galen's contemporary Aretaeus, like an animal inside an animal, all but alive.[57] That Galen had long ago dismissed this idea in favour of a restricted movement of the uterus caused by the constriction or weakening of the surrounding muscles and that sixteenth-century anatomists agreed with him did not put an end to popular ideas about it and its consequences, or the similar transference of human characteristics to other organs, such as the smiling spleen.[58]

It might be thought that discoveries made by the anatomists of the sixteenth century would have modified substantially opinions and ideas about the female body. The frontispiece of Vesalius's *Fabrica* proudly shows him demonstrating to a large audience an open abdominal cavity of a woman, a visual assertion of the superiority of his knowledge over what had gone before. This was visual rhetoric, for progress was in fact slow. The most significant collection of medical writings on gynaecology published in this period, first edited by Gessner in 1556 and enlarged by 1586 by Caspar Bauhin and still more in 1597 by Israel Spach (1560–1610), contained in its final form 20 separate treatises, none of which was specifically devoted to the female anatomy. Only a few illustrations on its opening pages, taken from Vesalius via Felix Platter, show the female body, but although Platter was the first anatomist to list and illustrate differences between the female and the male skeleton, Spach did not bother to include any images of the female skeleton.[59] Mercado in his work on women's diseases included in the same volume still believed in the (imagined) singularity of a cranial suture, the *sutura sagittalis*, in women that when blocked does not allow melancholic humours and spirits that have reached the brain to escape, and hence leads to perturbations or passions in the brain.[60] He, and his fellow writers, instead, followed traditional ideas about the workings of the female body, different in kind from that of a man, and were concerned almost entirely with diagnosis and treatment. They could also combine a variety of, to modern eyes, incompatible explanations. Van Foreest, for example, in book 29 of his *Observations* dealing with women's diseases, strongly rejected the notion of a wandering womb in favour of harmful vapours, while still believing in hysterical suffocation, as well as in the harmful effect of retained female seed.[61]

All anatomists were faced with a major difficulty, a lack of female bodies. Even if the rules for university anatomies stipulated that there should be a formal dissection of a female corpse every three years or so, this rarely happened. The Paduan statutes admit the difficulty, qualifying their insistence that there should be a male and a female body dissected annually with the phrase "or at least one of them". Female criminals were far less likely than men to be executed, the main source of bodies for official dissections, and those condemned for witchcraft faced burning far more often than hanging. Andrea Carlino lists no woman among the 19 individuals recorded as having been publicly dissected in Rome between 1556 and 1586.[62] Only one woman dissected by Vesalius was executed, a women who had sought to avoid this punishment by pleading pregnancy, a plea correctly rejected by the midwives who had examined her.[63] The corpse of another, a nun, was specially removed from her tomb in Florence by permission of the Duke and sent to Pisa for Vesalius to dissect and make into a skeleton.[64] He dissected

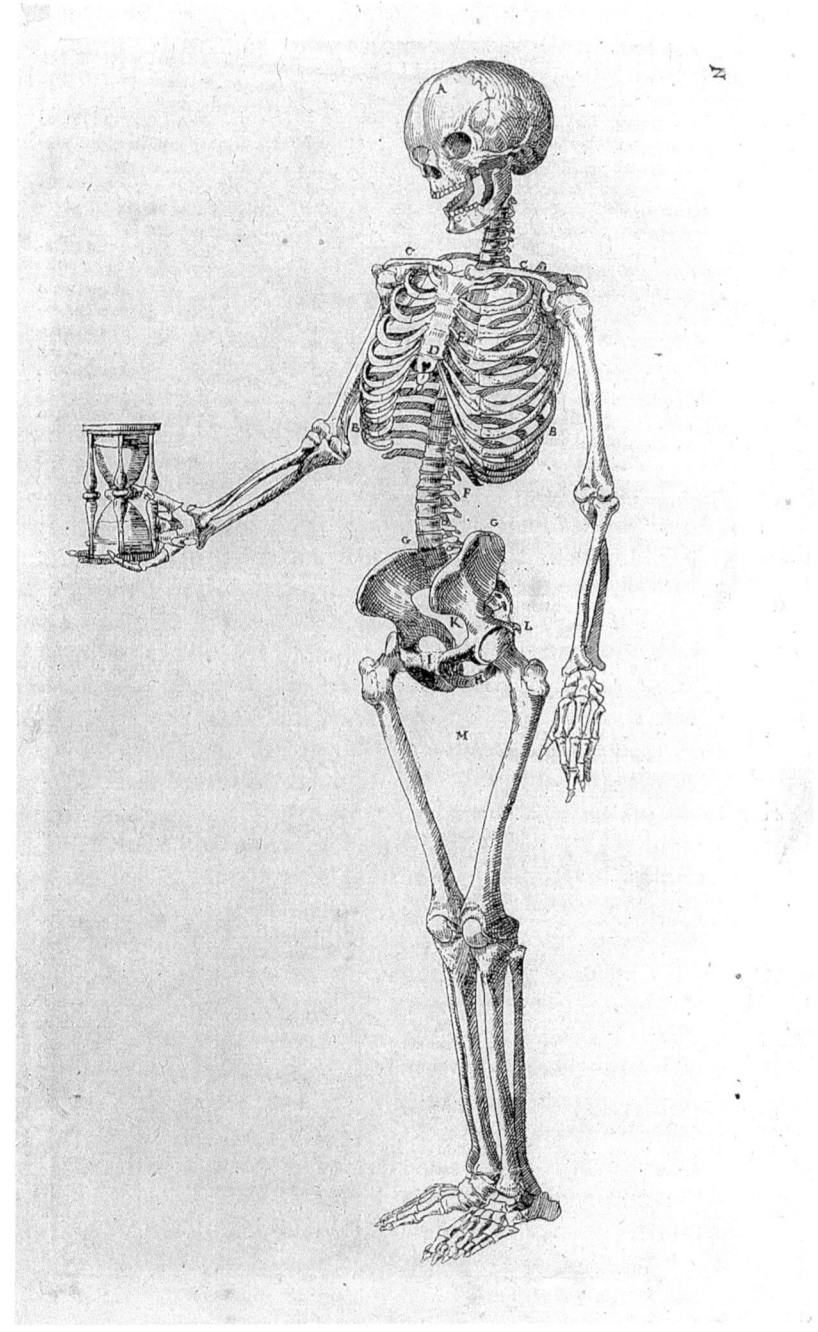

Figure 7.1 The skeleton of a woman, from Felix Platter's *De corporis humani structura et usu*, Basle, A. Froben, 1583.

three others in public displays. One of them, that of the mistress of a monk, had been obtained somewhat illegally by his students, like the body of a 6-year-old girl at Pisa removed from her tomb also by students. Others, probably dissected in private, were of disreputable or luckless women, a couple of prostitutes, a hunchback of 18, a woman beaten to death by her husband and two who had died in childbirth. Only one, a girl in the entourage of the Countess of Egmont, seems to have been dissected in an autopsy.[65] Realdo Colombo likewise proudly recorded his public dissection at Pisa, by special authorisation of the Medici Duke, of a woman condemned for killing her two illegitimate children by suffocation. The period between execution and dissection was small enough for him to show his audience, Valverde among them, the blood flowing from the uterus during her period.[66] Falloppia certainly dissected several female corpses and after his death one of his students, Georg Purkircher, in 1564, reported proudly how he had assisted at the autopsy of a teenager who had died of emphysema and had seen the clitoris just as his master had described, although he was unable to locate the hymen.[67]

But it was one thing to observe, and another to present the results of one's observations in a manner that was clear and convincing (and accessible) to others. Falloppia's *Observations*, which contain probably the best account of female anatomy at the time, are difficult to follow because they are couched in the form of a critical commentary on Vesalius, and Vesalius's largely dismissive response is still more so. The dispute between the two men, as well as uncertainties about the hymen and clitoris, will have hampered the formation of a clear understanding of the female reproductive system. Book V of the *Fabrica* is its weakest by far, its mistakes excused by its author on the grounds that he had little experience of dissecting women, although more than some had alleged, and that, when he did have the chance, he rarely could observe everything with as much care as he would have liked. Midwives, he complained, were extremely reluctant to admit any male to see the moment of birth, and his text does not give any indication that they had made an exception for him.[68] Portraying the internal organs added new problems, as can be seen neatly in the images in Charles Estienne's anatomy books. That of the external surface of the womb of a pregnant woman was drawn accurately by his artist from the dissection performed by the surgeon De la Rivière, but that of the two foetuses within it owes far more to traditional images than to reality. The small size of the wood blocks used by Estienne and his publisher meant that details of the external genitalia were almost impossible to discern, even if they had been drawn accurately.[69] In other artistic representations the visual conjunction between old beliefs and new discoveries is doubly striking. On the one hand, modern interpreters can see almost at a glance what to them are obvious errors. Beautiful and accurate as Leonardo's depictions of women's external bodies are, in those of the internal body he follows medieval precedent in drawing a multi-chambered womb and a direct connection between the womb and the breasts that would allow menstrual blood to pass upwards to form milk.[70] In a famous image he showed with great accuracy the position of the child in the womb, but the womb that surrounds it is more akin to the shell of a nut. Vesalius was no better. In the *Six Anatomical Plates*, and still more in the *Fabrica*, Vesalius improved on his predecessor Berengario in many ways. His plate of the abdominal cavity with the female urogenital tract was larger and more accurate than any previously published, but he still retained the idea of a connection between the womb and the breasts and his drawing of the uterus after it had been removed shows signs of a hurried dissection.[71]

Both Leonardo and Vesalius also held to the theory, ultimately going back to Aristotle, that the genital organs of the woman are a mirror-image of those of the male, one displayed externally, the other internally. So, for instance, the ovaries correspond to the testes, the cervix and vulva to the penis.[72] This relationship is displayed most clearly in the image of the uterus of a woman Vesalius had dissected at Padua.[73] But as Michael Stolberg and Helen King have trenchantly argued, this does not support the conclusion that Thomas Laqueur and others have drawn from it that all doctors from Antiquity until at least the late seventeenth century believed that there was only one sex, man, of which woman was but a poor imitation. Galen, as Vesalius and other anatomists knew well, had also stated that one could equally well say that the genitalia of a man were an inverted version of those of the female, and, if a comment recorded during his Bologna debates with Corti is his, Vesalius also pointed to differences between the two.[74] Nonetheless, because, as his text makes clear, he regarded the uterus as including what we would term the vagina and cervix, the 'long neck of the uterus', the penis-like image that occupies most of the plate emphasises far more than any words in his accompanying discussion or caption the inverse relationship between the male and female genitalia.[75] Their size and striking detail draw the reader's eye away from the womb itself, with the result that the image forcefully sends out a message that Vesalius may not have intended.

Given that learned doctors could reach such disparate conclusions from a limited amount of evidence, it is not surprising that Rabelais, a doctor himself, should have directed some of his sharpest satire against his fellow practitioners at their ideas about the female body. In his *Tiers Livre*, Dr Rondibilis is called in by Pantagruel as an expert to advise Panurge whether he should marry or not. After a long exposition on how one might reduce the perils of concupiscence, he concludes that Panurge and his putative wife are of a sufficiently sound temperament to be allowed to marry. But he is still concerned about Plato's view of the womb as a raging animal, likely to engender a host of ills from epilepsy and apoplexy to mere nasty smells. Galen, he reports, holds a different view to that of Aristotle, but, even with Galen's more favourable opinion, nothing, he concludes, can prevent a wife from cuckolding a husband, such is the ferocity of her hidden animal. Finally, he wishes to examine the urine and pulse of the lady, following an aphorism of Hippocrates, to see if she is pregnant, only to be rebuffed by Panurge,

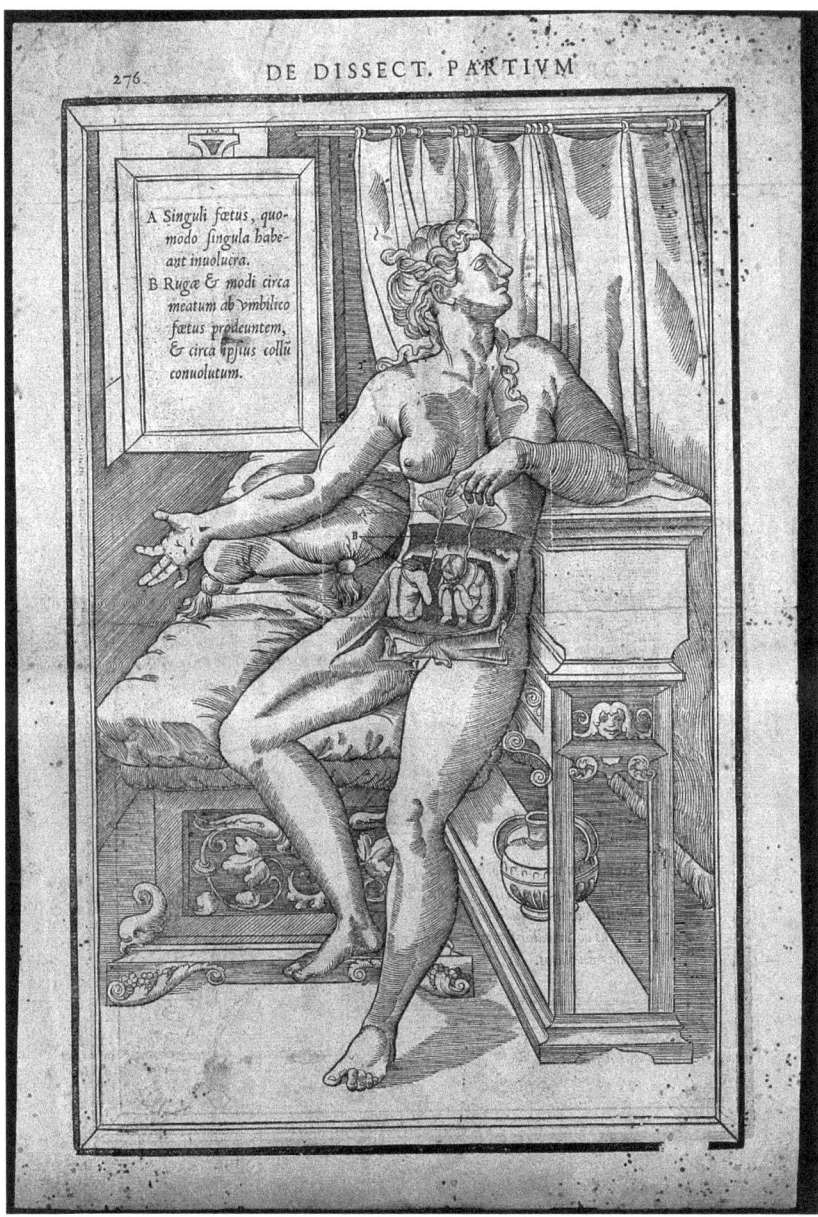

Figure 7.2 Twins in the womb. Although some of the drawings of a pregnant woman in Charles Estienne's *De dissectione*, Paris, S. de Colines, 1545, were made during the removal of a dead foetus, others are more fanciful. The details are also difficult to make out because they were engraved onto a small printing block which, as can be seen, was then inserted in an already existing larger block.

194   *People*

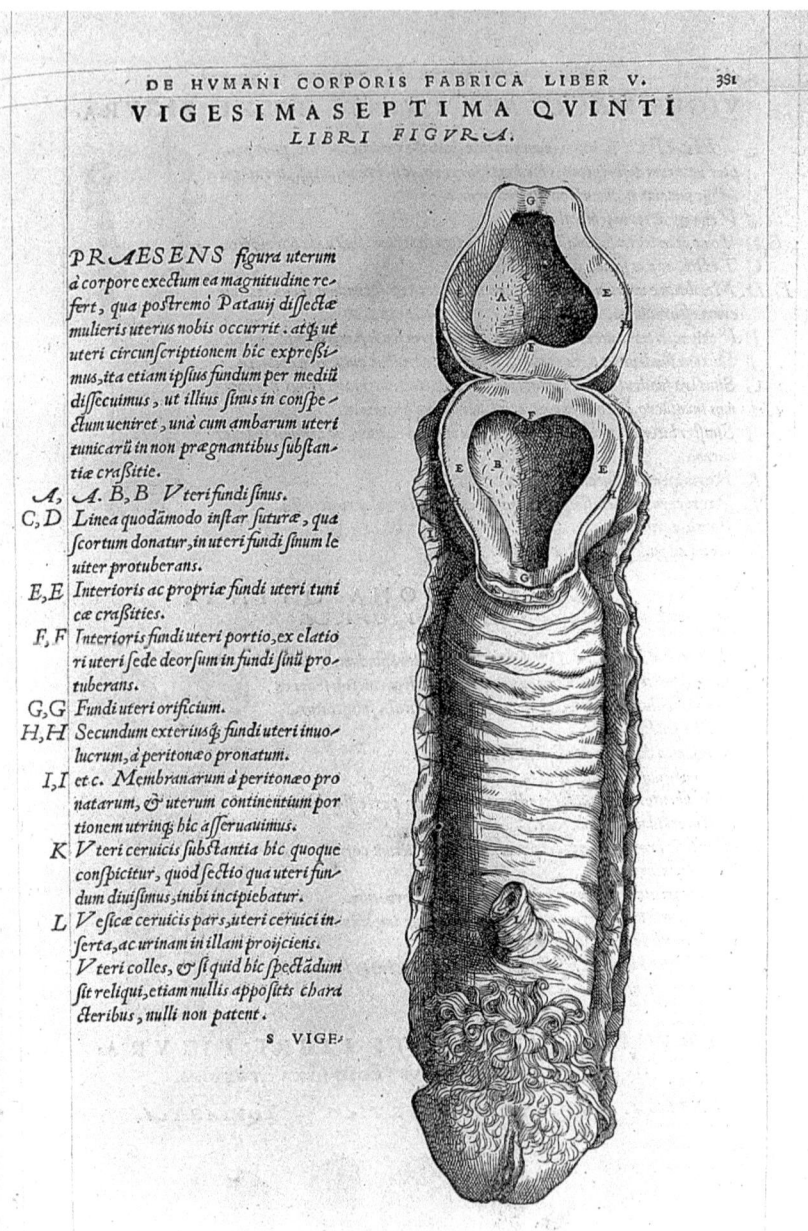

VIGESIMASEPTIMA QVINTI
LIBRI FIGVRA.

*PRAESENS figura uterum
à corpore exectum ea magnitudine re-
fert, qua postremò Patauij dissectæ
mulieris uterus nobis occurrit. atq; ut
uteri circunscriptionem hìc expressi-
mus, ita etiam ipsius fundum per mediũ
dissecuimus, ut illius sinus in conspe-
ctum ueniret, unà cum ambarum uteri
tunicarũ in non prægnantibus substan-
tiæ crassitie.*

A, *A.* B, B *Vteri fundi sinus.*

C, D *Linea quodãmodo instar suturæ, qua
scortum donatur, in uteri fundi sinum le
uiter protuberans.*

E, E *Interioris ac propriæ fundi uteri tuni
cæ crassities.*

F, F *Interioris fundi uteri portio, ex elatio
ri uteri sede deorsum in fundi sinũ protuberans.*

G, G *Fundi uteri orificium.*

H, H *Secundum exteriúsq; fundi uteri inuo-
lucrum, à peritonæo pronatum.*

I, I *et c. Membranarum à peritonæo pro
natarum, & uterum continentium por
tionem utrinq; hìc asseruauimus.*

K *Vteri ceruicis substantia hìc quoque
conspicitur, quòd sectio qua uteri fundum diuisimus, inibi incipiebatur.*

L *Vesicæ ceruicis pars, uteri ceruici in-
serta, ac urinam in illam proijcieris.
Vteri colles, & si quid hìc spectãdum
sit reliqui, etiam nullis appositis chara
cteribus, nulli non patent.*

s VIGE-

Figure 7.3 The uterus of a woman dissected by Andreas Vesalius, *De humani corporis fabrica*, Basle, J. Oporinus, 1543, p. 381 [481]. The image stretches
almost the full height of the very large page.

who declares that this is a matter for a lawyer familiar with the Justinianic legal regulations on inspecting the belly. The worthy doctor leaves, having pocketed a large fee. This satire is all the more piquant because Rabelais's notes on Galen show that he had reread some of his books on generation just before he put pen to paper.[76]

This confusion is attacked in a more sober way by Laurent Joubert, who devoted most of the first volume of his *Popular Errors* to matters concerning sex, pregnancy, childbirth and the care of the neonate. These four books are longer than all the others, although this may be because he changed his original plan and shortened the rest of his planned 30 books, which were to deal with all remaining aspects of medicine and health, in order to fit into a single volume.[77] His list of errors is very long. Is it a good idea to sit a woman in labour over a hot cauldron, or as some good wives do in villages near Montpellier put the husband's hat on the stomach? The last, he thought, may have originally been to symbolise the presence of the husband. There is no truth in the notion that a woman who gives birth under a full moon will have a son at the next birth; if under a new moon, she will next have a daughter.[78] Joubert remained sceptical about monstrous births in the shape of birds or animals, and even more so about the hobgoblins or harpies that would escape from the womb and fly around the room, but should not be killed, for that would result in the death of the woman. In his view these were so-called uterine moles, congealed blood expelled from the womb and almost certainly the result of a miscarriage.[79] Even if the story of a respectable midwife from Châtellerault who had claimed to have captured and smothered such a harpy were true, no harm came to the pregnant woman herself, who had beautiful children later.[80] He was not entirely opposed to women healers for he also had personal experience of the good that they could do. He acknowledges that some of the testimony offered by the official midwives in Béarn, Paris and Carcassonne had proved valuable, but considered that even midwives were ignorant about the anatomy of the uterus. He makes an exception for Mme Jeanne Massale, or Gervaise, whom he praises for never missing an official dissection at Montpellier when it was a woman who was being dissected.[81] He also dedicated his 1580 edition of the *Grande Chirurgie* of the medieval surgeon Guy de Chauliac to his mother, who had often assisted in bandaging the sick and poor and used an ointment for the nipples that had a great reputation through much of South and South-Eastern France.[82]

Women and Domestic Medicine

This example of Madame Joubert allows us to penetrate a little further into the world of women and their activity as healers.[83] A women writer like Louise Bourgeois was very much the exception, both in having access to the court and in publishing.[84] More often in the sixteenth century the voice of women can only be heard from two very different sources, the recipe books which they owned and the occasional deposition in a legal case. A rare example of such a deposition concerns Jean L'Escalier, a female 'empiric' practising around Angers in the 1560s and 1570s who was taken to court by the Angers Medical Faculty. She had been brought up by a wealthy benefactress who belonged to one of the leading families of France and from whom she learned her physic. She returned home, possibly after a period of foreign travel, and spent the rest of her life treating the poor and needy. Including those who had been given up for lost and left penniless by their doctors. She used oils and waters which she had distilled herself, and watched over her patients like a good physician, a type of medicine that, her lawyer claimed, needed no authorisation, for God had allowed the simplest of people to help those who needed it.[85] At the same time in Spain a Morisco woman Maria de Luna was practising medicine with great success, according to her son, Román Ramírez, when he testified before the Inquisition. She was the daughter of a distinguished healer, Juan de Luna, who had taught her all he knew. She gained a great reputation for her knowledge of herbs and her work as a midwife, and patients came to see her from miles around. She appears to have been illiterate, for she owned no books and any written recipes she might have had her son no longer retained in his possession. All his learning, like that of his mother, had been originally obtained orally, and he had to keep in his memory all the recipes and treatments that she had taught him. Indeed, the only book he owned was a copy of Laguna's Spanish version of Dioscorides that he had bought in Madrid around 1560, some 30 years before.[86]

An English healer of this kind, Margaret Hunt, similarly described her methods in 1528 when she was being examined before a legal officer of the Bishop of London. When visiting the sick, she first ascertained the name of the sick persons. She then knelt and prayed to the Trinity to free them from all ills and their enemies. They were then told to say for five consecutive nights five Paternosters, five Aves and a Creed, followed by three more Paternosters, three Aves and three Creeds. At bedtime they were to repeat one Ave and one creed in worship of St Ive, to save them from all envy. But she did not always rely entirely on prayers, for she also prescribed herbs for ague and for sores, remedies which she had learned from a Welsh woman, Mother Elmet. Seventy years later, Goodwife Veazy, an expert in the cure of "ringworm, tetter-worm and canker-worm", used prayers as well as applying a little honey and pepper to the afflicted part. For her services, she received the commendation of none other than Robert Cecil, Lord Burghley.[87]

These examples show that the range of women offering healing was almost as wide as that of men. All these women were well respected in their communities and enjoyed a great reputation for healing, but a lady with links, however tenuous, to the aristocracy who could afford the services of a lawyer in a complex suit enjoyed a very different status from that of a Morisco woman. For Maria de Luna, healing was a trade, for Jean L'Escalier it was part of her religious obligations to the poor and needy. Jean was clearly literate, possibly even in Latin, but Maria could read and write only with difficulty, if at all. We do not know how Jean learned her medicine, but Maria gained her expertise like an artisan within the family from her father. And beneath Maria, there will have been many women, like Margaret Hunt, who had learned their trade by association with other women in an oral tradition to which historians do not have access.[88] The description of Jean's practice fits neatly with that of Celestina, for she implies that, like her, she had a place where she could make her ointments and remedies, probably one much bigger than that of Maria. All three women were extending tasks that were the job of women within the home, such as cooking and treating minor ailments, to a wider community.

But there is a major difference in status between Jean and the others. Jean was on the fringes of the aristocracy, where a sense of obligation could extend beyond the immediate bounds of the house and family. By the end of the century, many women of this class in England were literate at least in English, and recipe books survive showing that they could copy, exchange and use remedies for treating the poor and needy.[89] Some of them, like Lady Margaret Hoby (1571–1633), may even have carried out minor surgery, although these will have been the exception, and, others, like their male counterparts, supported, and even practised, alchemy.[90] Lady Mary Herbert, Countess of Pembroke (1561–1621), was said by John Aubrey to be "a great Chymist" and to have spent a great deal of time each year in her own laboratory, as well as providing a yearly retainer for the Paracelsian Thomas Moffet.[91] Every gentry household was expected to have some basic instruments (as today) for dealing with minor injuries and ailments, and its still room could be used not just to produce refreshing drinks but also distillations that could be used to support the health of the family, something that was mainly the duty of the wife or mother.[92] The most celebrated of these Tudor ladies among historians was Lady Grace Mildmay (1552–1620), who had been taught medicine by her governess cousin, Mistress Hamblyn, who was herself well versed in both medicine and surgery. It was she who suggested to Grace that she should study closely William Turner's *Herbal* and Bartholomew Traheron's English translation of Vigo's *Practica* (which she supplemented with many other books). The detailed inventory of her still room shows a variety of bottles, apparatus and substances that could go towards the making of drugs on an almost professional scale. Aqua vitae and metheglin were made in batches of ten gallons a time, and to make oil of cinnamon required five pounds of cinnamon and five gallons of wine. This cost money. The over 150 different ingredients, including roots, herbs, spices, gums and purgatives, for one "most precious" healing balm came to ten guineas, a sizable percentage of her annual budget of £130 for running her household.[93]

But, as the example of Jean L'Escalier shows, similarly learned ladies from the upper and gentry classes were not confined to England. Anne de

Croy, Princesse de Chimay (d. 1539) and a member of the distinguished D'Albret family, selected "very special and singular recipes" in her notebook from the large collection that she had in her possession. Later owners, or members of the family, added further recipes in both French and Flemish.[94] Alisha Rankin has also drawn attention to such distinguished German aristocrats as Anna of Saxony, Dorothea von Mansfeld and Elizabeth von Rochlitz who took a detailed interest in medicine and pharmacy and provided treatments to many of those in need.[95] At the court of the Tyrol, the morganatic wife of Ferdinand II, Philippine Welser (1527–80), who had followed her mother in providing drugs and advice to women in Augsburg, had her own pharmacy in the castle at Ambras and collected together many recipes in a large volume.[96] These ladies were simply following in the footsteps of earlier male medical enthusiasts like the Palatine Elector Ludwig V (1508–44), who copied out in his own hand 13 volumes of medical recipes.[97]

But although such recipe collections often include some ascribed to or used by women healers, it is not always easy to decide whether an anonymous volume was owned or used by a woman, as Elaine Leong, the leading scholar of such books from the next century, admits. The spread of women's literacy in Europe, particularly from the 1550s, makes it likely that they were involved in their production, particularly when they contain advice on cookery or cosmetics, as in Wellcome WMS 634 (English), 639 (Flemish) and 659 (Italian), but the overwhelming majority before then were owned and written by men. Two notebooks in the Wellcome Collection and a third in the British Library coming from the same area a century or more apart and owned and used in the sixteenth century by the same owner show a typical mixture of much older recipes along with others supplied by friends or obtained through networks of genteel ladies.[98] Wellcome WMS 5282, written around 1450, was owned in the early sixteenth century by a surgeon, Andrew Wylkynson, before it passed into the hands of a country gentleman, Henry Dyneley (d. 1589). He had obtained British Library, Royal MS A.17.xxxii in 1560/1 and was already in possession of Wellcome WMS 244 by 1564. All show annotations by people living in the North Cotswolds and were clearly well used by the various owners. Henry himself announced on the flyleaf of this last manuscript that the letters HD alongside a recipe indicated that he had tried out and proved the worth of these medicines, oils and ointments. After his death, the book came into the hands of Sir Francis Dyneley, and was annotated further in 1592 by another Henry Dyneley with gardening information. At all periods additional material recording proven remedies was constantly being made at the foot or in the margins. Other notebooks of this type, written in a more practised hand, suggest that when a book became full or was in danger of falling apart, it was carefully recopied for further use.[99]

The miscellaneous contents of some of these collections are mirrored in cheap printed books, particularly in almanacs, such as the *Calendrier des*

Bergers, The Shepherds' Calendar, sold for 6 sous, where one might find weather information and advice on gardening as well as medical recipes and advice on when to let blood.[100] The same combination occurs in France at a slightly higher level in the books on agriculture written by physicians such as Antoine Mizaud, Charles Estienne, the earlier writer on anatomy, and his collaborator and son-in-law, Jean Liébault (c. 1535–96).[101] Their 1572 *Agriculture et maison rustique, Farming and the Country House*, went through several editions as well as being translated into German (1580), Italian (1591) and English (1606). Liébault's published works had a strong female bias. His first published medical work, a large compendium of practical guides to health in Latin, contained as its second part a Latin version of Rösslin's *Rosengarten, Rose Garden*. Five years later, in 1582, he brought out two huge volumes, one on gynaecology (called in a later edition *A Treasury of Secret Remedies for the Diseases of Women*), the other on cosmetics, both French versions of Italian works by Giovanni Marinelli (fl. 1563).[102] Neither these nor the *Maison rustique* could be classified as domestic medicine, except for the fact that their male reader would be expected to pass some of their information down to womenfolk or his servants. They were too large, too expensive and too learned for even the moderately literate, and were, like Guillemeau's and Louise Bourgeois's books on childbirth, almost certainly above the heads of many of the midwives they claimed to wish to educate.[103]

The later title of Liébault's book on gynaecology, a *Treasury of Secret Remedies*, places it firmly within the tradition of secrets discussed by William Eamon. Published around Europe and aimed at a literate male audience, these were miscellaneous compendia, usually in the vernacular, covering many aspects of household management, and especially giving advice on remedies and distillation.[104] To judge from the numbers that were published, they were extremely popular, being cheaply printed on poor paper and easily carried around the countryside for sale. The most famous of them, that written by Alexis of Piedmont, went through 70 editions between its first appearance in 1555 and 1600. It was clearly aimed at an audience of wealthy townsfolk and country gentry, interested in alchemy and in similar arts, who would be impressed by the account in his Preface of his travels as far as the Levant in search of enlightenment and expertise. Some of their authors were distinguished medical men, like Pietro Bayro, physician to the Duke of Savoy; others, like Fioravanti, were 'empirics' and others, like Alexis of Piedmont, may have masqueraded under a false name. Their recipes often required substances that differed from those available in pharmacies and ranged from exotica such as wild boar's teeth and the dung of a black ass (or, if not available, of a white one), to things commonly produced at home such as soaps, perfumes and hair dyes. Their confections were marketed as tried and trusted remedies against common ailments such as sores, eye problems, abscesses, stomach-ache and piles.[105] Others claimed to be written to help the poor, and at least some of their contents, once assimilated by a reader, could be passed on orally to non-readers or in a simplified form to those who could read only a little.

These books, intended for a literate but non-professional audience, constituted a substantial proportion of publications relating to medicine in the sixteenth century. Collections of remedies, short explanatory textbooks and guides to health formed well over 60% of medical literature in English printed between 1486 and 1604. Intended for laymen, they were priced relatively cheaply: Elyot's *Castel of Helthe* and T. C.'s *An Hospital for the Diseased* (1578) sold for 6d, Thomas Moulton's *The Myrour or Glasse of Helthe* (1531), a medieval compendium by a friar, for half that (far less than Vigo's *Surgery*, which cost 4s).[106] Few of the early authors were medical men themselves: Sir Thomas Elyot (1490–1546) was an aristocratic humanist who wished to bring to wider notice the new humanist medicine of the 1520s; others were schoolmasters or, like Andrew Boorde and Thomas Paynel (fl. 1528–67), former monks. John Caius wrote his first book on the English Sweat in English, but his second account, four years later in Latin, was changed considerably to fit the expectations of his intended international readership.[107] By the 1580s far more of the vernacular treatises were being written by members of the London Colleges, such as William Clowes, or those, like John Hester, who wished to publicise the new Paracelsian physic. Many authors expressed an intention to bring their knowledge to the lower classes, sometimes mentioning the poor in their titles, and directing their advice to common conditions encountered in every home, many of them, like ague, fever, coughs and sciatica, terms that covered a multitude of what to modern eyes are symptoms of a variety of conditions.[108]

Medical recipes can also be found in cookery books that were produced in ever larger numbers at the end of the century. These were frequently aimed at women as responsible for the management of the household, a major change from the treatises on household management of the previous century which were far more concerned with estate management. It is perhaps not surprising that the first printed collection of recipes by a woman and claiming to provide diets for the sick was produced in Germany, where female literacy was higher than elsewhere, in 1597. It branded itself as "a valuable new cookery book . . . not only for the healthy, but especially for the sick in diseases and accidents of all kinds, as well as for pregnant women, those in childbed and the elderly infirm".[109] Its author, Anna Weckerin (d. 1596/7), was the wife of a Colmar physician, Johann Jacob Wecker (see later, p. 295), and the mother-in-law of a medical professor at Altdorf, Nicolaus Taurellus (1547–1606), who saw her book through the press. But although some of its recipes are specifically listed as for the sick or the pregnant, and she emphasises that she had used them to help her husband in his practice, few give any indication of the conditions for which they are appropriate and are scattered among many ordinary recipes.[110]

Patients' Perceptions

Domestic manuals in the sixteenth century preached a modified Galenism, based on the humours and the six non-naturals (earlier, p. 97), and rarely contained any theoretical exposition or debated academic points.[111] The so-called *Salernitan Guide to Health*, which claimed to be written for an English King at Salerno, the famous medical centre of medieval Italy, was printed across Europe in many editions and languages from 1480 onwards, sometimes accompanied by learned commentaries like that of Curio and by other works on dietetics, sometimes in a small format on its own.[112] The German translation put out at Leipzig in 1505 by Melchior Lotter occupies a mere 20 pages. Around 1550 a Yorkshire parish priest Robert Parkyn copied the extremely popular versified medieval distillation of its contents by John Lydgate (1370–1451) into a page of his notebook alongside rules for a good death. Other similar handbooks of health proliferated, allowing almost everyone to be his or her own physician.[113] How far this translated into a theoretical understanding of illness is harder to assess. Literary authors across Europe expected their readers to understand at least the basics of the Galenic system although the depth of their involvement varied from author to author and genre to genre. Matthieu Malingre, the author of a morality play published in 1533, gives a leading role to a physician, who describes how he diagnoses a variety of diseases from urine and cures them by bleeding, explaining at the end of the play how Christ, the heavenly physician, works in a similar way to remove the deadly poison of sin.[114] The Evangelical princess Marguerite de Navarre (1492–1549) in her play *Le Mallade*, written only a few years later, took a more critical view of human healing. The wife of the sick man contrasts her own domestic remedies, including a boar's tooth, herbs and pigeon broth, with the expensive and dangerous individualist prescriptions of the Galenic doctor, but both are equally useless compared with belief in God.[115] The humour of Dr Rabelais is at times more specifically focussed on learned medical ideas, and Shakespeare expects his audience, and for his sonnets his readers, to be familiar with at least the outlines of Galenic medicine, and to appreciate his use of them in delineating character.[116] But Galenism also existed alongside beliefs in the stars, demons, witchcraft and the evil eye as causes of disease, and many people viewed the body less as gently oscillating between balance and imbalance to be controlled by proper diet than as something in constant flux and subject to blockages and violent eruptions. Paré's treatise on monsters, like that on prodigies by Conrad Lycosthenes (1518–61), combines descriptions of Siamese twins and foetal malformations with stories of monsters created by putrefaction or the influence of demons.[117] Similarly, Paracelsus in his treatise on miners' diseases carefully explains the association of various diseases with different types of mineral, yet elsewhere he explains the existence of the elves, demons and cobbolds who, so it was believed, were ready to kill or injure all who entered their underground domain as having been sent by God to guard and protect the treasures of the earth and ensure that they were discovered at the appropriate place and time.[118] Jacques Ferrand, who studied medicine at Toulouse at the end of the century, not only gave a very detailed description of the clinical signs of love melancholy, going back via Galen to Hippocrates and the Greek poetess Sappho, but adduced several examples of women who believed that they been raped in their beds by devilish succubi and incubi, something he dismissed as merely nightmarish imagination, although it might presage something worse to come, such as epilepsy.[119]

Going behind these treatises to reach patients' own perceptions and accounts of illness is even more difficult, for two reasons: the bias of the sources towards a small male elite and the lack of fit with the experience of illness in a modern Western scientific and technological society. There are obvious similarities: the sense of relief when a chronic pain, toothache for example, has gone away or even the simple pleasure of being able to leave one's bed and walk around a room, if only for a while.[120] Other reactions appear strange. Crato von Crafftheim was advised by none other than Luther himself to abandon plans to become a clergyman because of his weak health in favour of the much less strenuous profession of a doctor, perhaps wisely, for he lived until his mid-seventies.[121] It is also hard today to imagine what it would have felt to live in a society where plague, illness, harvest failures, especially in the last third of the century, and death were common occurrences. The statues of the many small children prematurely dead that adorn the base of their parents' tomb as weepers are a visual reminder of the huge toll on the new-born and the young. Even if they reached the age of 10, which between a quarter and a half of them did not, they were unlikely to live beyond 40.[122] Mauricius Heling, writing to a doctor friend in Königsberg, spent half of his letter informing him that his wife was safely delivered of a child before dying herself of an extremely dangerous disease, and the child or possibly an older sister died shortly after. As Heling laconically wrote, "Many are the tribulations of the just, from which the Lord frees us".[123] Apparently harmless conditions quickly turned fatal or defied the immediate ministrations of a healer. A woman in Delft whose minor injury to her arm had been treated by a local wise woman, Katerina in Forcipe (Forceps Kate or a geographical name, from the Hook?), suddenly became so ill that both a local surgeon and Pieter Van Foreest had to be called in. By then she was too weak to withstand surgery, and they had to place their hopes in a remedy taken from the book by another Dutch surgeon called Philip Hermann (fl. 1553). If this was the author of *Die peerle der chirurgijen*, this would have been a chemical remedy, for Hermann admitted that all his books were versions of Paracelsus's writings on surgery.[124]

Another Dutchman, Erasmus of Rotterdam, provides in his letters an excellent example of how a learned man might face up to different types of illness. In one of them he describes how in September 1518, he embarked on a journey from Basle to Louvain. He encountered problems right from the start. The sun was too hot, and he almost froze during the overnight stay in a village. The food made him sick, and he was roused too early from sleep to catch the boat, only to be kept awake by the noisy sailors when he tried to catch up on his sleep. Things improved somewhat when he took a horse from Strasbourg to Speyer and then a carriage to Worms and Boppard, although he found the smell of the horses nauseating. However, once he passed Cologne, he felt recovered and even pretty strong. His hopes were soon dashed. The wind and rain, and the sticky atmosphere, together with the shaking of the carriage, made him feel sick, vomiting so often that he could scarcely keep anything down – not that the food on offer was entirely palatable. He had to travel onwards from Aachen in a litter. He could no longer ride because of periodic ulcerations in the groin and struggled into Maastricht, playing down to his companions the extent of his pain in the kidneys. He felt shivery, and almost fainted. He was in constant pain from the corrupt blood that had gathered in his inguinal swelling. Once arrived in Louvain, he did not go to bed immediately, lest he give others the impression he had plague, but that night the swelling broke and the pain subsided. A surgeon was called in to apply an ointment but despite promising to return, he never did so, since he was convinced that Erasmus did indeed have the plague. This suggestion Erasmus strongly rejected, even after the surgeon's father came and examined him and repeated the original diagnosis. A Jew also was summoned, and reached the same conclusion, as did a further highly reputable surgeon. Finally, Erasmus called in a physician and recounted to him all his symptoms from the journey, emphasising the reasons why he did not believe that it was plague, but was the result of the climate, the food and the upheavals on the journey. At the mention of a swelling in the groin, the doctor became frightened, and left hurriedly after pocketing his fee of a gold crown, again promising to return after dinner, but sending a servant instead. Annoyed at the behaviour of all the medics, Erasmus committed himself to the hands of God. Two days later, he felt much better, and after a fortnight he managed to expel "black dead flesh" from the ulcer, just as the first surgeon had predicted. The swelling in the groin became bigger, but was not so painful, and Erasmus suspected that he had picked up something from one of the horses, for there were many horse flies around. Eventually the swelling became softer and finally disappeared completely. If this had indeed been plague, Erasmus reckoned he had conquered it by his own efforts and strength of mind, for half the trouble with illness, he declared, was caused by thinking about it (which is why he had allowed only a select group of friends to visit him, in case they caught his disease). His letter ends with an admission that in the end, when his illness was at its worst, he was convinced he was going to die, and, fearing neither the torments of living nor the terrors of death, he had placed his hope in Christ. Besides, at 50, an age reached by only a few, he had already enjoyed a good life and could not have complained if he had to die.[125]

This is a remarkable letter in many ways, for it shows a man of learning and status so fully in command of the ideas of contemporary medicine that he can defy his medical attendants while, at the same time, providing them with a description and an explanation for his condition that they can easily share.[126] His understanding of the body is structured according to the Galenic six non-naturals: the food and drink he had on his journey; his sleepless nights; the weather, too hot, too cold or too sticky and likely to cause plague; his exercise, riding, walking or riding in a carriage; his evacuations, both normal and abnormal; and his mental state. He is also in a far better position than any of the healers called in to decide what was wrong, for he knows his own body better than they. He also suspects, if in the end he rejects the idea, that he might have caught the plague; he is a little more sympathetic to the notion that his ulcerations may have been the result of bites from horse flies. He was also rich enough to be able to call on a range of practitioners, including a Jew, wherever he went, and he had little sympathy for the inhabitants of Louvain who should have known better than to put up with a gang of inferior and untrustworthy practitioners.[127]

Three years later, in the winter of 1521-2 Erasmus was afflicted with the first of what turned out to be a series of attacks of kidney or bladder stone. It lasted 20 days.[128] A further attack in spring. as the stone moved up and down the urinary tract, was so painful that he thought death might be preferable, considering also the political and religious disasters he saw around him.[129] In July he passed a huge stone, but the effort and the 15 days of pain he had suffered, along with a persistent headache brought on by the awful smell of the baths at Speyer, left him little more than skin and bones.[130] A further attack over Christmas 1523 left him despairing of life. His calculus returned again in the following May and then in July worse than before, and could not be shifted with turpentine, a remedy he often used.[131] Episodes like this continued from them on to the end of his life, despite changes of diet, visiting the hot bath (a favourite of Germans), taking healthy drinks of chamomile and parsley, and using a variety of remedies, including one devised by Thomas Linacre.[132] In August 1526, baffled by the conflicting arguments of his doctors, he consulted by letter another famous doctor and translator of Galen, Wilhelm Cop, the doctor to Francis I of France, about this and about chalky signs in his urine, fearing that this might portend some ulceration of the urine tract, a condition he had heard had been responsible for Linacre's death in 1524.[133] Despite further episodes of acute pain, Erasmus struggled on for the next 12 years until his death in 1536, preferring to treat himself and using his writing of books and letters as a way of distracting himself from the pain when he could. Other sufferers, and there were many, may not have been so patient.[134]

Erasmus's tolerance of pain is mirrored in what is an unusual series of documents from sufferers at the other end of the social spectrum, the rural poor of the hospitals of Haina and Merxhausen in Hessen. In order to apply to enter them, they had to first engage the services of an amanuensis who would copy down, sometimes in their own words, what they had told him about their conditions. Most had struggled on, perhaps for years, with the consequences of heavy labour or accidents, making their contribution as long as possible to the life of their family. Adam Bingel in 1577 described himself as a "poor, lame, old man without any means", who had always supported himself and his children through "hard, unpleasant and difficult work". When he could no longer do this, he turned to herding cattle, and was employed by a neighbour in this for several years. But now, after "a darned fall", he was completely "lame in one arm" and could no longer work at all. Even if they were to be admitted, petitioners like Adam hoped that they would still be able to carry out some useful activity in the hospital for this would give them a sense of status within their new community.[135] Keeping going as long as possible must have been the aim of many of the sick in general. A similar indication of the importance of keeping up appearances is visible also in Erasmus's description of his journey to Louvain, for on two occasions, at Maastricht and St Trond, he switched from a carriage to a horse in order not to give the impression that he was ill, and, once arrived in Louvain, he deliberately refrained from going straight to bed so as not to frighten or annoy his host.[136]

Sometimes it was not one's own illness but that of a family member that proved the last straw for the poor of Hessen. In 1579, Walpurgis, the wife of Hermann Kuzen of Hanau, applied on behalf of her daughter who had long suffered from epilepsy, which had left her "quite lame in the limbs". She was now suffering from cancer of the foot, an "abominable illness" which made her incapable of earning her bread, and the family were too poor to look after her and could find no one to maintain her. A similar case in 1596 concerned a 12-year-old boy who had also suffered from epilepsy, with up to two or three attacks a day. His disease had damaged "not only his senses and his reason", but it had left him unable to move or stand properly; he was like a small child. His parents, pious, industrious manual workers, were forced to leave him alone to go out to work, but now feared that he might fall into water or a fire and die as a result of this lack of care.[137]

Stories like these give a sense of the pressures that the sick themselves were under when making choices about what to do and whom to consult about their illnesses. Erasmus as a learned and wealthy individual could summon and choose between a variety of healers – and to disregard them if he thought he knew better about his own body – but most of the sick had not that luxury. The Cologne town councillor Hermann Weinsberg (1518–97), despite enjoying good health himself, recorded in his diary the trials and tribulations of his family, a further reminder how illness would involve the wider family, not least because of the financial constraints that it involved, especially if a breadwinner fell ill.[138] Not every family could, like Weinsberg's, call on a range of friends and acquaintances to supplement their own efforts. The rural poor in a village community, and possibly with a kind lady of the manor to assist, are likely to have been in a better position than a new immigrant to an already crowded city like London or Palermo, where living conditions were so bad that the population numbers could be kept up only by a constant influx of new immigrants from the countryside.

In the hierarchy of healers, women occupied an ambiguous position. The major providers of healthcare within the home and in most villages, they were respected for their knowledge of the diseases of women and children as well as of local herbs, which they could transmit informally to others in their networks. Some women, particularly among the highest social classes, might acquire an expertise, particularly in the preparation of remedies, that was equal and often superior to that of many physicians, and those midwives who were authorised to act in their communities had a certain recognised status within them. But such women were also regularly derided for their ignorance and credulity, condemned, like the village parson, for the damage they inflicted on those who sought their aid through their lack of understanding of the principles that were thought to govern all healing. Increasing literacy allowed more of them access to written medical material even if in this period the medical information provided in such handbooks was still largely written for the benefit of the male head of the household, who would then pass it on by word of mouth to his wife and servants. Conversely, the growing corporatisation of medicine excluded women more and more, or, like the widows of barbers, confined them to the least medical aspects of their trade.

If in the next century their voice becomes louder, through their own publications and through historians' recovery of their notebooks and diaries, it still uncertain how far the experiences and aspirations of these women can be extended back half a century or more to a time when female literacy was less common. The English historian of medicine Roy Porter was full of sympathy for those whom he considered overlooked by earlier historians, especially women, patients and the mentally ill, and in his many books he demanded that that they be given appropriate recognition. This chapter represents my limited response to the challenge posed by my erstwhile colleague. But there are still gaps in our knowledge, and, more often, the repetition of the same examples or the same conclusions gives the impression of a greater and more secure documentation for this period than is actually the case. Sixteenth-century patients and sixteenth-century women healers have one thing in common. Largely voiceless, frequently invisible and often dismissed as ignorant, both groups still remain among the great unknowns of medical history.

Notes

1 Estimates for female literacy suggest that only 5% of women could sign their name in the mid-1550s, almost all from the wealthiest classes. Numbers may have been slightly higher in Protestant countries than in Italy and Spain because of the need for all to know the Bible, but everywhere female literacy lagged considerably behind that of men.

2 Hurd-Mead 1938.
3 Bourgeois 1626; King 2013: 133–9.
4 This imbalance is particularly visible in the excellent surveys of Pelling 2003; Lindemann 2010; Leong 2018; Green 2008: 246–87 is an excellent study of gynaecological literature before 1600.
5 Wyman 1984: 24–6; Park 1985: 71–2; Green 2008: 294–6.
6 Wenkebach 1925: 57–60.
7 Andretta 2011.
8 Wyman 1984: 25–6; Brockliss and Jones 1997: 262; Broomhall 2004: 16–70.
9 De Moulin 1998: 69–70.
10 Wyman 1984: 26–7.
11 Wyman 1984: 29.
12 Kerwin 81–2; Clark 1964: 144 is more sympathetic to the College but notes that Walsingham was back with similar requests for others in 1584, 1586 and 1587.
13 The claim of the wife in Marguerite de Navarre's *Le Mallade* 1946: 14–15.
14 Pelling and Webster 1979: 187.
15 Wear 2000: 22.
16 Thomas 1973: 209.
17 Munkhoff 2014; Nolte 2020: 225–7.
18 Wyman 1984: 30.
19 Brockliss and Jones 1997: 268–9; Broomhall 2004: 71–95; Strocchia 2019: 179–216.
20 Kinzelbach 2014b; Nolte 2020.
21 Stevens Crawshaw 2014.
22 Munkhoff 2014.
23 Pelling 1996, 2003: 189–224.
24 Green 2008.
25 Marguerite de Navarre 1946: 31–2 (originally c. 1536).
26 Wyman 1984: 34; Brockliss and Jones 1997: 266–7; Pelling 2003: 189–224; Lindemann 2010: 122–3.
27 De Rojas 1970: 45, 53–7; a better English translation in De Rojas 1958: 28, 34–7.
28 Granjel 1980: 140–1 (interestingly the only discussion of women in his substantial book).
29 Eccles 1982: 108–14.
30 Green 2008: 137–8, distinguishing ecclesiastical supervision (from around 1300) from town appointments (a little later) and from formal licensing (early fifteenth century but in Southern Europe perhaps not till the sixteenth century).
31 Flügge 1998: 313–500 is an exhaustive study of German regulations.
32 Wiesner 1993: 82–3; Flügge 1998.
33 García Ballester 1993: 169.
34 Brockliss and Jones 1997: 265.
35 Flügge 1998: 383–415.
36 Flügge 1998: 264.
37 Wiesner 1993: 83–4; Flügge1998: 328–72; the English quotation is from Eccles 1982: 89.
38 Green 2008: 247, noting that it depended heavily on Michele Savonarola's *Practica* of around 1450.
39 Eccles 1982: 11–13; Whiteley 2019.
40 Sheridan 2010. She was anticipated in 1609 in writing a birthing manual for midwives by the surgeon Jacques Guillemeau, whom she may well have known.
41 *Ibid.*, 115. The image of the child lying transversally in the womb is common in medieval manuscripts, Jones 1984: 53.
42 Fischer-Homberger 1983: 53–61.

43 Davis 1975: 259–60.
44 Broomhall 2004: 214–31; King 2007: 38–9; Rankin 2013: 27–35 describe royal women discussing their ailments by letter and acting as go-betweens with physicians. For male surgeons and female autopsies, Green 2008: 257–8.
45 A full physical examination of a male patient was only a little more common.
46 Stolberg 2021b: 14.
47 Nutton 1990b: 141–3.
48 Vives 1555: 11 (originally 1538).
49 Stolberg 2021a: 317–47.
50 Green 2008: 267–87.
51 Maclean 1980.
52 Allen 1985: 85–126; Dean-Jones 1994: esp. 176–209; Connell 2016.
53 O'Rourke Boyle 1996: 98–100.
54 Nutton 2008d.
55 Maclean 1980: 30–5.
56 Maclean 1980: 38–9.
57 Maclean 1980: 40–1; Ferrand 1990: 263–6; Dean-Jones 1994: 65–76; King 1998: 216–18, 225–36; Flemming 2000: 294–303.
58 Pagel 1984: 135–7.
59 King 2007: 2–4, 26; Stolberg 2003: 277–84.
60 Maclean 1980: 4; Spach 1597: 895–7.
61 King 1998: 244–5.
62 Carlino 1999a: 95, 231.
63 Vesalius 1543: 539.
64 Vesalius 1546: 140–1, 2015: 166–9.
65 O'Malley 1964: 436, n. 7.
66 Carlino 1999a: 101, n. 84, 95, n. 94.
67 Purkircher 1988: 154.
68 Vesalius 1546: 139–43, 2015: 66–71; Kosmin 2018: 85.
69 Talvacchia 1999: 162–83; Cazes and Carlino 2003. For the continuation of medieval images of the foetus in the womb, Whiteley 2019.
70 King 2013: 51.
71 Vesalius 1543: 378–80, 478–80; Thiery 2014. Changes to the 1555 plates are minor.
72 Vesalius 1543: 281, 481.
73 Vesalius 1543: 380, 480.
74 Stolberg 2003; King 2013: 16–17, 49–64.
75 Kosmin 2018: 86–7.
76 Rabelais 1944: 414–19, 1964: 205–41; Screech 1958: 83–103: Antonioli 1976: 195–200, 244–9; Nutton 1988b.
77 Joubert 1587: sigg. Q 1r–8v, 1989: 245–68; the later books are presented in a revised and shorter form in Joubert 1587, 1995.
78 Joubert 1587: 149–51, 166–8, 1989: 170–3, 182–3.
79 McClive and King 2007.
80 Joubert 1587: 162–6, 1989: 181–2.
81 Joubert 1587: 199–200, 1989: 211–13, 209.
82 Davis 1975: 260–1.
83 Nolte 2020.
84 Perkins 1996; Bourgeois 2017: 1–57.
85 Brockliss and Jones 1997: 275–6.
86 García Ballester 1984: 82–3; a partial English version in 1985: 265.
87 Thomas 1973: 211, with other examples on 211–27.
88 Rankin 2013: 77–80, noting also the use of orality to protect secret remedies.
89 Leong 2018, but most of her examples fall after 1600.

90 Latham 2010.
91 Aubrey 1962: 297; for Moffet, later, p. 312.
92 For the development of ideas on healthy living, Cavallo and Storey 2013, 2017.
93 Pollack 1993: 26, 102–4, 128–9; Wear 2000: 54; Pollack 1993: 110–42 prints medical extracts from her papers.
94 London, Wellcome Collection WMS 222.
95 Rankin 2008, 2013.
96 Schloss Ambras, PA 1474; Stolberg 2021a: 487–8.
97 Heidelberg, University Library, Cod. Pal. germ. 261.
98 London, Wellcome Collection WMS 244, 5262; British Library, Royal MS 17.A.xxxii.
99 London, Wellcome Collection WMS 141, 634.
100 Brockliss and Jones 1997: 282.
101 Davis 1975: 205–6.
102 Liébault 1577, 1582a, 1582b.
103 Guillemeau 1609; Bourgeois 1626, 2017.
104 Eamon 1994. For the German tradition of the *Kunstbüchlein*, which might also be marketed as a recipe collection, *ibid.*, 112–16, although it often contained more artisanal information.
105 Eamon 1994: 124–47.
106 Slack 1979: 243–7; Richards 2012.
107 Caius 1552, 1556.
108 Slack 1979: 254–6, 263.
109 I have cited this from the second printing, Weckerin 1598; Wiswe 1970: 48.
110 Weckerin 1598: 40, 148, 153, 97, 133, 157.
111 Lindemann 2010: 11–30; Cavallo and Storey 2013, emphasising the role of the non-naturals in conserving health.
112 Curio 1553, the first of many printings, including English versions of the commentary in 1617 and 1634.
113 Mikkeli 1999; Hardingham 2005; for Parkyn's notebook, Dickens 1947: 59.
114 Malingre 1533.
115 Marguerite de Navarre 1946: 14–15, 26, 32; Broomhall 2004: 139–42.
116 Antonioli 1976; Schoenfeldt 1999: 74–95; Kerwin 2005; Pettigrew 2007.
117 Paré 1573, 1982; Lycosthenes 1557a, 1557b (the latter's title is subtly different).
118 Paracelsus 1941: 43–126; contrast 251–3, the conclusion to his book on *Nymphs, Sylphs, Pygmies, and Salamanders, and on the Other Spirits*.
119 Ferrand 1990: 308–10.
120 Newton 2018: 195–8, although the great majority of the examples in her book fall outside this period.
121 Gillet 1860: I,58; Gryllus 1566b: 2v.
122 Lindemann 2010: 30–40.
123 Clemen 1929: 26.
124 Forestus 1591b: 487–91, 1653: 4,144–5.
125 Erasmus, *Ep.* 867; Allen III, 393–401.
126 In 1527 a friend claimed that he knew far more about medicine than most doctors, and asked for his medical advice, *Ep.* 1811; Allen VII, 33.
127 For his later involvement with the Aldine edition and his own translations, see earlier, p. 108.
128 Erasmus, *Ep.* 1248, 1267, n. 7; Allen IV, 609; V, 32.
129 *Ibid.*, 1267; Allen V, 32.
130 *Ibid.*, 1302, 1342, 1422, 1452; Allen V, 96, 215, 405, 470.
131 *Ibid.*, 1408, 1422, 1466, 1487, 1489, 1534; Allen V, 381, 405, 496, 534, 537, 616.
132 *Ibid.*, 1558, 1603, 3106; Allen VI, 46–8, 157; XI, 299 for remedies *Epp.* 2057, 3106; Allen VII, 507; XI, 299.
133 *Ibid.*, 1735; Allen VI, 379–80.

134 *Ibid.*, 1342, 3106; Allen V, 215; XI, 299.
135 Gray 2001: 186–7, 2002, 2007.
136 Erasmus, *Ep.* 867: Allen V, 398–9.
137 Gray 2001: 231–2, 246.
138 Jütte 1988, 1991: 163–204; Lundin 2012: 57–60, 251; Nolte 2020: 222–3.

Beliefs

8   Learned Medicine

Learned medicine as taught in the universities of the sixteenth century was no static repetition of traditional dogmas, a series of quibbles over trivial differences. Rather, particularly in the second half of the century, there developed an increased emphasis on experience and experiment, of which anatomical dissection and medical botany were but two examples, while debates were more often concerned with new diseases and new methods of therapy than with textual minutiae.[1] Although many teachers in smaller universities concentrated on transmitting the basics of medical theory and practice with little thought of novelty, the students who travelled around Europe (earlier, pp. 127–33) were well aware that in places like Paris, Montpellier, Bologna, Padua and, at the end of the century, Basle, new ideas were being vigorously debated among friends, colleagues and students and transmitted quickly by letter or in print around the European intellectual world.[2] The overall structure of the courses on offer appears rarely to change, usually single hour lectures on a set text that was explained, commented on and, if necessary, criticised by a professor. The subject of his 'ordinary' lectures might be repeated later by others more junior and in competition with one another. John Caius noted ruefully that his lectures at Padua on Aristotle clashed with those by the anatomist Realdo Colombo.[3] There was frequently a division between the chairs in practical and in theoretical medicine. Lectures on practical medicine dealt with diseases and their treatment, some caused by imbalances within a particular organ (a chilled stomach or an overheated liver both had serious consequences) but more often by peccant material. This could be introduced from outside or produced from internal putrefaction, clogging up the natural movement of fluids such as blood around the body, and obstructing the workings of the liver, spleen and uterus or heating the urine within the kidneys to form hard stones.[4] Treatment usually involved removing the peccant matter by diet, purgation or even surgery, the subject of lectures by professors of anatomy.

Chairs in theoretical medicine were often more prestigious and better paid. These aimed to provide the student with a complete overview of medicine, beginning with the wider question of the role and purpose of medicine, before going on to explain the vocabulary of medicine and the workings of

DOI: 10.4324/9781003223184-12

the body as expounded by Galen – its elements, humours and their mixtures, faculties (the capability of each part of the body to perform its appropriate function), and the ways in which any imbalance or malfunction could
be corrected and health maintained. But there was often an overlap between
what was taught in practical and theoretical lectures, especially on fever,
and it was common for a professor of practice to proceed to a chair of
theory when it became vacant. This overlap, particularly in universities like
Padua, was increased by the opportunity to hear lectures that were listed
as 'extraordinary', that went beyond the statutory texts, or were given in
private on topics that interested the lecturer and that might combine both
theory and practice. They offered an opportunity for students to learn in
much greater detail about specific aspects of medicine, for example fevers,
drawn particularly from the lecturer's own experiences at the bedside.

The main introductory texts remained the same throughout the century
in most universities: Galen's *Art of Medicine* and the shorter *Method of
Healing, for Glaucon*, Hippocrates's *Aphorisms* and *Prognostic*, sections of
Avicenna's *Canon* on fevers and, from Book I, on some basic principles of
medicine, and Rhazes's *Medicine, for al-Mansūr*. All these were studied in
Latin, often from the 1510s in new and more accurate versions, and they
could be supplemented by other ancient texts, such as Hippocrates's *Head
Wounds*, other Galenic works, and, for medical botany, Dioscorides. By
the end of the sixteenth century sections from recent surveys in the Galenist
tradition, such as Fernel's *Medicina Universa*, were also used as the basis
of commentary. Anatomy was originally taught from Mondino's *Anatomy*,
but his exposition was replaced first by Galen and then from the mid-1530s
by more modern handbooks, like that of Guinter.[5] Teaching by means of
commentary did not necessarily mean simply repeating past conclusions.
It was flexible in that it gave the lecturer considerable scope for including
his own ideas and experiences (or for passing quickly over Galen's attacks
on ancient Methodists and Empiricists in favour of expositions of what he
considered more relevant modern debates). The texts that were chosen were
often relatively short, and, like the Hippocratic *Aphorisms*, and Galen's *Art
of Medicine* or his shorter *Method of Healing*, ranged widely over the whole
of medicine. Their basic principles of theory and practice, once learned,
could be extended and amplified by the lecturer.

The Impact of the New Galen

The full impact of the abundance of new material which was becoming
available in the Greek Galen was not felt until it had been translated into
Latin from 1526 onwards. The earlier syntheses of Symphorien Champier
(1471–1539), although more extensive than their predecessors, did not radically alter the picture, since they depended on his great knowledge of the
medieval translations of Galen in the earliest editions of the Latin *Opera
omnia*, and not directly on the Greek.[6] In the first decade of the sixteenth

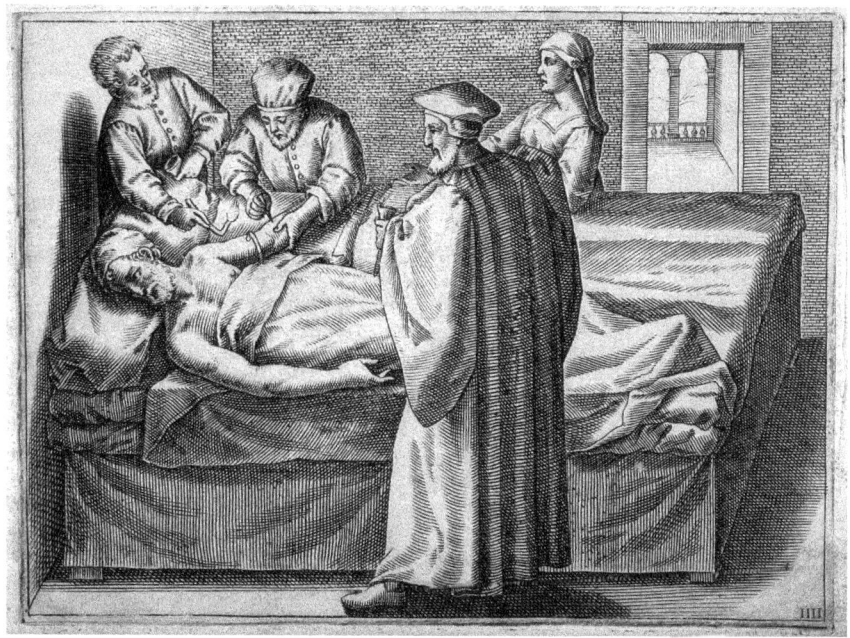

Figure 8.1 A physician superintends a surgeon bleeding a man's arm, helped by an assistant while a woman, possibly the patient's wife, looks on. Engraving by Bartolomeo Bonfadino, Rome, 1586.

century Leoniceno had shown in his short essays on *The Three Types of Teaching*, *De tribus doctrinis*, and *The Formative Power*, *De virtute formativa*, that medieval physicians had misunderstood what Galen had said on certain points, but his conclusions were of little concern to most practising physicians.[7] Manardi's demands for a greater clarity in terminology likewise focussed on specific problems and could be fulfilled only by the tiny number of physicians who knew Greek.[8] Among them was Pierre Brissot (1478–1524), a Parisian doctor, who in 1514 argued that the medieval practice of revulsive bleeding, letting blood from a site as far away from that of the ailment as possible, was contrary to the teaching of Hippocrates and Galen, who had favoured derivative bleeding from near the locus of the ailment.[9] Although he was supported by some of the Paris Faculty, others disagreed strongly, and apparently persuaded the Paris Parlement to ban derivative bleeding. In 1518, Brissot moved to Portugal, partly to study some of the new drugs arriving there, and used his controversial method at Evora during an outbreak of 'pleurisy'. This aroused the hostility of a former royal physician, Dionysius Brudus, the father of Manuel Brudus (see later, pp.), who sent him some extensive and detailed criticisms, to which he replied at length.[10] By late 1523 Brissot had returned to Paris, where he died shortly afterwards. His tract, seen through the press in 1525 by one of his friends, created a stir, not least because this was the first major change in therapeutic practice openly advocated by the new humanists. Until then, the innovations of the Hellenists could be dismissed as philological trivia, outweighed by the centuries of success using revulsive bleeding, but here was an instance where, so it was claimed, the new humanist Galenism was far more effective. That in practice neither method was so clearly superior to the other only fuelled the controversy, which lasted for a generation. Those who supported the traditional view even appealed to the Emperor Charles V to ban this novelty, while others like Professor Drivère at Louvain supported Brissot. In Italy Matteo Corti argued that choosing the appropriate method depended on whether the swelling was painful or not, a compromise opinion attacked by the young Vesalius as being based on a flawed understanding of anatomy. He argued instead that in all inflammations of the sides of the thorax blood should be let by opening the right axillary (basilic) vein.[11] Both sides continued to appeal to texts for justification, but the later contributors to the debate referred more often than their predecessors to their own experience with these procedures as a way of resolving the issue. Fifty years later, Laurent Joubert made no reference to this debate in his survey of ideas on bloodletting, emphasising merely that, when used carefully, removing blood was useful, although not the certain path to a successful cure that its advocates claimed.[12]

A far more serious attack on a major tenet of older Galenism was mounted by Manardi when he denounced the use of astrology in medicine. He may have inherited his hostility from Leoniceno, who, according to their pupil Brasavola, told his students to avoid making predictions if possible, for even the best of men could make a mistake when making a prognosis in a case of illness. Indeed, he had almost to be forced to make a prediction in both acute and chronic diseases, and one could not have dragged a word out of Manardi on the subject. Brasavola himself concluded, with apologies to Galen, that prognosis in acute diseases was hard, and in chronic ones even harder: he compared it to going on a journey without knowing what hazards one might find. Given Galen's emphasis on prognosis and its continuing importance in establishing a physician's reputation throughout the century, this reluctance is hard to explain unless these Ferrarese teachers simply feared for their reputation if things went wrong or had learned from their Greek texts of Galen's dislike of astrological medicine.[13]

Manardi's first (undated) letter denouncing astrology, *Ep.* II, 1, was published in 1521. Many of its arguments were taken over from Gianfrancesco Pico della Mirandola (1470–1533), but Manardi added further points of his own.[14] Astrology, he argued, no longer fit the new situation: neither the Ancients nor the Arabs were aware of the recent discoveries that made Aristotelian cosmology outdated. Besides, Galen, although well informed about the technicalities of astronomy, as he showed in *Critical Days*, was extremely sceptical about the use astrologers made of it and was very careful to distinguish astrology from what might be termed meteorological medicine, the belief that interactions in the heavens could change the weather and thus the environment in which diseases might flourish. Only a few years later, in 1529, he singled out Galen's involvement with astrologers as a mistake, a rare human error, appealing to his earlier letter and to Pico. It was an argument he developed further in another letter of 1532, *Ep. XV, 8*, but by then a text on astrology, *Prognostics from the Time One Takes to One's Bed*, had been published in the last volume of the Aldine edition in Greek as one of the treatises ascribed to Galen. There were disputes in Padua and Ferrara as to whether Galen had actually written this tract or ever believed in astrology, but its first Latin translator, Struthius, was proud to have discovered Galenic authority for what he saw as a well-respected and widespread procedure. After all, it was taught in major universities such as Paris as a normal part of medical education and practised even by bishops.[15] But his arguments could not prevail against the justified relegation of the tract to the section marked spurious in the subsequent editions of the collected works of Galen, even though a new translation, by the Florentine Jacobus Antonius Marescottus, was later produced for the Giuntine edition of 1565.

Other Galenists, such as Lange, joined in the argument along the same lines as Manardi, but it was an uphill struggle.[16] Several distinguished physicians, most notably Cardano, as we have seen (earlier p. 142), had a great reputation as astrologers, and Cardano's book of horoscopes (Figure 8.2) showed his technical skill to the full, allowing him to differentiate himself from mere common or garden astrologers.[17] Many of the teachers at Wittenberg, beginning with Melanchthon himself, also promoted the study of astrology as a way of demonstrating God's providence and the interaction between the world of the stars and the human body.[18] It also derived strength from the common belief that the workings of the universe, the macrocosm, were mirrored in, and influenced, those of the body, the microcosm or little world. But, increasingly, as Cardano himself explained, doctors restricted astrological predictions in medicine to showing the effects of the heavenly constellations on climate, in the tradition that went back to the Hippocratic *Airs, Waters and Places*.[19] Others, like Cardano's rival, Luca Gaurico, concentrated on instructing their readers how to calculate more accurately the Hippocratic critical days in order to treat their patients more successfully.[20] Books like Johann Virdung of Hassfurt's *Nova medicinae methodus*, *New Method of Medicine*, of 1532 which attempted to demonstrate a new way of curing disease by means of astrology, or Antoine Mizauld's *Planetologia*, *Planetology*, of 1551, described on its title page as "filled with astronomical, medical and philosophical material in order to show the relationship and harmony between the celestial and human bodies and between astronomy and medicine", were directed to a learned readership.[21] But by the end of the century, however, most physicians had rejected the astrological medicine they had inherited from the Arabs, and it comes as surprise to find a reissue

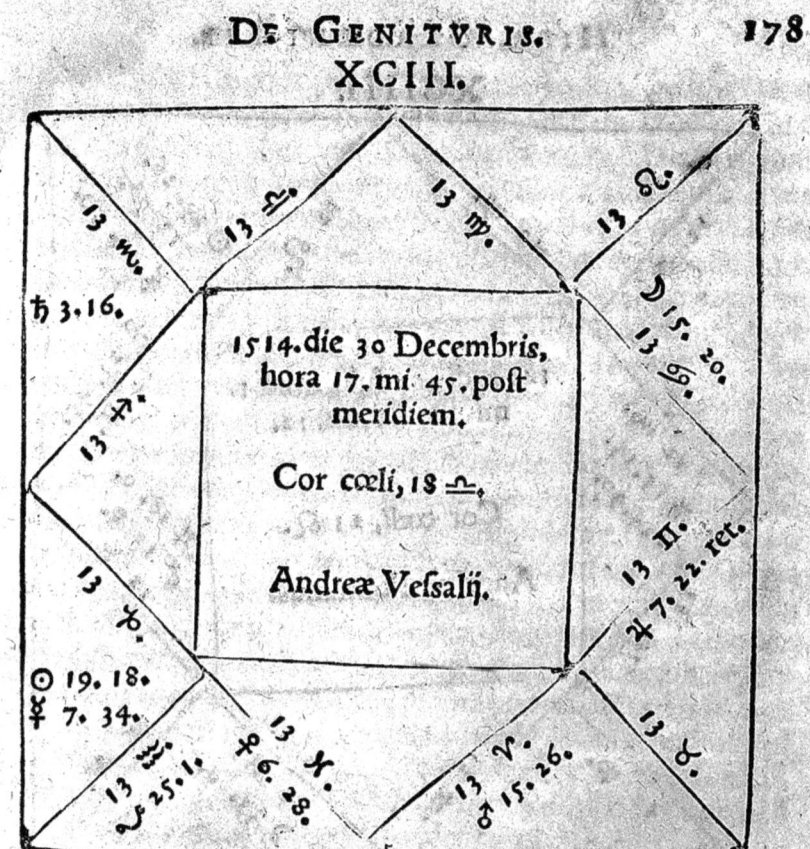

De Genitvris. 178
XCIII.

1514. die 30 Decembris, hora 17. mi. 45. post meridiem.

Cor cœli, 18 ♎.

Andreæ Vesalij.

H|c in dissectione corporū admirabilis, antiquisᴈ merito cōparandus, opus prima inuenta scripsit, sanè adeò egregiū, ut negotium penè totū absoluerit, celebris in uita, iam nunc Cæsaris medicus, & post fata etiam celebris futurus. Si genitura hæc sua est, ad amussim omnia conueniunt, nam Mars in quadrato Lunæ potentis in octaua, studiū & agilitatē manuū præstat, Mercurius in trino Iouis, & Venus in quadrato, ingeniū mirabile, & facundiam pro artis conditione, imo supra eam, decernunt. est enim medicus insignis. Luna in opposito Solis, memoriā & scientiā, & multos dat hostes, clarū etiam facit: quia nocturna est genitura. Saturnus cū corde Scorpij, in sextili Mercurij, ingeniū profundū, memoriā, studiū. Spica Virginis in corde cœli, gloriā ex arte, quantā quisᴈ alius. decet etiā animaduertere Martē aspicere Solē in sua exaltatione existentē, tū Lunā in suo esse domicilio, hæc gratiā apud Principes decernūt. illud solum deest, quod nullius Planeta horoscopi locū possidet, iuxta decreta nostra.   yy ij

Figure 8.2 Girolamo Cardano's horoscope for Andreas Vesalius, *Libelli quinque*, Nuremberg, A. Petreius, 1547.

of Virdung's book in 1584 along with the pseudo-Galenic *Prognostics*, the *Medical Mathematics* of Hermes Trismegistus and three tracts by Ficino. Its Venetian author, the learned astronomer and instrument-maker Giovanni Paolo Gallucci (1538–1621), also included his own commentary on Virdung's medical astrology and dedicated his book to a fellow enthusiast for astrology, the Bishop of Modena. At least one Italian reader made copious notes on the texts, except for that of pseudo-Galen, but it is unclear if he was a medical man.[22] Elsewhere doctors placed little reliance on the stars in their practice, although as the famous examples of the English astrologers Simon Forman and John Napier at the turn of the century show, the sick continued to seek their assistance, although mainly to learn the future outcome of their condition rather than to receive direct therapeutical guidance.[23] But even if these medical astrologers dealt more with prediction than cure, the fact that patients from all social classes sought their assistance was reason enough for the hostility of physicians towards them.[24] Nonetheless, the presence of many medical students at Galileo's classes in Padua may indicate at least a residual professional interest in the relationship of the heavens to mankind.[25]

Uroscopy and Diagnosis

A second element in late medieval medical practice that lost much of its independent authority in the sixteenth century was uroscopy, the diagnosis of illness by inspecting urine.[26] Although he had used uroscopy in his practice, Galen had never written a specific treatise on it, and it was left to his successors in Late Antiquity to bring together his scattered observations in a single work. The short treatise by Theophilus Protospatharius, c. 600, was turned into Latin soon after and was included in the Salernitan corpus of ancient writings, the so-called *Articella*, that was studied by every medical student. Both the Arabs and the medieval Western authors contributed their own synopses and guides to urine diagnosis and charts showing a circle of colours going from pure white to the deadly black and back again were extremely common in manuscripts of all kinds. The reader (for self-diagnosis from urine was also common) was instructed what conclusions to draw from its colour, consistency and contents, whether they were floating or gathered as sediment into the bottom of the flask. Patients expected their doctor to examine their urine. Michael Bäris, a physician at Schlettstadt (Sélestat in Alsace) in 1554 complained that he had been unable to eat until late in the evening because he had had to examine the urine of 15 different patients.[27] The urine flask or jordan appearing in illustrations identified the doctor, as indeed it continued to do well into the seventeenth century (Figure 8.3). But by then it might also indicate that its owner was a charlatan, a 'piss-prophet', whose patients were so foolish as to entrust themselves to his care or to expect an accurate diagnosis from urine that might have been brought along by others after a long journey. Humorous stories and

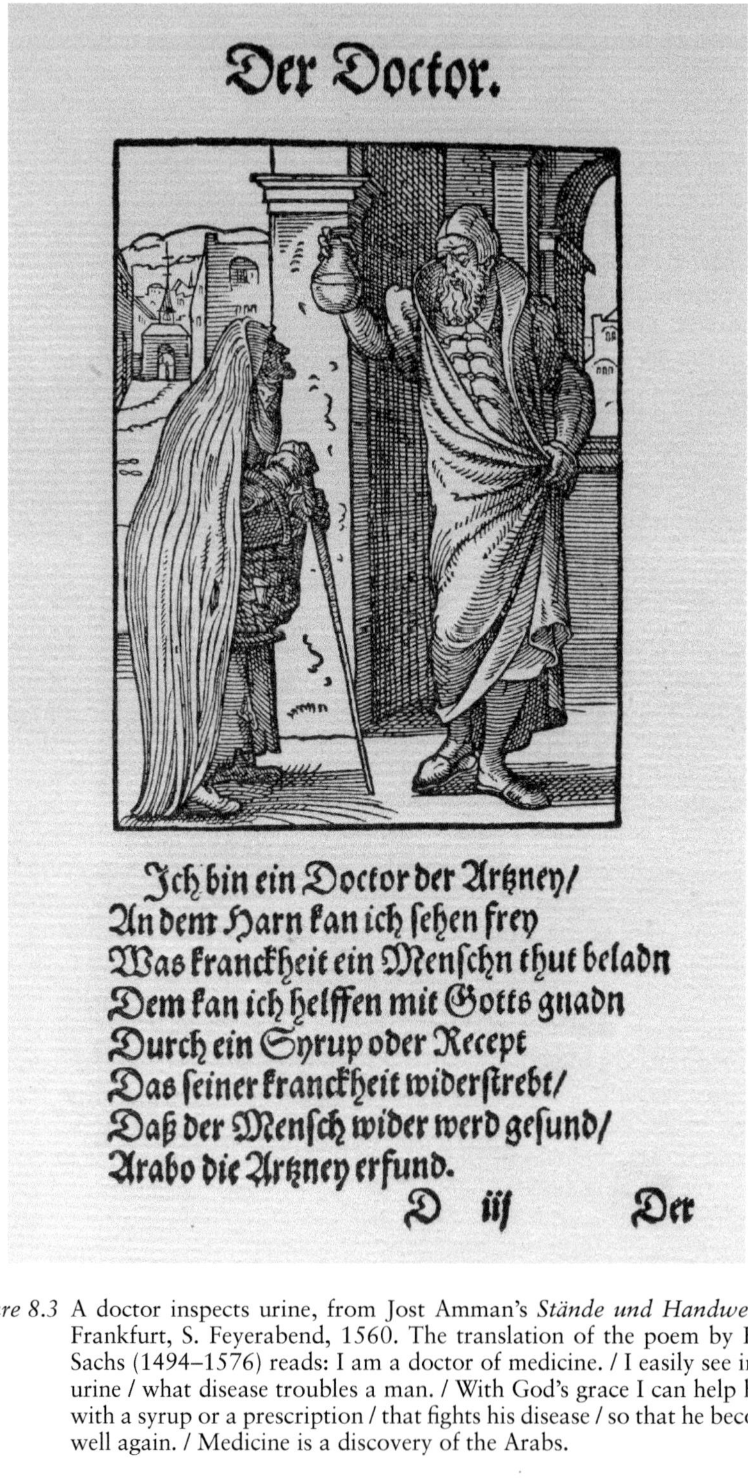

Der Doctor.

Ich bin ein Doctor der Artzney/
An dem Harn kan ich sehen frey
Was kranckheit ein Menschn thut beladn
Dem kan ich helffen mit Gotts gnadn
Durch ein Syrup oder Recept
Das seiner kranckheit widerstrebt/
Daß der Mensch wider werd gesund/
Arabo die Artzney erfund.

D iij   Der

Figure 8.3 A doctor inspects urine, from Jost Amman's *Stände und Handwerker*, Frankfurt, S. Feyerabend, 1560. The translation of the poem by Hans Sachs (1494–1576) reads: I am a doctor of medicine. / I easily see in the urine / what disease troubles a man. / With God's grace I can help him / with a syrup or a prescription / that fights his disease / so that he becomes well again. / Medicine is a discovery of the Arabs.

jokes about credulous or stupid patients who wanted a urine examination abound in both medical and non-medical literature, and go back a very long way to classical times.[28] Pieter van Foreest, in a vituperative denunciation of uroscopy, declared that it was impossible to draw any conclusion from urine that had been brought along in clogs or dirty flasks used to hold vinegar, oil, brandy, wine or Danzig beer that might have been in transit for days from Hungary to Holland. Nonetheless, he occasionally felt compelled to assent when asked to diagnose from a specimen already shaken vigorously in a flask of many colours, but he admitted that by this concession the "bright splendour of the profession" had been somewhat darkened.[29] Considerations of status, the desire of a physician to distance himself from the uroscopist and to avoid dealing with a patient's foul excrement, a major concern in Tiraqueau's discussion of the standing of the medical profession, may have contributed to a decline in a reliance largely on urine diagnosis among Galenists, although it was strongly advocated by Paracelsians.[30] But this change was also influenced by a shift in ideas on diagnosis brought about by the arrival of more Galenic material.

The error of medieval commentators who had interpreted the opening sentence of Galen's *Art of Medicine* in terms of a method of logical analysis was demolished by Leoniceno. Others followed him in seeking to establish a new method of therapy along the lines Galen had laid down in his large *Method of Healing* and in his shorter work of the same name dedicated to his friend, the doctor Glaucon.[31] Both were translated afresh direct from the Greek, the former by Thomas Linacre (Figure 4.2), and the shorter *Method* became a staple of university teaching. The leading exponent of the new method was Giovanni Battista da Monte, who taught at Padua from 1539 to his death in 1551. Not only did his students publish their transcripts of his lectures, but two of them produced their own more accessible summaries of them. In 1544 John Caius, while on his return journey from Padua, arranged for the publication in Basle of a version, emphasising method, that he published under his own name, to the great annoyance of Crato, who sought to defend the memory of his teacher by publishing his own summary there in 1555. Both books enjoyed a wide circulation and helped to differentiate the new Galenist therapeutics from their medieval precursors.[32]

Da Monte's method, which was followed by his colleagues and successors such as Bassiano Landi (d. 1562) and Antonio Fracanzano (d. 1567), reiterated the message of Galen that a true understanding of illness required both theory and practice together.[33] They were intertwined and demanded the full use of a doctor's capabilities in the investigation of illness and disease. Each patient was different, and the doctor had to find ways of determining that individuality in order to diagnose and to treat, for individuals responded differently to drugs and other therapies. One needed to conduct a full examination of the patient in his or her environment, noting as many of the signs of disease as possible and relating them to what was known about the body and its workings. Touching and looking beneath the clothing, particularly for female patients, was not always possible, for social reasons, but observation of external signs was essential, particularly in fevers, the third element in what came to be known as 'semiotics'.[34]

If uroscopy had to be defended against any suggestion of quackery, the taking of the pulse and drawing appropriate conclusions from it remained unchallenged as a central part of diagnosis, a mystery that was properly revealed only to the trained physician. In the absence of accurate measuring tools, claims for his interpretation of the pulse depended on the fineness of touch of the physician and on an ever more complex correlation of observations with disease conditions.[35] Artistic representations often have the physician examining a patient, often female, and diagnosing a range of conditions from pregnancy to fatal illness and even, following ancient precedent, love. Its basic texts remained the 16 books on the pulse by Galen, frequently summarised by such as Gessner and even reduced to tabular form by Caspar Bauhin in Basle. They were also given an exhaustive commentary by Leone Rogano (d. 1558) in a frequently republished tract on pulses and urines.[36] Along with his own short guide to pulses Bauhin also reprinted the 1555 guide to taking the pulse, the *Ars sphygmica*, *Art of the Pulse*, by Struthius, whose enthusiastic claim that this had been lost for 1200 years is as exaggerated as his earlier endorsement of Galenic astrology.[37] The third tract in Bauhin's compendium was an unpublished lecture by his Paduan teacher Girolamo Capodivacca (1523–89), who had said more about it in his (posthumously published) tracts on the method of practical medicine.[38] Similar claims were made by another Paduan professor, Ercole Sassonia (1551–1607), whose treatise on pulses was subtitled as "extremely necessary and useful for all students of medicine".[39] Colombo's discovery of the lesser circulation also raised questions about the relationship of the pulse to the heartbeat, a tricky question that was not resolved accurately until William Harvey in the next century.[40]

None of these recommendations on the best way to diagnose illness would have been unfamiliar to a well-trained Galenist, and not the least of Da Monte's skills lay in bringing together in a clear and informative way material from the whole Galenic corpus rather than simply the text on which he was lecturing. His reordering of the Galenic treatises in the greatly expanded 1541 edition of the *Opera Omnia* into different classes created a valuable didactic structure that emphasised the significance of the new semiotics.[41] His weakness, however, lay in his desire for completeness, a failing mitigated by his summarisers and by the compiler of his *Medicina universa*, *Universal Medicine*, which brought together selections from all his published writings and rearranged them into subject groupings.[42] In addition, he shared in a Paduan tradition of bedside teaching at the neighbouring hospital of San Francesco.[43] Although he had no formal position there, he used to take his students and colleagues there to demonstrate and to discuss openly the details of the case before them. His bedside consultations, which might also take place in the patient's house, were famous, being copied down verbatim by students (including interjections by the audience) and later published in ever larger editions from 1554 until 1583 to demonstrate in practice the medical logic that suffused Da Monte's teaching. The final edition included over 300 such cases and had been put together from the notes of four different students, including Donzellini and Crato.[44]

Together with his lectures, both formal and private, they show that he did not despise urine diagnosis, but that he was concerned to set out how one might distinguish carefully between the different types of urine and to show how these distinctions might be correlated with the range of possible diseases. Throughout he insisted on beginning with a precise description of the significant signs before moving to causes and the essence of the disease, and, if possible, the proximate causes. Other professors followed slightly different sequences, as they sought to distinguish between symptoms logically.[45] In this way they hoped to come to a precise and accurate understanding of the illness and of the appropriate cure by establishing a method that could be extended to cover every kind of ailment, including those that might require surgery. This emphasis on the importance of Galenic methodology recurs throughout the century. Along with anatomy, method was the one thing that the young doctors who set themselves up as a New Galenic Academy in Florence in the early 1530s insisted upon as distinguishing themselves from the Arabs and their more recent predecessors who had neglected Galen to follow an outdated methodology.[46] Sixty years later, the French royal physician, Nicolas de la Framboisière (1560–1636) published two books setting out his rules, or canons, for effective practice along the lines laid down by Da Monte. The first, in Latin for physicians, is subtitled an aphoristic method, *aphoristica methodus*, the second, in French for surgeons, instructs them how to practise surgery 'methodically' ('*methodiquement*'), beginning with the signs before proceeding logically to a cure.[47]

Arguing With Galen: Fracastoro and Contagious Disease

The new Galen did not merely impose a new overall method on academic medicine. The abundance of new material from the master himself revealed that not only was he a great experimenter and observer, but that he was also more hesitant about his conclusions than had been apparent in the medieval selection of mainly didactic texts. Even more importantly, it showed that Galen was often inconsistent, indeed at times openly self-contradictory. The long-lived imperial physician Julius Alexandrinus (1506–90) devoted over 300 pages to pointing out Galen's self-contradictions and Niccolò Rorario (fl. 1555) filled over 700: Andreas Laguna (1499–1560) in Paris contented himself with a mere 17.[48] All of them sought ways to reconcile the apparently divergent statements within Galen's writings. According to Alexandrinus when Galen in his first book on *Elements* asserted that none of them could be found in a pure state but a few pages later talked of pure elements, he was merely describing their appearance of purity, which, for the purpose of his argument, could stand for the reality. Likewise, when in the commentary on *Aphorisms* Galen declared that pure warm water did not always evacuate superfluities fully, he was not contradicting his oft-repeated statement that it always did, but was referring only to one type of evacuation, via the skin. The rare example of a slave who committed suicide by holding his breath did not refute Galen's opinion that breathing was an involuntary activity but was the exception that proved the rule.[49] Others contented themselves with pointing to the gaps in Galen's expositions. Lorenz Gryll, for instance, embarked on a study of taste because he had found no convenient exposition in Galen or among his contemporaries. The ten books of *Controversial Topics in Medicine and Philosophy, Controversiae medicae et philosophicae,* by the Spaniard Francesco Valles (1524–92) almost trebled in length between its first edition of 1556 and its third edition of 1582, as he explored a variety of alternative explanations for phenomena offered by Galen and his modern followers. Students still bought summaries and epitomes of Galen's works, and similar study aids, but they were also aware of new ideas that supplemented or developed what he had taught. Academic Galenism in the Renaissance, as Ian Maclean showed, was far from monolithic or closed to new ideas.[50]

Discussions of plague and contagious diseases neatly show the ways in which learned physicians used their ancient texts and their own experiences to respond to contemporary needs. Galen had said relatively little about the epidemic diseases of his own day, largely repeating the teaching of the Hippocratic *Epidemics* and *Airs, Waters and Places,* that differentiated a widespread condition, caused by bad air that affected large numbers of sufferers at the same time, from an individual illness that was the result of some personal humoral imbalance. This explanation for epidemic disease was accepted by almost all physicians, even if they were not entirely agreed upon what bad air was and how it affected the patient. Did it act like a poison or did the hot, sticky air induce putrefaction in the bodies with which it came into contact? If one drew up a list of those most susceptible with young, fat, pregnant women, whose bodily constitution was extremely hot and moist, at the top, why did many of those who had a similar humoral balance escape infection? Besides, this theory of deadly air was at variance with the policies of the Health Board administrators who favoured a policy of quarantine, segregation and the use of *lazaretti.* And if syphilis behaved like an epidemic in spreading quickly around Europe, its later classification as a sexual transmitted disease cast doubt on the idea that it was spread, let alone caused, by bad air.

Galen had also briefly suggested that the apparently random infection of sufferers with a similar humoral balance was due to the presence in their bodies of what he called the seeds of plague. This was a vague formulation that could indicate that these were residues within the body from which a disease could 'grow' or equally hint at something more specific in line with what some doctors who claimed to be followers of the Atomists Democritus or Epicurus believed. Typically, Galen, having raised this possibility in passing in three tracts written at about the same time, quickly rejected it, never referring to it in any of his later writings on epidemic diseases, and only a handful of medieval authors noted his belief in 'seeds'.[51]

But one important ancient author familiar to Renaissance humanists who did write at length about seeds in connection with disease was the Roman poet Lucretius in his poem *The Nature of Things*. In this poem, written about 56 BCE, he set out to explain the workings of the universe as the Epicureans saw it, one not based on Aristotelian elements but on combinations of atoms. In certain configurations they could form harmful seeds which putrefied the atmosphere and affected the individual either directly or indirectly by poisoning the water, crops or animals that were eaten. The seeds themselves could either arise from the ground or be introduced into the atmosphere 'from outside'. Other Epicurean authors thought that this also explained how diseases could be spread by touch or contagion.[52]

The Veronese Girolamo Fracastoro, himself a poet and philosopher as well as a doctor, knew his Lucretius well, and drew on him for his studies of diseases, which occupied him for over 40 years. He had begun writing his poem *Syphilus* (earlier, pp. 25–6) around 1520, and had finished a first draft in 1525, five years before it was actually published. A prose tract on syphilis, begun by 1525, was finished in 1533, shortly before he embarked on a treatise on contagion, which he had finished in draft by 1538. The treatise itself was published in 1546 (Figure 8.4), but he was still revising his ideas about the English Sweat in 1551.[53] These studies have earned Fracastoro a reputation as a precursor of modern bacteriology who believed in the specificity of disease types and whose ideas were unjustly neglected by his contemporaries. This accolade is not entirely deserved, for it neglects the context of his book and of almost all Renaissance writings on disease.

The three books of *Contagion and Contagious Diseases*, published in 1546, followed directly on in the same volume from his investigation into the Aristotelian concepts of sympathy and antipathy, although Fracastoro never spelled out the connection in detail.[54] Both sections attacked those who proposed an explanation for the workings of the universe in terms of 'occult' or 'hidden' qualities. To Fracastoro how it worked was in no way obscure or inexplicable, but abundantly clear and intelligible to those who believed in antipathy and sympathy, the doctrine that certain combinations of elements could attract or repel others. The actions of a magnet and the ability of lime or a sponge to soak up water demonstrated this clearly, and the receptivity of bodies to some diseases and their virulence once in the body were also examples of the same principle at work.

By 1538 Fracastoro had developed the theory that it was the elemental combination of what he called seeds, *semina*, or 'seedbeds', *seminaria*, that explained the ability of contagious diseases to infect and the way in which they did so. He posited three different types of contagion: by direct contact, at a distance and indirectly by fomites. The first two types were familiar, the

HIERONYMI FRACASTORII VERONENSIS.

DE SYMPATHIA ET ANTIPATHIA RERVM

LIBER VNVS

DE CONTAGIONE ET CONTAGIOSIS

MORBIS ET CVRATIONE

LIBRI   III

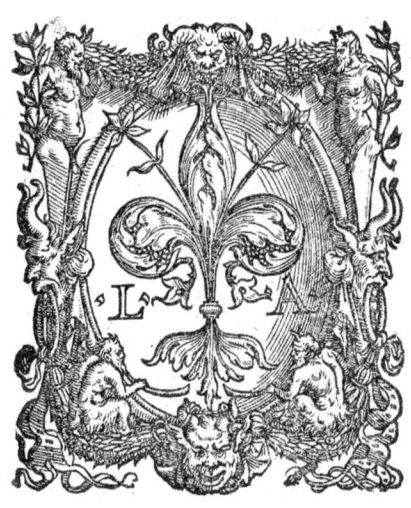

VENETIIS,   M D XLVI,

Figure 8.4 Fracastoro's study of contagious diseases, Venice, Heirs of Lucantonio Giunta, 1546, forms the second part of the book and depends on the theories of sympathy and antipathy explained in the first.

second exemplified by both bad air and the evil eye, something attributed to some animals such as the basilisk as well as to witches, but the third was not. The Latin word he chose, *fomes*, 'fomite' or 'tinder', had been used by theologians as a descriptive metaphor for original sin, which, like tinder, could remain inactive for a while before suddenly blazing up. Fracastoro's fomites could be transferred via wood or clothing, sometimes after a long period. The different combination of elements also explained why some diseases appeared to be transmitted by one type of contagion and why, once in the body, they could be attracted to one part rather than another. Phthisis, for example, did not attack the eyes, leprosy did not penetrate deep into the body unlike the relatively similar syphilis. His seed-bed metaphor also implied that, once in the body, these seeds could grow to poison or cause putrefaction in the parts to which they were attracted.

While accepting that contagion largely involved some kind of putrefaction of the humours and elements within the body, Fracastoro argued that his theory resolved the difficulty inherent in attributing contagion entirely to it, for that did not account for transmissibility. The seeds themselves did not have to be putrid, but it was their presence within the body that sparked off the putrefaction. Some seeds may have been engendered or already present within the body, but climatic changes outside the body could also produce the seeds of a new disease or, as with syphilis, later reduce its virulence and, in some instances, cause it to disappear entirely. It was an explanation that fitted both old and new diseases, localised as well as epidemic, and confirmed the utility of many of the practices of health administrators, notably quarantine and the burning of clothing and furnishings. Removing the seeds from both inside and outside the body, and preventing them from taking hold and growing, was the best way of dealing with these contagious diseases. It thus allowed space both for public health provisions and for the role of the physician in individual prophylaxis and therapy.[55]

Fracastoro was far from alone in discussing contagion in the relation to diseases such as plague, measles and syphilis, and many of his arguments, ideas and vocabulary can also be found in other writers. Even the rare word *fomes* was used by the Bolognese humanist and professor Filippo Beroaldo (1453–1505) in a well-known work on plague of 1505, but here only in the restricted sense of 'combustible' material already present in the body that could be activated to make a disease more dangerous.[56] Da Monte, who almost certainly knew of Fracastoro's ideas before their publication and who agreed with him in deprecating any belief in occult qualities or the effects of imagination, differed strongly over what he considered the unnecessary hypothesis of seeds. In his view contagion was a type of putrefaction, in which the distinction between such diseases related both to the degree of putrefaction involved and to the site of the major putrefaction, in ophthalmia the eyes, in scabies the skin, in pestilential fever the heart. His objections, although not published in print until much later, were known to

Fracastoro, who delayed his own publication until he had had time to study reports and transcripts of Da Monte's lectures.[57]

Da Monte's response was immediate. In his lectures after 1546 he repeated his view of the crucial importance of putrefaction, accusing Fracastoro of introducing unnecessary entities, "absurd *seminaria*", "figments of the Epicureans". Except for direct contact, and possibly contact by fomites, he argued that air was always involved in the chain of transmission, and that the notion of some residual seed of disease within the body could be explained more simply by the lingering presence of corrupted humours. The wide range of possibilities for the cause, degree and site of the putrefaction easily explained the differences between diseases, even before considering individual receptivity. It was no wonder, he declared, that Galen, who knew about seeds, gave up attempting to answer the question why this, rather than that, person should fall ill with a particular disease.[58]

Plague and Putrefaction

Given the importance of plague, syphilis and similar diseases, not to speak of the respect accorded to both Da Monte and Fracastoro, it is not surprising that the debate about contagion should have continued to rage widely across Europe for many years. All participants praised Fracastoro's ability as a doctor and philosopher, even as they took issue with many of his specific points.[59] Jacobus Sylvius in Paris resolved the problem of the differential spread of an epidemic by emphasising receptivity and subdividing the nine Galenic temperaments into an infinite variety, which he classified into more than 700 categories.[60] The Spaniard Valles (1524–92), praising Fracastoro as "a writer of no small learning and intelligence", agreed with him on the significance of sympathy and antipathy, and saw no difficulty in accepting an Epicurean view of bodily balance alongside that of Galen. He believed strongly in contagion, although in his exposition he made little distinction between bad air, something nasty within it or, more precisely, seeds or effluvia as the cause. Like Fracastoro, he disliked 'occult qualities', but he did not accept that every sympathetic disturbance involved seeds or effluvia, for there was also a limited place for imagination.[61] Others, like Da Monte's colleague Trincavella, understood the 'seeds' merely as a metaphor for the putrefaction itself.[62] Johannes Lange in his discussions of new diseases adopted Fracastoro's terminology, denouncing a belief in occult properties as "a vulgar refuge for those ignorant of causation". But he poured scorn on the idea of an infinity of new diseases, each with its specific form, and believed that putrefaction was not ubiquitous, for the seeds of plague might act like a poison, killing without putrefaction.[63] Valleriola in Arles had known little about Fracastoro in 1554, when he first wrote on plague, but four years later he described his ideas at great length and with a good deal of approval. Exactly how sympathy and antipathy worked, he could not say, although he favoured thin vapours as more likely candidates than seeds as vectors. Nor was putrefaction universal even in plague, for he had found it occasionally absent from some cases, and it certainly did not occur in rabies.[64] He did not go so far as Bassiano Landi in Padua, who conducted an experiment to show that putrefaction in the air could not be the culprit in plague. Having found that bread, milk, egg and wine exposed overnight to the sticky air of a plague season did not go off, Landi concluded that there was no such thing as a seed of putrefaction, and that the disease must have been caused by something else.[65]

The circle of correspondents around Crato von Crafftheim was also keenly interested in this European-wide debate on plague. In their publications, and in letters that circulated from Heidelberg to Vienna and on to Padua and back, they disputed with each other about a wide range of ideas about plague. Indeed, Crato's Frankfurt friend Caspar Hoffman wrote that there were now so many diverse opinions on the subject that he had begun to lose faith in his own, which he had planned to send him.[66] One of the interlocutors, Thomas Jordanus, as we have seen, put Fracastoro's ideas into practice in dealing with the Moravian outbreak of 1577, explaining how the nasty material on dirty instruments could cause infection and ordering the cleaning of the baths, and indeed their partial demolition, in order to destroy the 'seedbeds' of this outbreak.[67] Crato himself criticised Jordanus for a variety of mistakes, to which Jordanus replied in an appendix to the second edition of his book in 1583. Crato divided plague into two types, public and private: the latter, the result of bad regimen or bad air, was not contagious or dangerous except to the very few who were predisposed to it. Public plague derived from air containing lethal exhalations arising from putrescent bodies that might contain 'seedbeds' that multiplied and spread the disease widely, and a private plague might turn into a public one. Besides, he was not convinced that contagion always involved putrescence, and thought, *pace* Da Monte, his beloved teacher, that the two terms should be kept distinct. Elsewhere in an exchange with Mercuriale in Padua, Crato favoured putrescence more strongly, doubting Mercuriale's conclusion from his experiences in the Venetian plague that dry acrid vapours from the sick, which could in no way become putrid, could attack both body and brain on being inhaled.[68] A former student also reminded Mercuriale that in his lectures he had strongly asserted the universal presence of putrescence in plague. Other friends of Crato, like Peter Monau, placed the emphasis on sympathy and antipathy, which, as Mercuriale commented, was simply a fashionable way of referring to contagion, and something not believed in by the general public. Some of these epistolary contributions were short, others like Thomas Erastus's defence of his views against a Paduan correspondent, might run to several pages. Some exchanges of ideas stretched over several months, others elicited an immediate response.[69]

It would be easy to dismiss these debates as mere storms in an academic teacup, and to agree with Simone Simoni who in his plague tract bluntly dismissed as worthless any speculation about the causes of plague and the best way to achieve the ideal humoral balance that would prevent infection, topics that occupied hundreds of pages in the tracts of others.[70] For him, this was a mere waste of time, when what was needed was an effective method of treating the infection once it had arrived. But even if he was right that in time of plague one could not afford the luxury of a long academic disquisition, these debates about contagious disease were far from purely theoretical. Particularly during and after the great plague of 1575–8, they were based heavily on the experiences of those who had struggled to deal with hundreds of the sick. They raised important questions about infectious diseases, their virulence and their mortality. They sought to identify which groups were most at risk, and, if these were the poor and the artisans, what could be done for them since, unlike the rich, they could not withdraw to a country estate but had to consort with others in order to earn their living? The debate raised a variety of questions. Why were some regions less affected than others, or even managed to escape entirely? Could plague exist without apparent fever? And was a belief in occult causes in any way justified, when physicians took such pride in their understanding of what they could perceive by their senses?[71] By the end of the century Fracastoro's formulations may have fallen out of use largely because they had been subsumed into general discussions of contagious diseases, and many of the answers that he and others sought could not be found until the age of the laboratory.[72] But it is also striking how often they used their experiences to challenge simplistic or irrelevant formulations, and raised questions about transmission, isolation and receptivity that are still relevant in our modern Covid pandemic.

Modernising Galenic Theory: Jean Fernel

One of those who believed that contagious diseases were the result of some poison with a hidden origin was Jean Fernel (1497–1558), professor in Paris and the most celebrated of all French Renaissance physicians. He is known today for his alleged coinage of the term 'physiology', *physiologia*, the title of one of the major sections in his *Medicina, Medicine*, of 1554, although the term was already familiar to Galen and, as a classicising Latin word, it simply replaced the standard 'natural part of medicine', that Fernel had used in an earlier version of this treatise and continued to use regularly in the text itself. It was a term that encompassed all the parts of the body, including its anatomical structures, and was not confined to its functions.[73] From 1567 this revised version, along with two other parts dedicated to pathology and therapeutics, appeared under the title of *Universal Medicine, Universa medicina*, alongside his treatise *De abditis rerum causis, The Hidden Causes of Things*, first published in 1548, but probably composed before 1538 and circulating among colleagues soon after.[74] The *Universal Medicine* was not a revolutionary work but a restatement of Galenism in a modernised form. Although it diverged in some respects from what Galen had taught, it did not arouse the ire of the very conservative Paris medical Faculty, of which Fernel was a distinguished member, and became extremely popular as a compendium of all that was best in traditional medicine.[75]

The Hidden Causes of Things differed radically from the similarly titled work of Antonio Benivieni that had been published in 1507.[76] Benivieni, a skilled operator with the knife, had described a multitude of cases where he had been able to locate the cause of death by carrying out an autopsy, whereas Fernel was not concerned with dissection but with the hidden powers that were at work in the world and in the body. His book included ideas that he discussed further in his writings on physiology and pathology, and which had a wider relevance beyond the microcosm of the human body. Its first section, like Fracastoro's discussion of sympathy, derived ultimately from Aristotle, and was an exposition of the philosophical background to the specifically medical discussion in the second part. How much, if anything, he owed to Fracastoro is unclear, for Fernel mentions contemporaries by name only rarely. Both men were using the same classical and medieval texts and the same technical language, and Fracastoro was not among the moderns whose views on the origin of some childhood skin diseases in residual menstrual blood were attacked by Fernel.[77] Their divergences neatly show the flexibility of Renaissance Galenism in developing and applying the ideas of their master.

Fernel agreed with Fracastoro in denying that humoral changes alone could explain all diseases. Some were the result of deficiencies in the body's matter, but others were what he termed diseases of the total substance, or, in Aristotelian terms, involved altering the form that defined the individual thing or being.[78] Pandemic, pestilential and poisonous diseases attacked the body through their own total substance. Sometimes, as in scabies and phthisis, the source of the infection was obvious, contact with a sufferer who could transmit the poison, but in others the cause was hidden or occult (i.e. not immediately visible) but still coming from outside the body. This might be something ingested, like bad food, spread by some form of contact, as in rabies, or inhaled with the air. These airborne diseases Fernel divided into the endemic, caused by exhalations from the earth, the epidemic, the result of violent seasonal changes, and the pestilential, brought about by a hidden malignant quality sent down from heaven and the stars, and scattered like seeds (a metaphor that he also used to define the specific nature of these diseases). A pestilential disease was not the direct result of a general putrefaction, for that would attack more than one kind of animal, but the consequences of this seed-like, heavenly cause that produced the putrefaction that then corrupted the whole body.[79] These occult diseases, Fernel believed, were best fought by using a drug that also operated through its own total substance, particularly if it had been found to be a specific remedy against a particular disease. This was not an indulgent acceptance of any drug touted by a travelling salesman, but an appeal to the experience and skill of a trained practitioner who knew how to use the appropriate method of enquiry that would allow him to distinguish between different types of disease and also to adopt an experimental method.[80] An understanding of the workings of the universe and of occult powers in their relationship to the heavens was not in Fernel's view something magical but a type of rational learning that went back to Plato and, in particular, to his Neoplatonist followers in Late Antiquity. This belief in natural magic operating through hidden qualities was a typical Renaissance way of thinking. It was not opposed to reason, for it emphasised the ability of the true physician or philosopher to penetrate beneath the surface and see the interconnections that animated the world. What he saw was hidden only in the sense that it was not immediately perceptible to the untrained mind. The greater one's understanding, the clearer one's vision became.

Fernel reiterated these ideas in 1542 in his *De naturali parte medicinae*, *The Natural Part of Medicine*, which 12 years later became the first section in his major textbook of Galenic medicine, *Medicine*, of 1554 and its subsequent revisions.[81] He followed Aristotle and Galen in positing that the body was made up of simple parts composed from different proportions of the four elements and their qualities, which in turn made up the organs of the body. The overall mixture or temperament was more than the sum of the temperaments of the individual parts, but the result of a combination of the bodily fluids or humours affected by the organ and of natural, celestial and vital heat. But in order to live, the body as a whole required in some way to be animated.[82]

This animation was produced by the soul, which, as Galen had taught and Leoniceno had further shown, came from outside and was the power that shaped the foetus.[83] It was, Fernel argued, something immaterial, celestial in origin, and as such compatible with Christian doctrine and capable of being defended against accusations of Galenic materialism. The soul had its parts, which following Plato and Galen he termed natural, sensitive and rational, but they were contained within its unitary form, for the destruction of any one part inevitably led to the destruction of the rest. Each part in turn engendered a constellation of powers, or faculties, each of which was responsible for a particular bodily function, and which operated through spirits.[84] Although he had emphasised the role of the natural spirit, produced in the liver and responsible for nutrition and growth, Galen himself had said little about any other spirits, and it was Arabic authors such as Avicenna who had developed more fully the notion of a vital spirit, produced in the heart and responsible for energy, and a psychic spirit, produced in the brain, each with its own system of conduits, respectively veins, arteries and nerves.[85] To these Fernel added a sensitive soul or spirit responsible for sensation and imagination, while giving a special role to the vital spirit in controlling and preserving life.[86] This vital spirit he identified, at least in part, with divine heat, distinct from but also similar to the natural heat produced in the body in that both required air and an oily or fatty humour, akin to the medieval 'radical moisture', without which the heat would be extinguished and the body die.[87] In what could be regarded as a break from or a development within the Galenic tradition, Fernel regarded humours as secondary formations, in but not of the body, and he included alongside the traditional four Galenic humours and the oily humour an alimentary humour that formed and nourished the tissues and an aqueous humour that permeated all parts of the body and helped them to cohere.[88]

Fernel's schema depended on an extremely detailed knowledge of Galen and Aristotle. Like Avicenna's *Canon* centuries earlier it sought to harmonise Galen's inconsistencies in line with what could be observed or revealed by reason. It answered many of the objections to Galenic physiology raised by Christian theologians and, particularly in Northern Italy, by Aristotelian philosophers.[89] At the same time, by insisting that the body often worked through occult (i.e. not manifest) powers, he opened medicine to some of the Neoplatonist, some might term them 'magical', ideas on the workings of nature that were found in Italy especially among followers of Ficino, and, in a more strident form, among Paracelsians. His views in turn were attacked by a variety of physicians and philosophers, particularly over the vexed question of generation, but his elegant and lucid Latin and his apparent omniscience gave him an authority in academic circles (particularly north of the Alps) that is not easy to explain today.[90] But he raised important questions, and some of his suggestions, particularly of the role of heat, were taken up by subsequent, more empirical investigators in the following century.

Alternatives to Galen

Some, of course, still remained closely attached to every word of Galen. The Conte da Monte, a doctor from Vicenza (1520–87), defending Galen's views on fever, struck out at Fernel, Fuchs, Valleriola, Erastus and even Alexandrinus for their innovations, even though all of them could claim to be in the mainstream of contemporary Galenism.[91] But there were other ways of utilising the classical tradition of medicine. Giovanni Argenterio (1513–72), the first professor of medical theory at the revived university of Pisa in 1543, while vigorously attacking Galen's ideas in general, praised Hippocrates highly and condemned Galen for refusing to adopt many of the insights he had found in the printed Hippocratic Corpus of 1526.[92] Parisian teachers in the middle of the century often based their commentaries on unfamiliar texts in the Hippocratic Corpus to avoid the rigidity of Galenism and introduce their students to new areas of medicine, even if, as J.J. Scaliger pointed out in a series of devastating critiques of their interpretations of *Head Wounds*, their understanding of Hippocratic Greek left a lot to be desired.[93] Guillaume de Baillou (1538–1616), who served as Dean of the Faculty in 1580–2, modelled his studies of widespread diseases on the Hippocratic *Epidemics*, carefully describing the weather and climate at various times and seasons of the year and endeavouring to relate them to the diseases he encountered.[94] Elsewhere, writers like Caius and Gessner sought to incorporate new or forgotten classical texts relating to medicine into their books and lectures.

The most celebrated of these seekers after Antiquity was Girolamo Mercuriale, who in his lectures and writings strove to show the relevance of Classical Antiquity to modern problems.[95] His guide to students on precisely what and how to read mentioned only one modern author, the Parisian Jacobus Sylvius for his discussion of the best way of reading the works of Hippocrates and Galen in order.[96] Mercuriale was not against the Arabs: he commends Rhazes, Averroes and, his favourite, Avicenna, for their practical expertise, but it is the ancients who must be read diligently and have their most useful ideas, like those of any medical author, copied out in well-organised commonplace books.[97] He expected his students to read their texts in their entirety. Like Leonhard Fuchs and even Vesalius (no stranger himself to the writing of a student handbook), he condemned summaries and compendia as a waste of time and money, as well as dangerous, for they robbed the student of the chance to digest fully the original arguments, which were rarely presented in context, and were easily forgotten by a student who had not developed the discipline of thorough reading and note taking. Indeed, although a prolific commentator himself, he frowned even upon commentaries, with a few exceptions, for they inhibited the reader from making his own judgement on a difficult passage. It is striking also that his list of classical authors to be read goes beyond the obviously medical to include historians, geographers like Strabo and even poets, although, like some compilers of today's reading lists, he also betrays an awareness of the frailty of student enthusiasm and does not expect his recommendations to be followed in full.

It is this assemblage of material from a great range of ancient sources that distinguishes all Mercuriale's publications. He covered a broad range of themes from lactation through childhood diseases, rabies, plague, skin complaints, poisons and poisoning, cosmetics, and eye-diseases, to physical exercise, to say nothing of his editions and lectures on Hippocrates and Galen, or his letters and *consilia*.[98] Characteristic of them all is his bringing together of a wide variety of information which he then submits to a medical and philological analysis. This is shown in his most famous work, *De arte gymnastica*, *The Art of Physical Exercise*, first published in 1569 and then in much enlarged and revised editions in 1573, 1577, 1587 and 1601. That so many revisions were thought necessary testifies not only to Mercuriale's continued interest in the subject, but also the wide public of doctors and antiquarians eager to buy this magnificent work. Its significance was enhanced from the second edition onwards by more antiquarian detail and especially by the 21 woodcuts of ancient exercises designed by a distinguished artist in Rome, Pirro Ligorio (1510–83) on the basis of ancient works of art, ancient remains and inscriptions (not all of which are authentic).[99] Its aim, as Mercuriale explained to the Emperor Maximilian II in his preface to that and subsequent editions, was nothing less than the restoration of the ancient art of physical exercise or gymnastic, which had so enhanced the strength and martial vigour of the Greeks and Romans that they could conquer large parts of the known world. The new diseases of the sixteenth century were in part due to the failure of contemporaries to keep themselves fit, and this return to the past would thus benefit the present.[100]

The book has a simple plan. It opens with the longest of the six books, which brings together the evidence for the structures and personnel involved in physical exercise in Antiquity. He was helped by members of the circle of Roman antiquarians around Cardinal Farnese, who provided him with detailed plans of the baths in ancient Rome and with information about the ancient inscriptions of bath attendants and boilermen, as well as doctors and trainers, all of whom who were necessary for the baths to function. This was a remarkable reconstruction, not improved upon until the nineteenth century. It is followed by two books setting out the various types of exercise encountered in Antiquity, the first listing the exercises that were performed in an ancient gymnasium or the baths, the second others that were also thought to contribute to health, ranging from standing still, singing and bowling a hoop to martial arts, swimming and hunting. Book Four is the most theoretical, setting out Mercuriale's general rationale for exercise, as well as laying down rules for how it should be performed and by whom, almost all of which can be found in today's handbooks of exercise. He warns against over-exercise, specifying the need for a preliminary period of warming up and for what in his view is often neglected, a similar period of gentle exercise to cool down. The final pair of books follows the arrangement of Books Two and Three, explaining the effects and advantages of each exercise in turn. Singing or even shouting may be useful in chest conditions, while being pushed to and fro in a swing or taken for a gentle country drive may provide a little physical stimulation but also, and more important, impart a welcome sense of pleasure to those who are incapable of taking independent exercise themselves. Throughout, Mercuriale linked his ancient authorities with the games and physical activities he saw around him in Rome, Padua or Pisa, and, although aware of the very different circumstances of sixteenth-century Italy, he believed that there was a place for more forms of exercises than the fencing and riding engaged in by the wealthy.[101]

In one sense he was not breaking completely new ground, for exercise, as one of the six non-naturals, had often appeared in general treatises on the maintenance of health as well as in recommendations for individuals since medieval times, not least in the famous *Salernitan Regimen for Health*.[102] The importance of physical exercise formed the second part of the treatise on education, *De moribus ingenuis*, *True Morality*, written by the Italian humanist Piero Paolo Vergerio (1370–1444/5). When around 1505 the humanist Paolo Cortesi (1465–1510) wrote his description of the ideal cardinal and his court, he included a long section on the importance of keeping the cardinal healthy. The effects of too much food and wine, to say nothing of the emotional strain of life with the Borgias, could be mitigated in part by exercise with the small ball, as recommended by Galen in a treatise only recently published for the first time in 1490 in a translation by Niccolò da Reggio.[103] The new translation of Galen's *The Preservation of Health* by Thomas Linacre that first appeared in 1517 attracted further attention, and Galen's ideas on the importance of exercise were spread throughout the century in commentaries, treatises and even poetry as well as in vernacular treatises like Sir Thomas Elyot's *The Castel of Helthe*, Andrew Boorde's *The Breviary of Helthe* or Georg Pictorius's *Dialogi del modo del conservare la sanità*.[104] Elyot in particular took over many of his recommendations for forms of exercise, including football and dancing, as well as vociferation and singing, adding to the descriptions in Oribasius ideas of his own such as "romping in harneys" like a horse.[105]

Not all were convinced by Mercuriale. His friend, Andrea Bacci, who had read the book before publication, praised its erudition, but doubted whether its careful description of various exercises was of any value whatsoever in a modern society given over entirely to luxury and gaming.[106] The Savoyard Emilio Duso devoted a mere six pages and Julius Alexandrinus 26 to describing the same exercises as Mercuriale but without bothering to mention his name, concentrating instead on the general principles of healthy living.[107] But one reader of Mercuriale certainly hoped to put his ideas into practise and may well have done so; Richard Mulcaster, Headmaster of Merchant Taylors' School from 1561 to 1586, and later of St Paul's School, both of them schools founded in London to promote the new humanist learning. His educational manifesto of 1581 had a two-fold aim, to educate children "for their skill in their booke or health in their bodie".[108] Modern scholars have paid much attention to the first requirement, for which Mulcaster proposed regular school plays among other things, but have said less about the second. Of its 30 sections, which open the volume, 28 paraphrase exercises described by Mercuriale, who is praised as the first to bring to public attention the importance of physical exercise.[109] Although we know that some of Mulcaster's pupils did play games and practise archery, it is not clear whether this was in school time, and, like many of his other innovations, the emphasis on the moral virtues of games did not take hold in English public schools until centuries later. Indeed, when in 1864 John Blundell, a doctor from Kent, provided an English paraphrase of the whole of *De arte gymnastica* in one of the first modern investigations into the workings of the muscles, he declared in his foreword that England was only just beginning to take note of the gymnastics movement, already well developed in Germany.[110]

Learned Medicine in Practice

Some of this academic learning filtered down to the wider reading public in handbooks and guides to domestic medicine in the vernacular as well as in Latin. But, until recently, it has not been easy to gauge how much this was reflected in the day-to-day practice of physicians, or, to put it crudely, what those patients who were able to pay the doctor's fee hoped to get for their money. The objection that all pre-modern medicine was an exercise in harming, rather than curing, the patient, even if true (which is far from clear), is irrelevant here, for all types of pre-modern medicine were defective in the light of current conceptions of disease and pharmacology and it is only in the last century that medical intervention could be said to have cured many diseases.[111] The variety of patients who fill the many pages of Van Foreest's *Observationes* does not suggest that there was a general lack of faith in medicine, and his complaints about some of his colleagues' reluctance to treat the poor for less or, indeed, nothing indicate that it was a lack of means rather than any mistrust of doctors in general that led them to other and cheaper practitioners.[112] Information on what doctors actually did, as opposed to their theories, comes from two sources. Printed publications of case histories, whether in the form of letters or as specific collections, became common in the sixteenth century, many of them written by or to major figures in contemporary medicine. To find out what had been done before the accounts were redacted into a form suitable for a wider public, one must have recourse to manuscripts and the notebooks in which doctors wrote their own case notes. Neither has been fully exploited as yet. Studies on printed sources tend to emphasise particular clinical novelties without giving the wider context, while the major project by Michael Stolberg, the only large-scale investigation of manuscript case notes, concentrates on Germany.[113] The two complement each other, the latter revealing the immediate actions of the physician at the bedside or in the consulting room, the former often explaining and justifying the thinking behind them. Together they provide some answers to the questions implied at the beginning of this section.

Physicians were consulted on a wide range of conditions, from childbirth and mental illness to fever and gastric problems.[114] Mental conditions in the Galenic tradition were closely linked to the physical body, for the imbalance of bodily humours affected the brain. An excess of bile was thought to cause mania, while the most celebrated of mental abnormalities, melancholy, was the result of an excess of burnt and black bile. It was associated both with what today might be termed depression and with the rare quality of genius, a link that can be traced back to the Aristotle and his school in the late fourth century BCE.[115] It could be diagnosed from physical signs, which were sometimes interpreted physiognomically: a person's appearance both indicated the physical make-up and, as in the best-selling tract on physiognomy by Giovanni Battista della Porta (1545–1615), linked it with the wider animal world and the character traits associated with different animals.[116] Behaviour, too, provided important clues to which of its many forms this melancholy disease might be taking – laughing, weeping, hallucinations, silence or extremes of anger or, a favourite theme of poets and playwrights, the desperation of a lover. The exposition of erotic melancholy by the French physician Jacques Ferrand, first published in 1610, incorporated the conclusions of half a century of medical writing, and was in turn used in his later revisions by Robert Burton (1577–1640) in his masterpiece of erudition and wit, *The Anatomy of Melancholy*.[117] His description of this complex disease, and the equally complex ways in which doctors, philosophers and theologians sought to understand it, has its counterpart in art in the much earlier, and equally famous, portrait of Melancholy by Albrecht Durer (1471–1528).[118] That a German artist, a French physician and an Oxford don should devote so much effort to depicting this mental condition also demonstrates the varied ways in which the ideas of learned medicine could be transmitted to a wider public.

For the most part, doctors and their patients agreed that the cause of a mental disorder was usually something physical or, even if not, that it could be discovered in exactly the same way as they looked for the causes of physical diseases.[119] They examined carefully the patient's urine, blood and faeces (although some preferred not to get too close to these evil-smelling substances) and took the pulse. Both Georg Handsch and Van Foreest report detailed conversations with their patients, and also emphasise the importance of a proper examination, hardly surprising since both had studied at Padua. This thoroughness, they believed, was one of the things that distinguished the 'elite' physicians from lesser healers. How much attention they paid to prophylaxis is less clear from the nature of these case histories, but Galenic demands for continuous familiarity with one's patients and their habits would have been best served (and financially rewarded) if a physician enjoyed an appropriately high status and moved within the same social circles as his patients. Treatment consisted primarily in terms of evacuating whatever noxious matter was thought to be at work in the body, mimicking or assisting it in its natural modes of evacuation in order to restore the balance of the body. Hence the use of purgatives, clysters, bleeding (with due caution), sweating, particularly with guaiac in syphilis, as well as diet and drugs. Visiting baths and mineral springs was only just beginning to be adopted in England for medical treatment, one of its early advocates being the well-travelled cleric, William Turner, but was common in Italy and Germany.[120] Heavy bleeding or purgation was reserved for the most extreme cases, when prostration was thought to allow the body's own forces to work against the small residual amount of harmful or peccant matter.[121] The rationale behind these therapies, namely the need to restore the balance within the body and to strengthen it to resist further harmful changes, was accepted by everyone, even if there might be disagreements over its application in an individual case.

The actual bleeding, like surgery, was usually performed by a barber or a surgeon (Figure 8.1). Van Foreest condemned fellow physicians who knew little or nothing about surgery, but his own direct surgical interventions were confined to emergency bandaging. Instead, he insisted that the overall management of the case was his job (something he claims was accepted by almost all surgeons), since the process of recovery was at least as important as the actual surgical intervention.[122] Similarly, the preparation of drugs was something to be left to apothecaries, but doctors were expected to understand how they worked and what to prescribe for each patient. Drugs that were claimed to work for most or all conditions and in every case, no matter what the humoral balance, age or sex of the patient, were always suspect, even famous panaceas such as theriac, and those who touted them risked the opprobrium of being dismissed as charlatans.

A university-trained physician had two major calling cards. He claimed to know better than his competitors how the body worked (or was generally thought to work) and he could appeal to experience. By the middle of the century he would have seen a dissected corpse and may have joined in the private dissection classes of his teachers, accompanied them on their visits and discussed cases with some of the most famous practitioners in circumstances that were likely to be superior to those he would encounter when beginning to practise anywhere outside a major city. This, as we have seen, was one of the frequent justifications for the *peregrinatio* to Italy, France and elsewhere, and was clearly accepted by many of those who were his prospective employers.

But this experience was also available via books, and there would have been few physicians in 1590 who had not a collection of tens of volumes, some of them very substantial. Their humbler competitors could not have afforded such a library, relying at most on small, practical handbooks. The learned physician had been trained from school how to identify and copy down matters that would be significant, and Mercuriale was not alone in advising his medical readers how to do this. Several medical commonplace books survive, not to speak of the thousands of books that, like those of Thomas Lorkyn (earlier, p. 76) bear marginal notes or underlinings that reveal the interests of their reader or, since books often circulated, readers.[123] The development of indexes also facilitated access to individual passages in large books, like Matthioli's *Herbal*, and several owners compiled their own indexes. How this material might then be deployed is nicely illustrated by Van Foreest in his *Observationes*, although not every physician was as wealthy, learned and well-established as he was in Delft and Alkmaar. But it was an exceptional, and perhaps unlucky, practitioner who did not have some books, and, like that of the local cleric, who might also have some medical expertise, his learning would be regarded as superior to that of his patients and, in a small town, of less academic competitors, whether local or merely transient.

Van Foreest's method of exposition remained the same throughout his many volumes: he would begin with a detailed account of the case, usually one of his own but occasionally taken from the existing literature, explaining the nature of his patient and why he or she had chosen to come to him, and following the case through to its conclusion. Sometimes, he included other similar cases that he had diagnosed and treated similarly. A few cases chosen at random from his two books on diseases of the genitals in both men and women indicate his methods and the range of patients he treated. In *Observationes* XXVIII, 3–4, he mentions his treatment for the suppression of menses of a peasant girl, a nun and the wives of two citizens of Delft, giving a spread of ages and class. This *Observatio* is then followed by a *scholium*, an exposition frequently many times the length of the case history, in which he explains the rationale behind his therapies. He moves in order from questions of diagnosis to discussing causation and finally treatment. In these chapters, his main sources are the Greeks, particularly Paul and Aetius, who are far more informative than Galen (who says relatively little about women) and Hippocrates, but also late medieval authors such as Niccolò Falcucci (d. 1412), Valesco de Taranta (d. 1418), Matteo Ferrari di Grado (d. 1472) and Marco Gattinaria (d. 1496) as well as others more recent such as Amatus Lusitanus and Donato Altomare (1506–62). He justifies his reliance on them by saying that he does not care whether the author is a Greek, a Latin, an Arab or a Jew, as long as he has found their practical advice to be sound.[124] For treating *post partum* pain, he recommended using a decoction of flowers of chamomile in beer, justifying this by cases he had met in Holland and Rome, and then adding other possible therapies from the medieval author Gilbertus Anglicus (fl. 1250), the humanist author Alessandro Benedetti and his Delft colleague, the 'distinguished doctor', Johann Tiengius.[125] Another important source was what he termed the *Harmonia gynaeciorum*, a large compendium of writings, both ancient and modern, on gynaecology, first published at Basle in 1566, in an enlarged form in 1586–7, and finally in a volume over a thousand pages long in the even more capacious edition by Israel Spach in 1597.[126]

Van Foreest's book on the sexual problems of men is more substantial. In an explanation that is four or five times the length of the actual account of satyriasis, *Observationes* XXVI, 10, he adds references to the *Practica medicinalis* of Lionello Vettori (d. 1520?), his Bolognese teacher Padoani and Guillaume Rondelet, professor at Montpellier, the "most important of the moderns".[127] All these scholars were working within the Galenic tradition, and Van Foreest continued to add references to similar modern literature well into the 1580s, if not right up to his death a decade later. It is this learning, and the way it was employed to explicate the data of experience, that set the learned physician above the humbler practitioner, with whom Van Foreest often enjoyed good relations, and still further above the so-called empirics. These, he alleged, even if successful, could not understand, let alone explain in what might be termed 'scientific' terms, why their therapy had worked, and if it failed, simply walked away from their even more distressed patient.

This chapter has presented a relatively favourable view of learned medicine and its practitioners in the sixteenth century. It was not always a bastion of conservative Galenism rigid in its rules, out of touch with patients or their diseases, and, like Shakespeare's Dr Caius, speaking a technical language that few could understand (a medical habit still to be found today). But any attempt at generalisation is fraught with caveats. The printed evidence on which I have relied, written by the doctors themselves, is naturally biased in their favour: their theories are always convincing, their therapies successful, unless thwarted by circumstances and individuals beyond their control. Case notes, however, suggest that there was a general similarity between the way in which all practitioners worked, subject always to the constraints of where they practised and what materials they had to hand, and seem to indicate that they shared many of their ideas about how the body functioned and even their therapies with the wider community they served. Most of those who have been cited here, although from different parts of Europe, represent an elite within a medical elite, working in substantial and prosperous communities and, at least occasionally, attending a monarch or local magnate. Georg Handsch may not have made an enormous amount of money as doctor to Ferdinand II of the Tyrol, but he may well have preferred security and status, and certainly enjoyed a greater income than if he had returned from his Italian studies to practise in provincial Bohemia or even to stay on in Prague.[128] Innsbruck, the capital of the Tyrol, was no backwater, and its position on the main trade route between Italy and Germany allowed him access to a wider range of medical materials and information than doctors in most other parts of Europe. Not everyone was so fortunate, as we have already seen in our survey of careers of civic doctors, but one may hope that those who sat at the feet of Brasavola, Da Monte or Fernel and who are mere names in a matriculation register or tax record at least attempted to put into practice some of the wise injunctions of their teachers.

Notes

1 Maclean 2002; Pomata and Siraisi 2005; Favaretti Camposampiero and Scribano forthcoming.
2 For Basle, Benkert 2020 and later, pp. 292–4.
3 Caius 1570c: 14v, 1912: 86; Nutton 2018a: 66; Baldo 2014: xliii; Stolberg 2021a: 39–47.
4 For medical practice, see later, pp. 236–40.
5 Nutton 2017a; for a reversion to Galen, see later, p. 264.
6 Copenhaver 1978: 52, 112–17.
7 Leoniceno 1506, 1508; earlier, p. 101.
8 Earlier, p. 102.
9 His date of death (traditionally 1522) is excluded by the evidence of a correspondent of Erasmus, *Ep.* 1407: Allen V, 378–80. Brissot quotes Galen in Greek, but his knowledge of Hippocrates comes largely through Galen, and his scanty references to Galen's venesection tracts suggests a limited acquaintance at best.
10 For the circumstances of this book, see the prefaces to Brissot 1525; Friedenwald 1939.
11 Driverius 1532; Corti in Brissot 1539; Vesalius 1539: 56; Eriksson 1959: 255–73. Cf. also Turinus 1545.
12 Joubert 1587, 1995: 77–88.
13 Nutton 2020a: 64–9; Maclean 2002: 303.

14 Manardi *Epp.* II, 1, XII, 5, and XV, 8: 1556: 30–2, 125, 150–62; Zambelli 1965.
15 Struthius in Galen 1536: 112v–13v. For Paris, Morel 1528: sigg. C ii v.; C iv v.; E ii v.–iii v.
16 Siraisi 2013: 43–4. In general, Newman and Grafton 2001.
17 Cardano 1555; Grafton and Siraisi 2001.
18 Kusukawa 1993.
19 Siraisi 1997: 124–31. For Paracelsus, later, p. 286.
20 Gaurico 1546.
21 Virdung 1532; Mizauld 1551.
22 Virdung 1584. Notes in London, Wellcome Collection, EPB 3077.
23 MacDonald 1981; Traister 2001; Kassell 2005; Hadass 2018; Stolberg 2021a: 154–9. Thomas 1973: 343–4, 375–7, 420–2 is classic.
24 Forman practised medicine and astrology for more than 20 years before he obtained a medical licence from Cambridge University.
25 Galileo, cited by Stolberg 2021a: 24.
26 Stolberg 2015.
27 Stolberg 2021b: 9–10.
28 Stolberg 2021b: 45–6, 132–4; Nutton 1996; Hart 1623 is a vigorous English translation of Forestus 1591a.
29 Forestus 1591a: 71–9, 174; Nutton 2006.
30 Tiraqueau 1561: 426–7; for Paracelsians, later, p. 294.
31 Leoniceno 1508; Nutton 1996. For medieval diagnosis, Loviconi 2020.
32 Caius 1544; Crato 1555, both based on the lectures in Da Monte 1554a. In general, Ongaro 1981.
33 Ferretto 2012.
34 For this trilogy, Valles 1588; for 'semiotics', note the addition of the word to the 1581 republication of Gessner's *Enchiridion rei medicae triplicis: I. simiotice, hoc est quae signa ex pulsibus et urinis dijudicat.*
35 Stolberg 2021a: 69, 177–80.
36 Gessner 1581 (originally 1555); Bauhin 1602; Rogano 1560.
37 Struthius 1555; Grisignano 1543 is based substantially on medieval authors on the pulse but may have attracted only local interest.
38 E.g. Capodivacca 1596.
39 Sassonia 1604.
40 Harvey 1628; Bylebyl 1985.
41 Even if the different ways in which libraries bind the individual classes complicate consultation.
42 Da Monte 1587; note the summary of his ideas on urines, Da Monte 1552.
43 Ongaro 1994 refutes the notion that Da Monte invented this bedside teaching; Klestinec 2010; Stolberg 2015.
44 London, Wellcome Collection, WMS 567 (of 1536–7); Da Monte 1554b, 1583; Hieronymus 2005: 1379–85. See also earlier, p. 89.
45 Maclean 2002: 294–301.
46 aa.vv. 1533. On this group, Ferretto 2012: 42–3.
47 La Framboisière 1595a, 1595b. Cf. 1609; for Paré's identification of the rational with the methodical surgeon, Houchon 2003.
48 Alexandrinus 1548; Rosario 1572; Laguna 1554.
49 Respectively, Alexandrinus 1548: 7v–8v; Rosario 1572: 221–4; Laguna 1554: 473.
50 Gryllus 1566a; Valles 1556, 1582; Maclean 2002; Ferretto 2012 gives other examples.
51 Nutton 1983.
52 Nutton 1983: 8–10.
53 Nutton 1990d: 199, note 7.

54 Fracastoro 1546; Pennuto 2008.
55 Nutton 1990d.
56 Beroaldo 1505: B, vi, v.
57 Da Monte 1554c: 78r–80v, 217v–27v, 1554c: 170r–5v, 1558b: 379–81.
58 Nutton 1990d: 208–14.
59 Gryllus 1566a: 50r, using his theories unusually to explain flavours.
60 Deer Richardson 1985: 178.
61 Valles 1556: 70r–v.
62 Trincavella 1586: 19v; cf. 146r–55r.
63 Lange 1589: 610–21.
64 Nutton 1990d: 215.
65 Nutton 1990d: 219.
66 Wrocław, University Library, Ms. Rehdiger 243, fol. 12v; *Ep.* 7.
67 Earlier, pp. 31–3.
68 Agasse and Pennuto 2016: 152–3, 216–29.
69 Nutton 1990d: 211–15; Siraisi 2013 20–3.
70 Simoni 1576.
71 Nutton 1990d: 224: Cohn 2010: 161–202.
72 Nutton 2011, discusses some later French theories.
73 Nutton 2012b; cf. Cunningham 2003.
74 Fernel 1560, 1567; (tr. Forrester and Henry) 2005; for the date of composition, *ibid.*, 12–13.
75 For his influence, Brockliss and Jones 1997: 128–33; Gryllus 1566a regards his ideas as a significant (if at times misguided) extension of Galenism.
76 Benivieni 1507.
77 Fernel 1567: 40, 2005: 586–7.
78 Deer Richardson 1985.
79 Fernel 1567: 94–114, 2005: 536–629. The definitions appear at 1567: 102, 2005: 575.
80 Fernel 1567: 133–6, 2005: 720–35.
81 The title repeats the standard term for the first section of medical textbooks, contrasting the natural body in health, with the six non-naturals, earlier, p. 97, and lead to the preter-naturals, disease and illness.
82 Fernel 1567: 91–4, 127–8, 2003, 190–3, 252–5; Hall 1975: 193: For Fernel's later summary, 1567: 23–6, 2005: 208–21.
83 Hirai 2011: 64–76; Bigotti 2019: 51. For the problems of reconciling the Galenic soul with the unitary soul of: Christian theology, Nutton 1990b; Bigotti 2019.
84 Fernel 1567: 154–9, 2003: 302–11.
85 Temkin 1977: 154–61.
86 Fernel 1567: 184–6, 2003: 356–63.
87 Fernel 1567: 129–31, 285–7, 134–6, 2003: 256–60, 508–12, 264–9.
88 Fernel 1567: 134–6, 2003: 264–9.
89 Nutton 1990b; Lines 1922.
90 Deer Richardson 1985; Hirai 2011; Bigotti 2019.
91 Conte Da Monte 1591 (ed. 1, 1580); cf. the comments of Peter Monau to Dudith, Dudith 2002: 306.
92 Siraisi 2001: 328–55. For Renaissance doctors, as for Galen, the historical Hippocrates was responsible for most of the Greek texts circulating under his name.
93 Lonie 1985; Nutton 2006.
94 De Baillou 2021.
95 Arcangeli and Nutton 2008.
96 Durling 1990.

97 Rinaldi 2006. For the persistence of Avicenna, Siraisi 1987; its price was higher in Padua in 1567 than in Venice, earlier, p. 72.

98 Mercuriale 2008: 809–60. This edition and translation, based on the 1601 edition, also contains a major biographical study by Jean-Michel Agasse; Kavvadia 2015, 2021.

99 Vagenheim 2008.

100 Mercuriale 2008: 2–7. Earlier humanists had also advocated a unity of physical, mental and moral education. Hale 1994: 194.

101 Céard *et al.*1990, esp. 295–376.

102 Curio 1553 is but one of the more than 40 sixteenth-century printings in several languages. In general, Mikkeli 1999: 14–96; Maclean 2002: 251–8; Cavallo and Storey 2013, 2017.

103 Cortesi 1510: LXXVIv–VIIr.

104 Elyot 1534, 1541; Boorde 1547; Pictorius 1550 (originally in Latin in 1549). For other authors, Agasse in Mercuriale 2008: 922–35, 1105–7z.

105 Elyot 1541: 48–53.

106 Bacci 1572: 446–51.

107 Duso 1582; Alexandrinus 1575.

108 Mulcaster 1581, 1887.

109 Mulcaster 1887: 71, 129–30.

110 Blundell 1864: pref.

111 *Pace* Wotton: 2006.

112 Nutton 1996: 247, although this did not mean that he favoured a universal levelling of fees.

113 Stolberg 2021a; cf. also Stolberg 2019, 2020, 2021b.

114 Stolberg 2021a: 160–220.

115 Arikha 2007: 113–72; Lindemann 2010: 44–5.

116 Della Porta 1586.

117 Ferrand 1610, 1990; Burton 1624; Gowland 2006.

118 The theme of the classic account by Klibansky *et al.* 1964.

119 Stolberg 2021a: 280–1.

120 Turner 1562; Palmer 1990b; Harley 1990: 48–9.

121 For debates over the value of bleeding in plague, Cohn 2010: 15–18. Cf. modern coma therapy in extreme cases of infection.

122 Nutton 2017c.

123 Durling 1990; Blair 2010.

124 Forestus 1599: 20–35, 1653: 3,282–5; on the value of his authorities, 1599: 31, 1653: 3,284.

125 *Id.: Obs.* LXXXI: 1599: 561–5, 1653: 3,401.

126 Aa.vv. 1566, 1597. On the latter edition, King 2007. Which edition Van Forest was using is unclear.

127 Forestus 1597: 69–72, 1653: 233–4.

128 Stolberg 2021a: 1, 2020.

9   Anatomy – the Touchstone of Modernity

The Classical Background

The study of the human body by means of dissection has always been controversial. Social and religious taboos, a physically based conception of the integrity of the individual as well as the degrading implications of being dismembered, to say nothing of the difficulty of obtaining a suitable corpse, have militated against the practice far more than any legal regulation. Indeed, some legal restrictions have been more concerned with the status of the dissector and the appropriate burial of the body than with any attempt to forbid dissection itself. From Classical Antiquity onwards, there have been reasoned objections to human anatomy on the grounds that the information gained from it could be more easily obtained by means other than deliberately cutting into a dead human body – by analogy with dissected animals, from surgical practice or, in today's medical schools, from working with models, digital simulations and TV presentations. Others argued that the constant repetition of the same dissection added little or nothing to what had been gained from the initial mapping of the human body. In their view a knowledge of the basic structures of the body was all that was needed by a doctor who was to deal with illness and internal changes within the body and who might prefer to leave the bloody business of surgery to 'mechanics' more adroit but less learned than he. Besides, since, in most pre-modern medical theories, illness was in general believed to be the result of constant alterations in the balance of the living body, what was revealed in a dead body, inert and divided into its constituent parts, was irrelevant to everyday medical life. Consequently, knowledge of the internal structures and organs of the human body remained for centuries partial and limited in application, while the actual practice of human dissection, the investigation of a human corpse by means of a knife, effectively disappeared for long periods. Even when, by the late sixteenth century, the dissection of a human corpse became more common, it was as a focus for pedagogy, and even entertainment, rather than for investigative research.[1]

Galen believed that Hippocrates too was himself an anatomist, something denied by modern scholars, who place the origins of Western anatomy

DOI: 10.4324/9781003223184-13

in the fourth century BCE with the experiments on animals and birds of Aristotle and his contemporary Diocles of Carystus. Human dissection as a research endeavour is first clearly identified with Herophilus and Erasistratus, both active around 280 BCE, the former certainly working in Alexandria in Egypt, the latter probably so. But although there was a tradition of skeletal anatomy, extremely useful for surgery, in that city that lasted at least until the second or third centuries CE, nothing further is known for certain of experimentation on the Herophilean model after 250 BCE, until a certain Marinus reintroduced it "in the time of [Galen's] grandfathers" around 100 CE. He and his pupils, several of whom became Galen's teachers, had to rely for their fuller understanding of the human body on comparisons with animals such as pigs and goats, supplemented by a few chance observations of corpses or aborted foetuses.[2] This revival spread to the major Greek cities of the Roman East, and also to Rome itself, where public anatomical displays around 155 CE by doctors such as Lycus of Macedon attracted large crowds, while sceptics warned ignorant bystanders not to be led astray by flashy instruments and smooth patter.[3]

Galen is the pivotal figure in the history of pre-Vesalian anatomy[4] (Figure 4.2). Passionately interested in dissection since his early days as a medical student, he assiduously sought out all the information he could find from those who had been trained at Alexandria. He made his early reputation in Rome with his public anatomical displays, and although he soon gave these up, he claims to have continued dissecting privately for the rest of his life. In his view, the whole of medicine depended on an understanding of the structures and workings of the body, in its widest sense including what today would be called 'physiology', and he was particularly proud of his remarkable investigations into the brain and the nervous system. Although he knew a little about the internal organisation of the body through his work as a surgeon and chance observation of corpses, he relied otherwise entirely on animals. He was aware of the limitations of animal anatomy, suggesting which animals might best be dissected to gain optimal results – the hyoid bone, for example, was best observed in large animals. But, at the very least, experimenting on animals could resolve disputed questions either directly or by ruling out some alternative solutions, and give insights into the way the human body functioned.[5] In short, without anatomical knowledge through dissection, medicine was fallible and incomplete.

This message he transmitted in a variety of books. Some were short summaries of his results for students; others, like his books on vivisection and on dissection (both now lost in their original language), were meant for his fellow practitioners. Still others, like his treatise on the *Opinions of Hippocrates and Plato*, were intended to demonstrate how his anatomical discoveries could contribute to philosophical debates, confirming the Platonist view of the body as comprising three interconnected systems based on the brain, the heart and the liver.[6] Galen encapsulated all his findings in the 15 books of *Anatomical Procedures*, of which the last five and a half survive today only in Arabic.[7] (There were rumours in the Renaissance that a complete copy in Greek had survived in a remote library, but none has yet been found.)[8] They constituted a remarkable manual of dissection, in which Galen gave very detailed (and often surprisingly accurate) information as to how and where to cut. More influential was another large treatise, the 17 books of *The Usefulness of Parts*, explaining his anatomical discoveries for the benefit of Aristotelian philosophers. In it he demonstrated the function and use of the individual parts of the body, ending with a hymn to the purposeful design of the Creator, or Nature. It was a powerful statement of the value of an anatomical understanding of the human body, written in a way that was accessible to non-medics.[9]

Medieval Anatomy

Galen's achievement, great though it was and rightly praised by modern anatomists, also contributed to the near demise of anatomical dissection precisely because of the extent and apparent finality of his discoveries. Christian writers like Nemesius of Emesa (fl. 350) eagerly seized on Galen's discoveries to support their ideas on the relationship of body and soul, but by then practical dissection had vanished almost entirely, even at Alexandria.[10] For the next millennium, the tiny handful of references to dissection are either quotations from Galen or, very occasionally, refer to the dismemberment of opponents' bodies in war.[11] Galen's writings on anatomy were copied in Greek and later translated into Syriac and Arabic, but only a few short summaries for students appear to have been frequently studied. The sheer length of the larger treatises discouraged their copying by hand, especially when their overall message could be obtained more easily and at less cost from other books. The more specialised anatomical works, like the treatises *The Voice* or *Problematical Movements*, were equally rarely copied. Neither in Byzantium nor in the Islamic world did the possession of Galen's anatomical works stimulate empirical investigation and his view of the body went almost unchallenged.[12] Criticism of it was rare: Abd al-Laṭīf's rejection of some of Galen's osteology and Ibn al-Nafīs's arguments in favour of the circulation of the blood are both exceptional and, equally important, had no direct effect on medicine as it was taught or practised.[13]

The fate of *The Usefulness of Parts* exemplifies the change from Galen to Galenism, and from an empirically minded and intellectually sophisticated approach to a dogmatism that left little room for doubt. Its message was well known, and it was among the earliest of Galen's works to be translated into Latin in the twelfth century as *De juvamentis membrorum*. Even so, this was not a complete version of the Greek, but omitted almost all the details of how to carry out the dissections on which its conclusions were based. It confirmed the importance of anatomical knowledge and the purposefulness of Creation (teleology) but in a way that did not require further dissection, let alone encourage readers to pursue the investigative procedures advocated by Galen.[14] The later more faithful translation by Niccolò da Reggio in 1317 was read by only a handful of specialists, if at all. Galenic empirical anatomy had become book anatomy, something to be read rather than practised in imitation of the master.

Signs of a renewed interest in dissection begin to appear in Western Europe from the early thirteenth century in the Po valley, where surgeons were often employed to carry out autopsies, sometimes at the request of the families of the dead.[15] Some of them also wrote their own short guides to anatomy for students. At Salerno in Southern Italy, whose teachers had become became increasingly familiar with Galenic medicine, one of them, Copho, wrote around 1100 an anatomy of the pig to help in understanding the human body. A beautiful manuscript of this treatise, now Wellcome Collection, WMS 290, which was commissioned by a London surgeon around 1450, ascribes its authorship to Galen.

A few of Galen's anatomical texts were available by 1270 in the new universities to supplement the Latin summaries of anatomy derived from Arabic handbooks. Students in Northern Italy, Paris, Montpellier, Erfurt and Oxford could buy from a university stationer large codices containing many Latin translations of Galen, sometimes including a short selection of anatomical writings passing under his name. Most commonly copied was the abbreviated version of *The Usefulness of Parts*, but several included Galen's *Problematical Movements* and the very fragmentary summary of *The Voice*, the former emphasising the relevance of anatomical information to resolving difficult medical questions, the latter describing the vocal organs.[16] None of them, however, explained in detail how to dissect, presenting Galen's conclusions rather than the methods by which they had been reached, and none can be considered popular, for they were read, if at all, only by senior teachers. But they helped to reinforce the idea that some knowledge of anatomy was essential for the understanding of Galenic medicine.

It was some time before this aspiration was realised within a medical Faculty, not least because of the gulf, both social and intellectual, between physician and surgeon. Physicians prided themselves on their understanding of the body's processes in health and illness, which were mainly detectable through the body's fluids and in which the organs and structures of the body provided at best a framework for the (in their view more significant) humoral changes to take place. Fractures, dislocations, wounds and the like they left to the 'mechanical' surgeons. It is not surprising then that the first university anatomy did not take place until around 1316, when Mondino de' Liuzzi (c. 1270–1326), a professor at Bologna, persuaded the authorities to allow him to dissect a corpse in front of his students.[17] In his *Anatomy* he several times refers to his own earlier experience as a dissector, but during his lectures he left the actual cutting to a surgeon while he explained to the audience what they were watching. His successors, who used his lectures as a textbook on which to comment and add their own observations well into the sixteenth century, often introduced a third member of the team, a junior professor, who read out extracts for his superior, called the *ostensor*, to expound further.[18]

Mondino based his book heavily on Galen as found in the early medieval Latin versions, but, unlike Galen, he began with the internal organs of the body, which were most likely to putrefy, and ended with the bones. He broke new ground in allowing intending physicians to see a corpse, but his purpose was essentially didactic, to relate what they had learned in lectures about the basic organisation of the body to what was visible before them.[19] He gave them little encouragement to go away and dissect for themselves. Besides, the circumstances of the actual dissection did not make it easy for the audience to identify smaller structures, and an annual anatomy or two could do little more than reinforce what had already been taught. Luke Demaitre rightly notes that "familiarity with the shape and substance of organs was less important than an understanding of their functions in the larger scheme of nature".[20]

Although the example of Bologna was soon followed by Padua, dissection was slow to catch on elsewhere. Vienna in 1404 was the first university north of the Alps to institute an annual dissection, but even there it was at first sporadic. Although a dissection took place in Paris in 1407 and there is an odd story of the vivisection of a condemned criminal being allowed there in 1475, regular dissections do not seem to have taken place there until a little later.[21] The requirement in the statutes of the medical Faculty of Rostock, shortly after 1433, and in the revised statutes for the University of Tübingen in 1497 for an annual dissection implies that the notion at least was already becoming common in Germany, even if it was far from being reliably realised in practice.[22] Permission had, of course, to be obtained from both civil and religious authorities, who insisted that the corpse be treated reverently and given proper burial, and sometimes ordered proceedings to begin with a special Mass. In 1452 in Vienna after the civic authorities had insisted on the most scrupulous adherence to legal and religious regulations, the Faculty decided to hold the dissection behind closed doors in their own premises to avoid any protests.[23] It was not always easy to comply with the requirements of the statutes for an annual anatomy, let alone for an anatomy of a woman every three years or so. A letter of the University of Pavia to the Duke of Milan around 1464–5, begging him not to burn a woman convicted of witchcraft, explained that they had not been able to hold an anatomy for several years, and that of a woman for many years before that, because of a shortage of appropriate bodies.[24] Things might also go wrong at the last moment. The 1441 dissection at Vienna had to be abandoned when the criminal selected for dissection survived his hanging and recovered in hospital.[25]

The Triumph of the Hellenists

The initial response to the arrival of Greek manuscripts of Galen's anatomical writings in Italy was primarily linguistic, as has already been noted (earlier, p. 102) and focussed on the clarification of terminology. They were first introduced to a wide readership in 1501 by Giorgio Valla (1447–1500) in a huge encyclopaedia with an uninformative title, *De expetendis et fugiendis rebus, Things to Look for and Avoid*. Nine of its books, 24–30 and 47–48, dealt with medicine, based principally on Celsus and two late Greek excerpters of Galen, Aetius of Amida and Paul of Aegina, which Valla read in manuscripts in his own library. Later printers, particularly in Germany, broke his large work into separate and more manageable sections, each with their own title. That dealing with anatomy, *De humani corporis partibus, The Parts of the Human Body*, was reprinted several times, the last as late as 1585, and provided the general reader with an insight into the new medicine.[26] This new Hellenised anatomy was first introduced into a medical textbook in 1502 by Alessandro Benedetti (1452–1512), who had travelled in the Greek world and owned a few Greek manuscripts. Provocatively he gave his work a purely Greek subtitle in transcription, *Anatomice*, a direct challenge to the earlier tracts with very unclassical Latin titles such as *Anothomia*.[27] The friend of leading humanists such as Merula and Ermolao Barbaro, Benedetti had begun his work in Venice in the 1480s, making use of Galen but also of the lexicographical information provided by ancient writers such as Celsus, Rufus of Ephesus and Pollux. His *Historia Corporis Humani sive Anatomice, An Enquiry into the Human Body or Anatomy*, was an elegantly written and beautifully printed survey, disguising what was a traditional Galenist exposition under a new vocabulary. It came under immediate attack from Gabriele de Zerbi (1445–1505), the leading anatomist at Padua, who countered the claims made for the new terminology by stressing his own considerable expertise with the knife.[28] Improvements in terminology, in his view, contributed little to the understanding of the body compared with knowing how and where to cut. The very appearance of his much larger book, printed in 1502 in double columns in the older Gothic script with many abbreviations, contrasted with the modern Roman lettering of Benedetti, and the detailed record of his many observations was a deliberate reproach to the Hellenists, few of whom were themselves expert dissectors. Like Antonio Benivieni (c. 1440–1502), whose *Some Remarkable Hidden Causes of Diseases and Cures* recorded his experiences with the knife in both autopsies and cures, Zerbi had long been involved with all types of surgery as well as presiding over the annual anatomy at Padua. His murder at the hands of brigands in modern Albania called forth various jibes at the manner of his death, portraying it as appropriate revenge for a life spent dissecting dead criminals, and his book was similarly scorned as outdated. It was Benedetti's shorter work that was more often reprinted, even if the Pavia editors of the 1517 reprinting felt it necessary to revert to the older medieval spelling and format familiar from Zerbi.

By far the most significant of the new writers on anatomy was Jacopo Berengario da Carpi (d. 1530), professor at Bologna and the author of two books on anatomy, a short introductory manual and a much longer and more innovative commentary based on his lectures on Mondino.[29] Both were illustrated with a small number of images, those in the *Commentary* largely tucked away at the back and intended more as schematic aide-mémoires than as a careful delineation of the body. Berengario relied heavily upon the Greek Galen in his criticism of Mondino, almost certainly through his knowledge of Chalcondylas's translation. But although he cited Galen more than 1500 times and believed that he had rediscovered the path that Galen himself had followed, he was no slavish Galenist. He preached what he termed an anatomy of the senses, *anatomia sensibilis*, encouraging others to see for themselves and to trust in what they could see and find. His own wide experience of cutting open bodies, both human and animal, in public and private, as a surgeon and at formal university anatomies, revealed that Galen had made several errors, not least in his description of the veins and in his belief in the existence of a *rete mirabile*, a vascular network at the base of the brain where psychic *pneuma* was produced.[30] Berengario's commentary is arguably the best account of the human body before Vesalius's *Fabrica* because of its depth of detail and its constant injunction to follow the author's own example of practical investigation. His much smaller *Introduction* is clearly written and a major improvement in accuracy over Benedetti despite its brevity.

The publication of the Aldine Galen in 1525 and, even more, of the Latin versions of the newly printed anatomical treatises changed everything. Within little more than a decade, anatomical lectures were being delivered to enthusiastic audiences and anatomical textbooks written by eager Galenists around Europe.[31] Matteo Corti (1475–1544), the best paid medical professor in Europe, expounded Galenic anatomy at Bologna and Pisa while someone else (in 1540 Vesalius himself) dissected the body in front of him and his audience.[32] Around 1538 François Rabelais was explaining to an admiring audience in Lyons the wonderful work of the Creator visible in a dissected corpse.[33] At the same time, at the new Lutheran university of Wittenberg, Philip Melanchthon insisted that students from all faculties should attend his course of lectures on the soul, half of which were taken up with an account of the human body based on the most up-to-date research on the new Galen.[34] He was guided in this by his friend, the distinguished Galenist Leonhard Fuchs of Tübingen, who agreed with him about the need to improve on Benedetti's book, which Melanchthon had found skimpy and puerile.[35]

Nowhere was the change so swift or so overwhelming as in Paris. Although a regular anatomical dissection had been held for 40 years or so, the subject attracted little attention, and remained entirely medieval in concept. Recent Italian authors seem to have been little noticed or read. A good picture of the attitudes of the Faculty of Medicine in the decade before 1533 comes from a series of eulogies that reveal a great deal about the hopes and interests of graduating doctors. While most of them remained resolutely fixed on the traditional skills of the physician in diagnosis (including uroscopy)

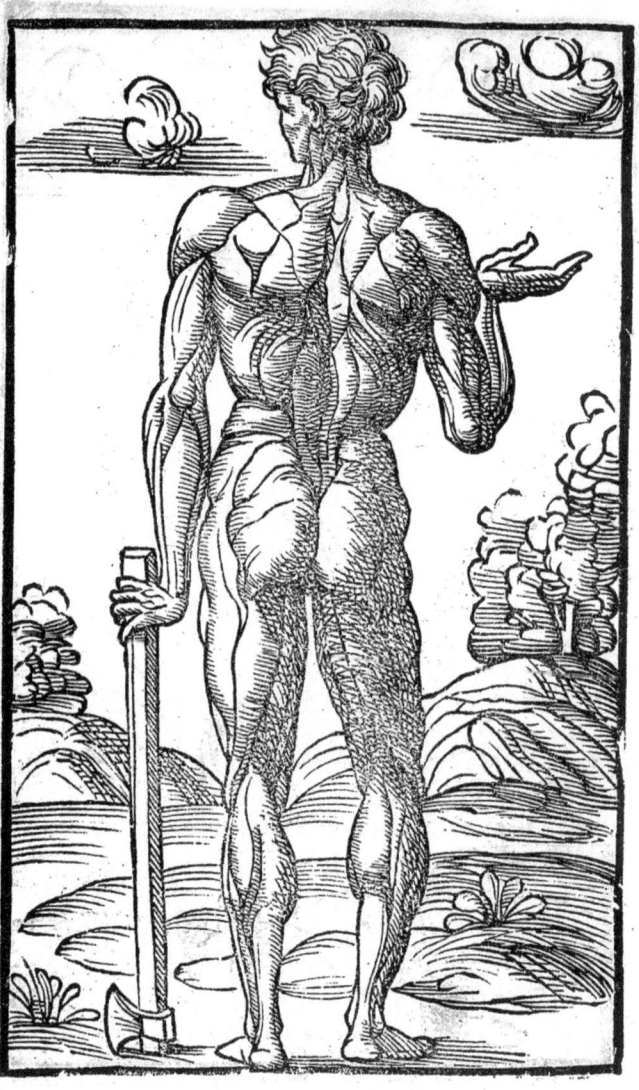

CHæc ē qn
ta figura: i q̃
a tergo uidē
tur oēs mu-
ſculi ſub cu-
te imediate
locati:q̃ præ
ſtat iuuamē
ta prænarra
ta / medicis:
& iſte figure
etiam iuuát
piĉores in li
neandis mē
btis.

Figure 9.1 The back muscles, from Berengario da Carpi's *Commentary on Mondino*,
Bologna, H. de Benedictis, 1521. In his caption Berengario expresses the
hope that his illustrations will aid artists in drawing the limbs.

and therapy, a small minority appreciated the lectures on surgery given by
Professor Tagault, and a similar number showed themselves to be experts
in medical astronomy, casting horoscopes to predict and control the course
of an illness (a specialty also of Louvain at this period). Of anatomy there is

not a word. If there were anatomical demonstrations, they seem to have had little or no impact on those physicians who attended them.[36]

But by 1533 when Vesalius arrived to begin his medical training, the situation was already changing.[37] Paris had become the most important centre for the translation of the newly printed works of Galen. Supported by the printer Simon de Colines, Jacobus Sylvius, Guinter and others embarked on a long series of new and more accurate Latin versions, including, in 1531, Guinter's translation of *Anatomical Procedures*. Two members of the Faculty, Andreas de Laguna (1499–1560) and Guinter himself, swiftly produced their own textbooks, in which they referred to their own experiences (and those of Tagault) in carrying out dissections.[38] Charles Estienne (1504–64), assisted by the surgeon Étienne De la Rivière, was also embarking on a remarkable project to produce a lavishly illustrated treatise on anatomy, available in both Latin and French, but, although it had been largely written by 1539 and many illustrations drawn during actual dissections, a variety of disputes delayed publication until 1545[39] (Figure 7.2). There were also private dissections in addition to the formal university courses, in both of which Vesalius, as he commented in his notes, acted as assistant to Guinter by doing the cutting. When he left for Louvain in 1536, he was succeeded in this task by the Spaniard Miguel Servet, famous today for anticipating Harvey in his arguments in favour of the circulation of the blood.[40] The most celebrated of the Parisians, Jacobus Sylvius, although not allowed to lecture in the Faculty halls until early 1536, taught elsewhere to great acclaim. The French author Noel du Fail describes how students from all disciplines clambered over walls and through gardens to get front seats at his lectures on Galen, when they had the opportunity to see the great man bring in freshly dissected portions of animal bodies to illustrate a particular point.[41] Vesalius heard him teach and would have learned more from him about the revived Galenic anatomy that Sylvius was to expound in his later *Introduction*.[42] It was an exciting time to be a student, especially as the new information offered a great range of alternatives to the dogmatic Galenism of the Later Middle Ages. It was now possible to be both modern and traditional at the same time.

Andreas Vesalius and the *Fabrica*

Almost from the moment the *De humani corporis fabrica*, *The Constitution of the Human Body*, appeared in print at Basle in summer 1543, readers acknowledged its significance.[43] Writing in March and again in early August, Hieronymus Gemusaeus (1505–44), professor of *Physice* (Natural Science) at Basle and one of the editors of the 1538 edition of the Greek Galen, pronounced it a remarkable achievement.[44] Its author, a young and ambitious Fleming, Andreas Vesalius (1514–64), had had since childhood a passionate interest in dissection. Educated at Brussels and Louvain, he moved to Paris in 1533, where he served as dissector for Guinter's lectures in 1535–6.[45] He returned to Louvain to complete his first medical degree with a dissertation updating Book IX of Rhazes's *Ad Almansorem*, a typically humanist enterprise, before going to Padua to take his MD in 1537.[46] Immediately on graduation, he was appointed professor of surgery there, with the task of presiding over the annual formal dissections. For his first course in December 1537 he recommended Guinter's textbook as the best available, but for the following year's course he produced his own revised and unauthorised edition as well as a collection of six anatomical plates to serve as an independent visual aid.[47] From the moment of its publication in 1538 he started making corrections in his own copy of the revised textbook in preparation for a new edition, but within a few months he began to use the book for a different purpose, as a help towards the preparation of his masterpiece, the *Fabrica*.[48] He also astonished his audience by dispensing with the traditional assistance of a surgeon to dissect and another teacher to read out the relevant text, and doing everything himself, an innovation that was not universally followed for several centuries and, indeed, was soon abandoned in Padua.[49] The appearance of the *Fabrica* in 1543 only confirmed the reputation that he had already established in Padua and elsewhere as an independent-minded and very skilful anatomist. A student at Bologna in 1540, Baldasar Heseler, recorded in some detail the comments that Vesalius made when invited there to act as dissector, to the delight of the large and enthusiastic audience, if not always to the satisfaction of the lecturer, Matteo Corti.[50]

Vesalius left Padua in 1542 to see the *Fabrica* through the press in Basle, and it was on his way back to Padua the following year that he was granted an audience with the Holy Roman Emperor, Charles V. His reward for presenting him with splendid copies of both the *Fabrica* and its shorter summary, the *Epitome*, was an offer to become one of the Emperor's household physicians. He accepted, accompanying the Emperor on campaign, before returning briefly to Padua to give his final series of anatomical demonstrations.[51] Imperial service from June 1544 restricted, but in no way prevented, his involvement with human dissection, at least at first. Vesalius continued to revise his views, replying to some of his critics in his *Letter on the China Root* of 1546, and making plans for further editions.[52] Oporinus, his publisher, was already announcing a second edition of the *Fabrica* in 1552, although the complete revision did not appear until 1555. Much of the new information contained in this edition derives from dissections, autopsies or surgical interventions he had carried in Italy or Brussels. (The most famous of his cases was his later unsuccessful attempt alongside others, including Paré, to treat Henri II of France after he had been fatally injured in the head during an tournament in 1559, and a recent discovery has revealed Vesalius's own account of his later treatment of Don Carlos of Spain following an accident.)[53] Shortly afterwards, he moved to Spain where he treated the Netherlanders at the court of the new Emperor Philip II and where his access to bodies was limited. Nonetheless, his annotations in his copy of the 1555 edition show him still adding new material, sometimes taken from others, but mainly the result of wrestling with the difficulty of expressing in words the 'feel' of bones, in preparation for a third edition which was never published.[54] His final book, which was handed over to a Venetian printer just before he set out in 1564 on his fateful voyage to the Holy Land, was a reply to the criticisms of another anatomist, Gabriele Falloppia.[55]

Vesalius's publications, lectures and notes allow historians the rare possibility of reconstructing the development of the ideas of a major Renaissance doctor at various points in his life, from the lectures he heard as a student in 1536 and his work in Padua before the *Fabrica* until shortly before his death. We can read his published works as well as the marginalia that give insights into his private thinking. One might even say 'public thinking', for Guinter's lectures of 1536 were taken down by an auditor and the printed version includes comments that can only have been made by someone standing by the dissected corpse and with a facility with the knife, something Guinter admitted he did not have – in other words, the young Vesalius, Guinter's dissector.[56] Letters and reminiscences by colleagues and students also fill out the picture of an ambitious and charismatic individual almost obsessed with getting things right – and, according to an English cleric, a gossipy companion at dinner.[57] His enthusiasm for anatomy more than satisfied the eagerness of his students, and those who were officially in charge of the organisation of the formal dissections supplemented the authorised bodies of executed criminals by securing others by both fair means and foul. The body of the recently deceased mistress of a monk at Padua was snatched from her tomb, and the skin flayed before it was handed over to Vesalius to prevent it being recognised by her lover, who might otherwise have made an official complaint.[58]

The *Fabrica* broke new ground in very many ways as well as providing the most detailed account of the human body yet written.[59] Its oft repeated message, that the structures of the human body could be discerned and understood only through the dissection of human bodies, has rightly been seen by today's anatomists as a landmark in the development of their subject, while its sheer size, the clarity and beauty of its images and the remarkable dialogue that it created between the text and the visual representations of parts of the body, ensure its status as a treasured possession of many institutional libraries around the world[60] (Figure 7.3). It remains, as it was from the start, a luxury production, which caused difficulties later for its publisher when the second, revised edition of 1555 did not sell as well as the first, and it is this that may have inhibited Vesalius's plan for a third edition.[61] Vesalius was well aware of this, hence his simultaneous publication of a much shorter and less elegantly printed *Epitome* of both the first and second editions, aimed at students.[62]

Until the recent appearance of English translations, less attention has been paid to his text than to his images, despite the substantial number of corrections he claimed to have made to traditional accounts.[63] His osteology, myology and, to a certain extent, neurology are remarkably accurate for someone dissecting without any technical aids to observation, and he made many discoveries throughout his life about all the major internal organs.[64] In his annotations to the 1555 edition, he altered his view of the position of the lens in the eye from the middle of the two chambers to towards the front, a correction later made also by Felix Platter, and drew a new (and more accurate) representation of the *levator palpebrae* muscle of the eyelid that he had earlier classified as a cartilage.[65] He recognised the problems raised by anomalies such as the absence of the optic chiasmus in an executed man or the extension of the gall bladder into the stomach of a papal oarsman he had autopsied.[66] Most of his findings were corrections to what Galen, and after him Mondino and Berengario, had said. Having in his first edition accepted Galen's view of a permeable septum in the heart, with some reservations, he was far more doubtful about it in the second. He similarly later took a stronger position against the notion of a *rete mirabile*. Some problems continued to exercise him for years.[67] Galen and Guinter had stated that water was found naturally in the pericardium at all times, but Vesalius knew that some anatomists denied this.[68] Matteo Corti, for instance, in his comments at the 1540 Bologna dissection argued (correctly) that when it did, it was a sign of some illness or malfunction, an opinion rejected by Vesalius in his subsequent lecture.[69] In 1543 he produced a number of examples from his own dissections on animals and human corpses to show that he had often found it, once in the heart of a man that was still beating when he examined it. Although he was not entirely certain, he thought that the fluid might be a natural lubricant, but he rejected any idea that it was transformed out of natural spirits into fluid at the moment of death.[70] In 1555, however, he removed both his comment about there being more water in men and women with a more humid temperament and about it collecting at various places in the bodies of criminals left in the sun on French gallows. Any suggestion that this might relate to the tricky theological problem of the water flowing from the body of the crucified Christ was also excised.[71]

Most of Vesalius's 'discoveries', such as his rejection of the seven-boned sternum, the divided jawbone or the placement of the kidneys, were rejections of Galenic anatomy as transmitted by texts, whether Galen's own or as interpreted by modern writers from Mondino onwards. Although Niccolò Massa (d. 1569) was right to point out that many others besides Vesalius were also finding mistakes in Galen, Vesalius had gone one step further by insisting that these errors were systematic, and the result of Galen's reliance on animal dissection.[72] Vesalian anatomy was, at least rhetorically, still a Hellenist anatomy, for in his preface he claimed to be restoring the lost Alexandrian anatomy of Herophilus, Erasistratus, Andreas and Marinus that had been overwhelmed by that of Galen thanks to the laziness of the medical profession.[73] Vesalius continued to profess his admiration for Galen and for what he had done, quoting extensively from him, but the whole tenor of his book gave out a different message. There was frequent criticism of Galen's views, as well as a constant assertion of the importance of human dissection, beginning with the visual imagery of the title page (showing the dissection of a woman even to her womb, the ultimate of human secrets) and the frontispiece (showing Vesalius dissecting a human arm, an allusion to the first pages of *The Usefulness of Parts*) and continuing almost to the arguments in the final pages.[74] Whatever the achievements of Galen, Vesalius was asserting that his anatomy was in every way superior.

But to see the achievements of Vesalius solely in terms of Galenism and anti-Galenism is misleading. The new anatomy of the 1530s was a Galenic science and strongly supported by Galenists, even if they were not themselves dissectors. Indeed, 'anatomical dissection' quickly became the new shibboleth. It was Vesalius's knowledge of Galenic anatomical writings that persuaded Giambattista da Monte to entrust him with the revision of their Latin versions for his new Giuntine edition, and John Caius tells us how, as good medical philologists, he and Vesalius worked together on manuscript material provided by Gadaldino to check readings in the Greek.[75] He was welcomed at meetings of a circle of humanists in Venice called the *Infiammati*, and, only a few weeks before the publication of the *Fabrica*, the Galenic translator Janus Cornarius, later one of Vesalius's most vehement critics, was sending his best wishes to him in Padua (although the fact that Vesalius had already been in Basle for a year or so hardly indicates an intimate friendship).[76]

At the same time, the greater one's acquaintance with the human corpse, the more likely it was that divergences between Galen's words and what was visible in a human corpse would become apparent. Berengario in 1521 had already identified several mistakes in Galen's description of the body, and still more were revealed 15 years later by the Venetian Niccolò Massa and independently by Guinter, despite the title of his 1536 textbook proclaiming that it was written 'according to Galen'.[77] Massa, some of whose lectures Vesalius had attended, grumbled that no one found Vesalius's claims particularly surprising since the scholars among his readers were well aware that Galen had largely dissected animals, and Galen himself had admitted that some of his conclusions were no more than plausible and provisional. Had he himself not been encumbered by other duties, both personal and professional, Massa was sure that he would have beaten Vesalius in the race to produce a modern textbook of anatomy.[78] Guinter himself provides the best proof that Galenists were happy to adopt a good proportion of Vesalius's corrections, for in his 1539 revision of his textbook he adopted almost all of his pupil's improvements, for example on the true pericranium (to the annoyance of Vesalius who, in his later notes, insisted on his own priority), and provided a much more accurate description of the muscles of the leg than Vesalius himself.[79] Vesalius was pushing on a door that was already open.

Reactions to the *Fabrica*

Immediate reactions to the *Fabrica* were divided. Few opponents went as far as Sylvius who insisted that Galen had dissected precisely and accurately: it was the heroic Roman body that had degenerated over time. Many others pointed out Vesalius's misunderstandings and mistranslations of Galen.[80] John Caius filled the margins of his editions of Galen with denunciations of the linguistic deficiencies of 'Wesalius', and carefully collected all the passages that demonstrated Galen's knowledge of the human body.[81] Cornarius angrily erased the name of Vesalius from his copy of the *Opera Omnia Galeni* with such force that the black ink spreads over the page and the indentations of the pen are still visible many folios later.[82] Others, like Colombo, Falloppia and Ingrassia, were quick to indicate in their own anatomical publications mistakes in his interpretation of the human body while accepting much of what he said.[83]

Of greater weight, at least for the moment, were accusations of impiety, disrespect towards his teachers and even deceit.[84] They did not lack foundation. His opponents were well aware that Vesalius in his own dissections had used dogs far more often than human corpses, and, significantly, a plate of a pig ready for dissection was tucked away towards the end of the *Fabrica* in Book VII, with acknowledgements that pigs were vivisected in Bologna and Padua at the end of his demonstration.[85] Indeed, Bartolommeo Eustachi openly questioned in 1563 whether Vesalius had properly described the human body because of his great reliance on animals.[86] Contemporaries did not need the modern Spanish scholar Juan José Barcía Goyanes to list the many places where Vesalius adopted Galen's conclusions, his order of dissection (beginning with bones), and even his words, all without acknowledgement.[87] Indeed, without including large chunks of Galen, almost unchanged, particularly in the later, more physiological books, Vesalius could not have written the *Fabrica* at the speed he did.[88] Even more than Galen had done, Vesalius concealed his debts to his contemporaries, except for the names of a few friends and students who provided him with information – and some of these disappear from the second edition of 1555.[89] Complaints about possible plagiarism were circulating in Padua within weeks, and caused Georg Agricola in distant Chemnitz to hope that Vesalius could explain everything, especially as he was one of the few scholars capable of adding something to what the ancients had written.[90] No wonder, too, that Parisians were annoyed at what they saw as an unjustified slur on Galen, for they would have remembered how in his unauthorised revision of Guinter's textbook Vesalius had placed his name on the title page in larger capital letters than that of his teacher. Vesalius, they knew, was a man of enormous talent, but also of vaulting ambition. As a Paduan colleague told his students in 1550, he was full of "a spirit of contradiction" and it would have been more acceptable to scholars if he had been more modest in his criticisms of Galen.[91]

Others less well acquainted with Vesalius personally took a much more favourable view. The book had sold out in Leipzig by the end of 1543, and several copies survive that were purchased within a few months of it going on sale.[92] Melanchthon and his colleagues at Wittenberg rightly saw

Vesalius as continuing a programme of anatomical research that Galen had begun but could not follow through himself. Not only did Melanchthon read his own copy of the *Fabrica* from beginning to end, inscribing in it a poem in its praise, but he also revised the medical section of his treatise on the soul to accommodate the new Vesalian anatomy.[93] Several of his pupils owned their own copies, some even presented by Vesalius himself, and Wittenberg maintained a tradition of frequent dissection that lasted well into the next century.[94] This message was transmitted to other Lutheran universities such as Jena and Greifswald, as well as in suitably abridged form to pupils in schools. It was almost an in-joke when from the 1570s Wittenberg publishers chose the head of Vesalius for the male figure in the cheap anatomical sheets (Figure 9.2) that students were encouraged to buy when attending lectures on Melanchthon's *De Anima, The Soul*.[95] What Vesalius himself would have thought of this *jeu d'esprit* can perhaps be deduced from his furious reaction to the unauthorised takeover of his images by the Flemish printer Thomas Geminus in London and by the Spaniard Valverde.[96]

Valverde's publication also shows how swiftly Vesalian anatomy was also adopted in Spanish universities except for Barcelona.[97] A similar development took place in England. Geminus proudly proclaimed that his illustrated compendium of anatomy depended on the *Epitome* and was cheaper and far less prolix than the *Fabrica* itself. Its plates, if not the whole book, had been strongly commended in 1544 by Henry VIII, although his absence on campaign delayed final approval and publication until the following year.[98] John Caius, who was appointed by Henry VIII to teach anatomy to the barber-surgeons in London on his return from Italy probably in 1545, was passionate in his advocacy of dissection, even arranging for two annual dissections to be carried out a year in his new Cambridge College in addition to those organised by the university. He was no Vesalian, but even he could not avoid praising his old house-mate in his *Autobibliography, De libris suis*, although he cunningly singled out instances where Vesalius in his second edition of the *Fabrica* had accepted corrections that he had suggested.[99] More telling, perhaps, is the comment of a young Fellow of King's, Christopher Langton (1521–78), in 1547 that "whoso is wyllyng to haue a particular rehersa[l] of all the partes, let him seke Gallen or Vesalius. For they haue written hole bokes and greate volumes of them".[100] Not long after this, the Cambridge anatomist Thomas Lorkyn (1528–91) obtained a copy of the 1555 edition, which he annotated copiously during a long career as a teacher of anatomy.[101]

The trajectory was not always upwards. Although at least three Oxford Colleges bought copies of the *Fabrica*, and the revised university statutes of 1549 required that a candidate for a licence in medicine had to provide evidence that they had 'made' (i.e. attended) two anatomies (as well as effecting three cures), there is no record of any arrangements being made for a formal anatomy, and in the revised statutes of 1564 all mention of anatomy disappears.[102] But in general, as Girolamo Donzellini wrote to Mattioli in

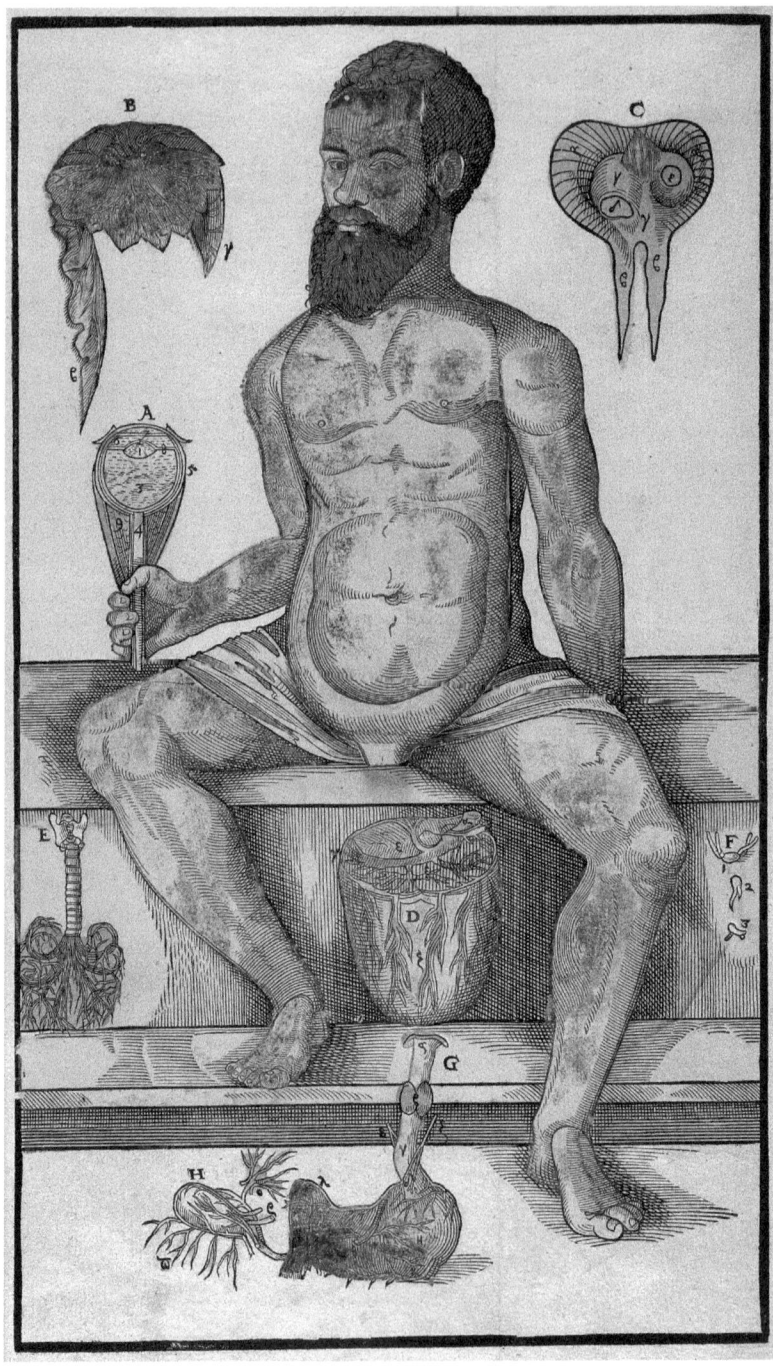

Figure 9.2 An anatomical fugitive sheet, Wittenberg, S. Groneberg, 1573, intended for students attending lectures on Melanchthon's *The Soul*. The head resembles that of Vesalius.

the late 1550s, although there might still remain in Italy and elsewhere some opponents of Vesalius, they were few in number and, like the monsters slain by Hercules, no longer formidable. Like Leoniceno, Manardi and Mattioli himself, Vesalius had triumphed over his initial detractors, and, like Copernicus, he had been brave enough to challenge orthodoxy and reveal new truths.[103] But at the same time, many recognised that he and his compeers had done what Galen had wanted to do but had been prevented from doing so by a lack of human corpses.

Anatomy After Vesalius

But it would be also wrong to credit Vesalius alone with the impetus towards dissection that meant that, when new universities were founded, one of the first university buildings to be built was a place to hold a dissection, as at Helmstedt in 1578 and at Leiden in 1594. Other universities, like Padua or Bologna, replaced previous temporary theatres with a more permanent one or abandoned the large and cold church where, as Vesalius's frontispiece implies, the annual winter anatomy was held for a purpose-built building.[104] Gisbert van der Horst arranged for a skeleton of a young woman, who had bequeathed her body to the hospital of S. Maria della Consolazione in Rome, to be preserved in the hospital for the benefit of students.[105] Such anatomists as the Ferrarese Giambattista Canano, the discoverer of the palmaris brevis muscle and the valves in the veins, or the Savoyard Leonardo Botallo (1530–87), a surgeon and anatomist who is wrongly credited with the discovery of the foetal duct that bears his name, did not need Vesalius to tell them how to dissect.[106] Realdo Colombo (c. 1515–59), colleague and later rival of Vesalius in Padua before moving to Rome, was never slow to announce his own discoveries such as the transit of blood from one side of the heart to the others via the lungs, even when others may have anticipated him.[107] Colombo's description of the ossicles in the ear can be paralleled in the accounts by Gian Filippo Ingrassia, professor of anatomy at Naples and Palermo, and by the Spaniards Pedro Jimeno (1515–51), Luis Collado (fl. 1548–72) and Juan Valverde, and his claims for his primacy in discovering the clitoris would have been disputed by Estienne and Falloppia.[108] The list of discoveries by other dissectors in the sixteenth century is substantial, and many universities, particularly in Italy, often had a distinguished series of anatomists. Famous names such as Falloppia, Eustachi and Fabricius of Aquapendente (1533–1619) lectured at Padua, while Bartolomeo Maggi (1477–1552) taught anatomy at Bologna well before a specific chair in anatomy was created in 1570. Its first holder was Giulio Cesare Aranzi (1530–89), who carried out detailed investigations into the hippocampus and choroid plexus in the brain and into the heart valves, describing the so-called Nodules of Aranzio. Other Bolognese teachers like Costanzo Varolio (1543–75) and Gaspare Tagliacozzi (1545–99) were also authorised to carry out dissections, although not at the same hour as the official professor.[109] north of the Alps, Basle, with Felix Platter and Caspar

Bauhin (1560–1614), attracted many students from further afield, eager to see the Vesalian tradition carried on with both public and private dissections[110] (Figure 7.1). Even today, Basle children are taken on Sunday afternoons to the Anatomical Museum to see the skeletons dissected by Platter and by Vesalius himself. Further north, Wittenberg had a flourishing school of anatomists led by such distinguished scholars as Salomon Alberti (1540–1600) and Johann Jessen (1566–1621) that lasted until 1601 when Jessen departed for Prague, angered about the lack of support for dissection after a brush with the civil powers.[111] Elsewhere, guilds of surgeons, as in London in 1540 or in Amsterdam in 1552, were also granted permission to carry out formal anatomies for teaching purposes.[112]

An interest in dissection was not confined to the medical professions. Pa'ez de Castro, the agent of the Spanish ambassador to Venice and noted bibliophile Diego Hurtado de Mendoza, was reading the *Fabrica* alongside Galen shortly after its appearance.[113] Many references to the anatomy of the human body can be found in a variety of literary genres, and the list of non-professional owners of the *Fabrica* speaks for itself.[114] Vesalius's famous title page to the *Fabrica* depicts a large and very varied crowd, not all of whom appear to be doctors or even fully engaged in the anatomy taking place before them. Distinguished spectators and friends attended John Caius's 'public' anatomies for the surgeons in London, one of whom, probably the Member of Parliament Thomas Marrow (1516–61), was in the audience regularly for almost 20 years.[115] The pulling power of a public dissection as a gory spectacle should not be forgotten. When in 1574 an Italian exile Antonio Pigafetta, who was working as a physician in Heidelberg, offered to demonstrate that blood circulated from one side of the heart to the other via previously unknown channels in the outer covering, a large crowd gathered in the square before the university. When he failed in his first attempt, he was encouraged to try again on the following day, with the same result. He left town with his tail between his legs and this spectacular disaster was still being talked about decades later.[116] At Bologna the public dissections were so popular that tickets were on sale to the general public as part of the festivities of Carnival.[117] As such they formed part of a new culture of observation that developed from, but did not entirely as yet replace, an older tradition that emphasised the body as one of the wonders of Nature.[118]

But however exciting Vesalius's programmatic assertion that the human body should be investigated only by dissecting humans might be, it faced two very different objections: that it was irrelevant to the day-to-day activities of a physician and, secondly and harder to rebut, that it was an ideal impossible to achieve because of a shortage of bodies.[119] Vesalius's anatomy at Bologna in 1540 had required three corpses of executed criminals and six dogs, one of which was vivisected to show the body in action.[120] Dogs were easy to get hold of, and, to judge from the number of anatomists who wrote on the anatomy of the foetus, so too were dead human foetuses, the result of abortions, miscarriages, failed caesarean sections or death in childbirth. But as Andrea Carlino showed from his study of the records of the Roman confraternity responsible for the religious aspects of a public execution and subsequent anatomy, finding suitable criminals for official demonstrations was no easy matter. It was preferable to avoid those with local links and to dissect instead those who came from a long way away, since the threat of revenge from angry relatives was less.[121] When Vesalius arrived in Pisa to conduct a dissection in 1544, a letter was sent to the hospital of S. Maria Nuova to see if suitable bodies could be found among people who died without relatives. If found, they were to be procured and transported in the utmost secrecy.[122] Besides, if finding a male body was difficult, finding a suitable woman was even more so. No wonder that Vesalius placed his dissection of a woman at the centre of his title page, possibly of the woman who had unsuccessfully feigned pregnancy in order to avoid hanging.[123] But even when all the relevant authorities, state, ecclesiastical and university, were in entire agreement, the provision of a corpse might founder on the unwillingness of the keeper of the town jail to release the body of an executed criminal or on the interference of "importunate busybodies". That was why no university dissection could take place at Wittenberg in the two years before 1587, except for the dissection of a child delivered dead, despite the strong support of the Elector and the town authorities.[124] And, no matter how supportive civic officials might be, zealous anatomists would always complain that what they were offered was never enough.[125]

One way out of the dilemma was to proceed extremely carefully in any attempt to integrate human and animal anatomy. Volcker Coiter (1534–76) in Bologna and later in Nuremberg dissected a wide range of animals, from salamanders and unicorns (!) to hedgehogs and chickens, in addition to carrying out formal human anatomies and a number of autopsies. He claimed to be the first since Aristotle in the fourth century BCE to dissect hen's eggs systematically to discover the development of the embryo, although he may well have been anticipated in this by Falloppia and by another Bolognese anatomist Aldrovandi, although their investigations were not published until later.[126] But although Coiter is often called a comparative anatomist and was careful about the differences between human and non-human material, that honour is better applied to the long-lived Hieronymus Fabricius of Aquapendente. In Andrew Cunningham's phrase, he developed an "Aristotle project", dissecting and analysing the various organs of a large range of animals to investigate the relationship between anatomy and function. It was backed up by a new anatomical credo: observation was merely the first stage in understanding any specific organ. It needed to be supplemented by an enquiry into its actions and a specification of its usefulness (a good Galenic term for function) until everything had been finally clearly and authoritatively demonstrated.[127] This method and this interest in comparisons Fabricius transmitted at Padua to his most famous pupil, William Harvey, whose innovative work on the heart and circulation and substantial but less successful investigation of generation depended on an even larger series of dissections of animals.[128]

Whether there was in fact a decline in investigative human anatomy at the end of the sixteenth century, as some have suggested, is difficult to determine.[129] The death of Falloppia from plague and the murder of Bassiano Landi in quick succession in 1562 were a blow to anatomy at Padua in the short term, for their immediate successor, Francisco Lendinara, was considered a nobody, but its reputation revived again under Fabricius of Aquapendente, who held the anatomy chair from 1565 to 1604.[130] Precise statistics are hard to come by, and any impression that there was less dissection activity taking place is vitiated by the natural tendency of historians to emphasise novelty and discovery as well as to minimise the difficulties in obtaining bodies at any period. Besides, for obvious reasons, there is little information about private, supplementary anatomy lessons, although these may have not involved more than handling bones, inspecting a skeleton, and dissecting an animal together with occasional participation in an autopsy.[131] A German student in February 1564 described how he was able to dissect the corpse of a teenage girl who had died of emphysema. He located the clitoris, as Falloppia had taught, but not the hymen, absent, he asserts, for obvious reasons, but his attempt to create a skeleton for himself out of the bones was a disaster.[132] Vesalius's achievement did accelerate a trend to a greater interest in human dissection that continued into the next century, particularly in Northern Europe. But there were always those who remained sceptical. The false but widely believed story that Vesalius had travelled to the Holy Land in penance for some anatomical crime testifies the continuing widespread suspicion of those who cut up bodies, and even those who practised it themselves had doubts about its value.[133] In his own book on surgery, Leonardo Fioravanti, who had studied medicine at Naples and Bologna, repeated the same accusations that had been levelled against the practice 1500 years earlier by Cornelius Celsus: it was cruel, taught students to treat bodies like chunks of pork, contributed nothing to therapy, and gave misleading information about the body (which was always changed in death, as he had observed many times). In short, it was a subject best suited to artists and sculptors. Nonetheless, despite his qualms, he devoted much of the second book of his *Surgery* to explaining what the surgeon should do if called on to dissect at an anatomy.[134] He praised professors of medicine like Prospero Borgarucci (1540–78) in Padua, for their interest in dissection, for it was an excellent thing, indeed essential, for all to know something about the great handiwork of the Creator, but at the same time, he warned against placing exaggerated hopes in its value for medicine.[135]

In one country, Spain, a definite decline can be clearly observed. Except at the university of Barcelona, the younger Spanish medical anatomists quickly followed the Vesalian model, and Valverde's abbreviated version enjoyed considerable success. But by 1570 Vesalian anatomy seems already to have been on the way out, and it was effectively ended during the 1590s, when the new statutes at Salamanca, followed later by those of Alcalá, made Galen's *The Usefulness of Parts* the only book prescribed for the anatomy course as "this contained all that a physician might need". From the 1580s onwards the dominant figure in Spanish medicine was Luis Mercado (1520–1606), who used his position as *protomedico* after 1592 to impose a heavily Galenist, if not medieval, curriculum on Spanish medical schools. Indeed, one could call it a Mercado curriculum, for he insisted on his own writings or those of which he approved as the sole textbooks for study. Indeed Mercado thought anatomy an irrelevance and asserted that in Spain good medicine had been practised for 200 years without recourse to dissection, forgetting that Vesalius had once been widely taught, at Valencia, Salamanca, Alcalá and even his own university of Valladolid.[136] One might argue that this retreat from Vesalius is but one example of a process whereby, as its historians acknowledge, Spain, at this period, was in the process of withdrawing from the mainstream of European academic life.[137] But Spain was not alone in returning to Galen at the end of the century. Both Freiburg and Ingolstadt modified their statutes to include more Galen, while Catholic Würzburg in its foundation statutes of 1587 specified that Galen's *The Usefulness of Parts* should be used at the annual anatomy, and Lutheran Jena based its teaching about the body in 1591 on the same book and on Avicenna's *Canon* I, 1.[138] At Padua Fabricius in his lectures often referred to Galen, emphasising his notions of utility and purpose far more than any strictly Aristotelian teleology. This was not antiquarianism, but the result of a debate about the purpose of anatomical information for physicians, for whom Galenic functional anatomy was more relevant to their needs than Vesalian descriptive anatomy, no matter how numerous Galen's errors.

But in general the relatively swift replacement of Galenic anatomy by that of Vesalius is no surprise, any more than the fact that, by 1600, Dioscorides was being superseded by more modern botanists describing a wider range of plants than those from his largely Mediterranean world. Galen's insistence on the need to understand the structures and workings of the human body through an active participation in dissection provided the stimulus to new discoveries that also revealed his own avowed limitations. At the same time, artists and printers emphasised the significance of the visual in new ways and to a wider community than ever before. Volcker Coiter's title page proclaimed that his plates of the principal parts of the human body, illustrated with new and most artistic drawings, would be of the greatest of help to "philosophers, physicians and especially all devotees of anatomy".[139] The crude anatomical fugitive sheets (Figure 9.2) and the somewhat more sophisticated collections of images by Jacques Grévin deserve as least as much notice in this regard as Leonardo or Vesalius, whose *Six Anatomical Plates* and *Epitomes* contributed to this popularisation, if they did not begin it.[140] Starting in Italy, and from the 1530s spreading rapidly around Europe, this new emphasis on dissection and what it revealed about the body exemplifies many of the characteristics of Renaissance medicine, and not least its novel ways of intertwining classical and modern ideas. Those who, even after 1543, continued to include Vesalius in a list of distinguished Galenists or to bracket the two men together for their "hole bokes and greate volumes", whether measured in size or in quality, were not wide of the mark.[141]

Art and Anatomy; Before and After Vesalius

No one in Basle in 1541 could have predicted that within two years, two local printers, Michael Isingrin and Johannes Oporinus, would have produced two of the masterpieces of printing, in terms both of content and presentation. While relatively little is known about Leonhard Fuchs's relationship with Isingrin, Vesalius was a constant presence in Basle during the preparation of the *Fabrica*, providing both detailed specialist guidance and the reassurance of a family friend.[142] Everything in the book, from its size, the quality of both print and paper, and the witty depictions of putti playing at being anatomists in the opening letters of each section, to the actual typographical layout, bespeaks a work of art as well as of anatomy.[143] This was not surprising since Vesalius had been brought up in the art-loving milieu of the Burgundian court and knew many artists in Venice, Including Jan Stephan van Calcar (c. 1499–1546), who illustrated and probably paid for the publication of the *Tabulae anatomicae sex* in 1538.[144] Vesalius also illustrated his lectures with sketches and references to the plates of the *Tabulae* and some of his own schematic drawings may well figure in the *Fabrica* itself.[145] In a *consilium* of 1538 he drew the instruments that he hoped would be made to help in curing the patient's urinary problems.[146]

The contrast between Vesalius's use of images as an essential part of his argument differs completely for what had gone before. Medieval illustrations of the human body were designed less as representations than as aids to remembering words.[147] A common set of five (or nine) pictures are found in a variety of contexts, ranging from lavishly illuminated codices to small charts designed to be folded into little booklets that could be attached to the belt of a travelling practitioner. They were keyed into a text, often in Latin but also in a variety of vernaculars, including Welsh, to serve as a visual representation of the verbal description of the body, its parts, its ailments and the influences of the stars upon it. Although few, if any, of the images are realistic, continuing a centuries' old tradition at several removes from the actual observation of the body, they continued to be reproduced well into the sixteenth century. Printed images long remained largely schematic, mainly because of technical restraints, and even when new images were drawn to illustrate a particular anatomical point, they were few in number. Those prepared for Berengario's commentary (Figure 9.1) were scattered throughout a very large book, and although Giabattista Canano (1515–79), had planned for a substantial number, drawn in greater detail than ever before, to accompany his book on muscles, only a few appeared when it was finally published, probably in 1541, and the rest appear to have been lost.[148] Scholars have carefully noted individual realistic representations in pre-Vesalian books, and the illustrations that accompanied Dryander's 1536 short tract on the anatomy of the head show a marked improvement in both technique and accuracy, but it is not until 1538 and the publication of the *Tabulae anatomicae sex* that new ground was really broken.[149] Although its images mainly followed medieval tradition, they were both larger in size and supplemented by much material from Vesalius's recent dissections.

The disjunction between anatomical illustrations in books and what artists were painting or drawing before the late 1530s is far from easy to understand, since artists had been studying the human form and depicting it realistically for at least half a century.[150] Pollaiuolo, Verrocchio and Donatello, to name but three, were interested in the accurate portrayal of limbs and the body's musculature, further inspired by the newly discovered remains of antique statuary.[151] By the late 1480s, Leonardo da Vinci (1452–1519) was making his first surviving set of exquisite anatomical drawings of both animals and humans, concentrating on surface anatomy, especially skulls, legs, arms and feet, and had formulated a very ambitious programme of drawing and three-dimensional modelling that would cover the whole of human life from conception to grave.[152] But, as with so many of his challenging ideas, he was soon distracted by other topics, and it was probably not until sometime after 1506, when he had moved to Florence, that he renewed his interest in dissection. In a memorandum of around 1508, he records that he had personally dissected ten corpses – in a much later letter, he mentions at least 30 – including both a centenarian at the hospital of Santa Maria Nuova and a 2-year-old child, whose bodies he noted were almost totally different. His detailed depiction of his findings, particularly of the vascular system and the muscles, was unsurpassed at the time, even if it also involved a fair degree of imagination, as in his representation of female genitalia and a child in the womb. He was particularly interested in the workings of the body, where his engineering and mathematical knowledge enabled him to understand the mechanics of the hand and arm in a way that was not achieved by others for a century or more. His artistic skills also suggested to him different ways of cutting into the spine or the skull, and of inserting wax into the ventricles of the brain to produce a three-dimensional object that could be easily drawn.

Many scholars have discerned a change in the character of his anatomical drawing in the period immediately after his move from Florence to Milan in 1508 and have plausibly associated it with a young Galenist and medical teacher at Pavia, Marcantonio della Torre (d. 1511), with whom, according to Vasari, he collaborated for a while.[153] As the professor charged with leading the annual anatomy, Della Torre will have been able to help Leonardo in obtaining bodies for dissection. In turn he will have benefitted from Leonardo's expertise with the knife, for his own knowledge is likely to have been based far more on books than on anatomical practice. Paulo Giovio, a student at Pavia at the time, later recalled that Leonardo had dissected in the schools, almost certainly at Pavia, and strong evidence has been recently provided for Leonardo's reliance on someone with a remarkable knowledge of at least the Latin Galen.[154] Martin Clayton and Ron Philo argue that Della Torre's influence can be seen in the 240 drawings and 13,000 words that make up Anatomical MS A, datable, they argue, to 1510–12. Above all, they credit him with not only encouraging Leonardo to perform many dissections but also with imparting a new rigour and enabling him to achieve a balance between detail and coverage that is absent from most of his earlier anatomical drawings.[155] Both men also disagreed strongly with those, like Mondino, who merely summarised the complex organisation of the body and thereby hindered progress in dissection.[156] Although Leonardo wrote that he hoped to have finished "*tutta la notomia*", "all the necessary dissection", by spring 1510, that does not by itself imply that he was planning a book, let alone that it was the volume of anatomical drawings seen by Antonio de' Beatis in 1517.[157] The notion that Leonardo and Della Torre were planning an illustrated book on anatomy is implausible, for none of the existing drawings from this period fits a commentary either on Galen's *De usu partium* or Mondino's *Anatomia*, the two texts most studied as an introduction to anatomy, and well-illustrated anatomical treatises and atlases still lay some way in the future. Even sketches made in lectures to illustrate disputed or difficult points in a dissection were unusual 25 years later, if we are to believe Vesalius's claim in the preface to his *Tabulae anatomicae sex*. This is not to deny the quality of Leonardo's drawings of the bones and muscles, or the way in which, in his last series of drawings on the heart and the lungs, around 1513, he tried to portray the body as a system in motion, writing in terms of its activities and functions.[158]

The question whether Leonardo's anatomical drawings had any direct impact on later artists is problematic. Some artists in Florence or elsewhere may have seen at least some of them when they were in the possession of his friend Francesco Melzi, and his example may have in some way inspired the artists of the *Fabrica*.[159] Certainly by the 1530s many artists of the calibre of Raphael and Michelangelo were drawing dissected limbs, and a print from the 1540s shows the studio of the Florentine sculptor Baccio Bandinello (1493–1560) littered with skeleton parts. Others like the anonymous artist who drew images of an articulated skeleton in the late 1540s, now in the Wellcome Collection, attended dissections.[160] Michelangelo joined Realdo Colombo in at least one at the house of a friend, while Vasari reports that the sculptor Angelo Montorsoli (1507–63) helped medical friends in Genoa to carry out many human dissections. Vasari himself was informed in advance by Vidus Vidius of a dissection that he was soon to perform and that would greatly interest him.[161] Many distinguished artists also drew images for anatomists' books. Girolamo da Carpi (1501–56) worked with Canano at Ferrara on the illustrations for his book on muscles, and Michelangelo may have assisted Colombo in Rome, although the promise of the frontispiece of his book, showing an artist sketching alongside the dissection table, is not born out by the book itself, which has no pictures.[162] Certainly by 1560 Michelangelo was convinced that no architect or artist was worthy of the name unless he had a knowledge of the anatomy of the human body.[163] Perhaps aware of what was taking place in Italy, both Charles Estienne in France and his dissector, the surgeon De la Rivière, engaged an artist to draw the dissections for their 1545 book.[164] To judge from style alone, Vesalius employed several artists for the *Fabrica*, including Calcar, although the belief that his master, Titian, was among them rests on a misunderstanding.[165]

By 1560, artists were even more frequently involved with anatomists, particularly in Italy, although few went so far as the Paduan anatomist Giulio Casseri (1552?–1616), who employed a German artist to live in his house and draw his dissections.[166] The artist Alessandro Allori (1535–1607) kept a room in the cloisters of San Lorenzo in Florence for the purposes of dissection and was allowed to keep body parts there from at least 1570.[167] Allori, like Giulio Romano (1499–1546) and other mannerists, delighted in depicting the body and its parts dismembered or writhing in strikingly unusual poses, while sculptors produced so-called écorchés, small sculptures of a body that had been flayed.[168] Allori was a leading member of the Florentine Academia del Disegno, whose members changed its statutes within six months of its foundation in January 1563 to ensure that they should all attend the annual anatomy.[169] Their anatomical interests, which they transmitted to their pupils, are neatly portrayed in an allegorical print by the Flemish painter and long-time resident of Florence, Jan van der Straet, Stradanus (1523–1605), which shows young painters and sculptors working from both human and animal specimens, carefully posed as skeletons or as corpses (Figure 9.3).[170] Alas, almost all trace of a book on anatomy for artists by the Bolognese Bartolomeo Passavanti (1529–92) has now vanished, but it is no wonder that the doctor Leonardo Fioravanti, writing in the 1560s, should have thought that dissection and its results were more relevant to the needs of artists than to those of physicians.[171]

Vesalius's concern for the visual impression created by his images in the *Fabrica* also broke new ground in many different ways. His images, some, like the series of muscle men set in a landscape of the Euganean hills, occupying the whole of a very large page, permitted greater clarity as well as the representation of, for example, the spinal vertebrae from several different angles and with shading to provide an illusion of three-dimensionality.[172] The contrast with those in Estienne's *Anatomy* is marked. His earlier images were cut into a small wood block which was then inserted into an existing larger one that had originally been used to illustrate, among other themes, the loves of the gods as described in salacious poems by Ariosto (Figure 7.2). The resulting image is too small to be totally decipherable, although, as Bette Talvacchia suggests, the connoisseur might well have appreciated the titillation of seeing the naked body in such a witty or, as some might consider it, a pornographic, context.[173] Estienne attempted to link this visual

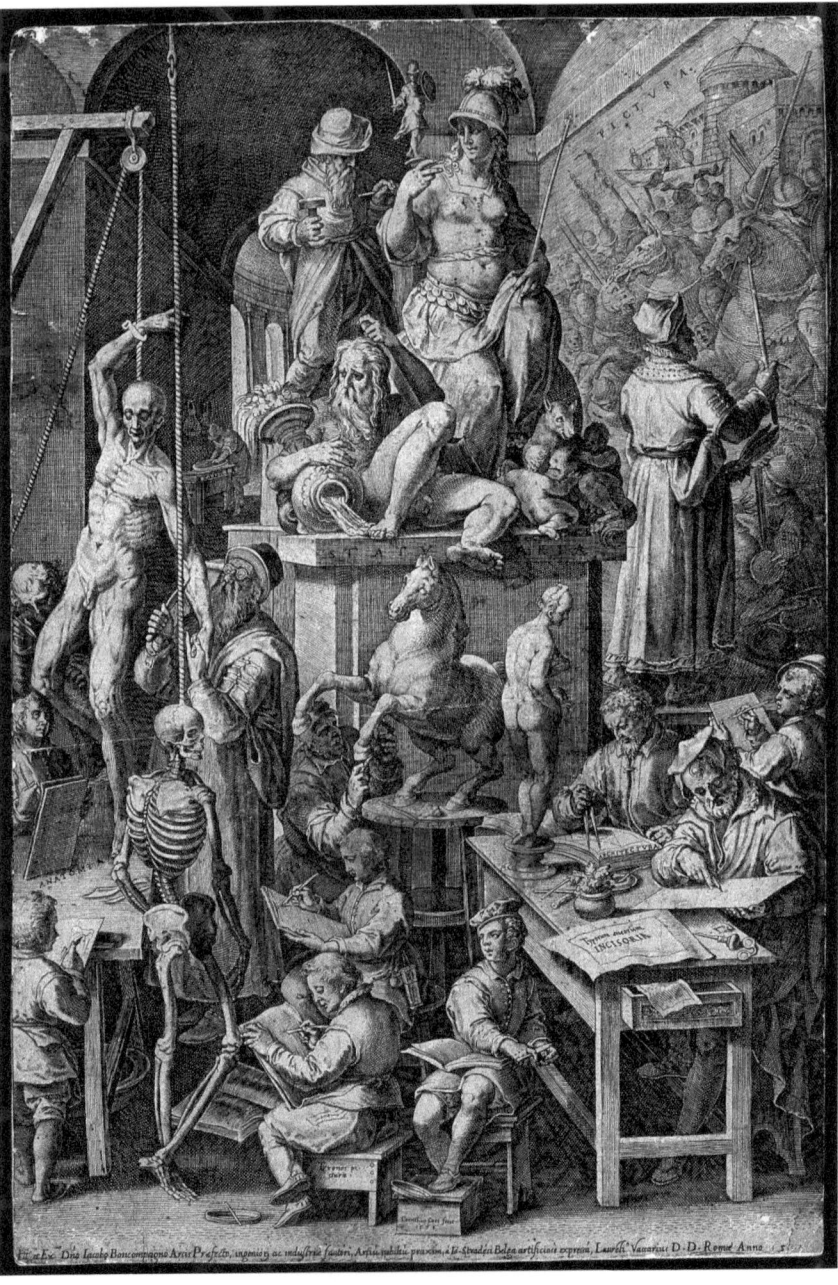

Figure 9.3 Artists drawing from life. A 1578 engraving by Cornelis Cort after
Stradanus.

information with the message of his text, but he was neither as consistent nor as thorough in the dynamic interplay of text and image as Vesalius, whose reader is encouraged to move from one to the other through the aid of a complex system of lettering that joins the picture to the actual words on the page, and to use his eyes as well as his mind while reading. Vesalius's own corrections to the 1555 edition show how his eye was able to pick out the slightest of details, and he expected his readers to do likewise.[174]

No other anatomist until Fabricius at the end of the sixteenth century used images in such profusion or in the same way. Costs and debates over the value and reliability of images of plants drawn from life will also have contributed to the reluctance of publishers to include more than a few plates in an anatomical treatise.[175] The 400 or so folio pages of Archangelo Piccolomini's *Anatomicae praelectiones, Anatomical Lectures*, contain a single large illustration, a portrait of the author and four small Berengario-like ones.[176] Significantly, the 1552 Lyons edition of the *Fabrica* was published by Jean de Tournes in a much smaller format, in two volumes, and with only four much reduced illustrations of skulls, and that of 1568 was also reduced in size, with its images redrawn more crudely.[177] Colombo's treatise appeared without any of its planned illustrations, while those of Eustachi (1520–74) had to wait until 1714 before appearing in print. However, images were not entirely neglected.[178] The unauthorised use of many of his images by the Fleming Thomas Geminus in London and the Spaniard Valverde de Hamusco in their anatomy books aroused the wrath of Vesalius, not least because Valverde's book quickly became very popular and was translated into a variety of languages, including French, Dutch and Italian.[179] His *Vivae icones partium corporis humani, Representation of the Parts of the Human Body Drawn from Life*, printed from the exquisite copper engraved plates still to be admired in the Plantin Museum in Antwerp, was the sixteenth-century equivalent of the modern selection by Saunders and O'Malley, privileging images over the text.[180] Much less expensive than the *Fabrica* and far less cumbersome than the *Epitome*, books like this could be brought to a lecture by students or used as a memory aid afterwards.[181] Even more successful in this role were the cheaper anatomical fugitive sheets, discussed earlier (pp. 72–3, 265), the Renaissance continuation of the medieval visual guides to the body and a reminder of how traditional ways of seeing and representation coexisted alongside the very different approaches exemplified by Vesalius and, still more, by Leonardo's drawings, which, however, remained largely unknown in private ownership.

Paradoxically, it may have been artists who benefitted most from the Renaissance re-evaluation of anatomy, for it provided them with possible patrons and encouraged them to improve their knowledge of the structures of the human body. Dissection certainly played a greater formal role in universities than it had done before 1500, and it became a shibboleth to distinguish the new medicine from the medieval. But the progress of anatomy was not always upwards. Individual faculties like that of Wittenberg rose and fell, and social pressures, allied to a feeling among some teachers of the irrelevance of anatomy to everyday medical practice, militated against it. Although seeing a corpse, and even cutting into it themselves, was popular with students, and public displays attracted crowds, such performances, like their medieval predecessors, aimed simply to reinforce the message that could be gained from books. More detailed instruction took place in private lessons or in attending an autopsy, about which far less is known. Vesalius may have changed the view of the human body as Copernicus had done for the universe, but one must be careful about accepting uncritically nineteenth-century and later views of the significance and role of anatomy in the sixteenth century.[182]

Notes

1 The preface to Celsus's De medicina 23–44 (Celsus 1971: I, 12–25) contains a classic exposition of arguments for and against 280 dissection, and was well known to the Renaissance, earlier, p. 100, and cf. later, p. For entertainment, Ferrari 1987; Hurren 2011 shows how many of modern preconceptions about the teaching of anatomy date only from the mid-nineteenth century.
2 Nutton 2013: 77–9, 120–3, 130–41, 219–21.
3 Mattern 2020.
4 Rocca 2003, 2008; Boudon-Millot 2014, 250–6; Nutton 2020a: 57–63; Salas 2020.
5 Nutton 2011: 10–17.
6 Although Plato himself had favoured the gut, not the liver, Nutton 2020a: 73, n. 73.
7 Galen 1956, 1962.
8 Caius 1570c: fol. 7v.; Nutton 2018a: 59, 70, n. 70.
9 Galen 1968.
10 Sharples and Van der Eijk 2008, esp. 11–14, 20–5.
11 The evidence assembled by Bliquez and Kazhdan 1984 shows the extreme rarity of dissection in Byzantium: two instances are exceptional examples of wartime cruelty, the rest quotations from, or allusions to, Galen.
12 Savage-Smith 1995.
13 For Abd al-Laṭīf (d.1231) and Ibn al-Nafīs (d. 1288), see Pormann and Savage-Smith 2007: 60, 46–8.
14 French 1979; Savage-Smith 1995.
15 McVaugh 1998; Park 1994, 2006.
16 Nutton and Bos 2011; Nutton 2022.
17 Mondino de' Liuzzi 1992.
18 Bylebyl 1990; Rumberg 2011.
19 Mondino de' Liuzzi 1992.
20 Demaitre 2013: 13–15.
21 Jacquart 1998: 225; Nutton and Nutton 2003.
22 Michel 2015: 305 (requiring attendance at an anatomy before graduation, and the costs to be paid for by those attending); Pielmeyer 1981: 46–52. Permission had already been given by Pope Sixtus V in 1482 for an anatomy every three or four years of a condemned criminal at Tübingen, Schultz 1986.
23 Schrauf 1899: 56–8.
24 London, Wellcome Collection, WMS 5265.
25 Schrauf 1899: 21.

26 Valla 1501; Branca 1981: 55–68; Ieraci-Bio 2017.
27 Benedetti 1502; Ferrari 1996, 1998; Giacomelli 2021.
28 Zerbi 1502; French 1999: 81–91. Although both anatomical books were printed in the same year, both men knew each other's arguments much earlier. For Zerbi's work on medical ethics, Tait 2020.
29 Berengario da Carpi 1521, 1522; tr. Lind 1959. See also French 1985.
30 His teacher, Alessandro Achillini (d. 1512) claimed to have seen the *rete* in 1503, but also raised questions about what exactly it was: Achillini 1521; Lind 1975: 61.
31 For artists, see later, pp. 266–72.
32 Eriksson 1959; Nutton1987b.
33 Antonioli 1976: 288–9; Fontaine 1984; see also above, p. 138.
34 Lutherans also strongly believed in the physical resurrection of the body.
35 Melanchthon *Ep.* 1182: 1977–: 1430. In his earlier *Physics* he had taken his medical information from Benedetti and Berengario.
36 Nutton 2003.
37 Typically downplayed by Vesalius 1543: iii.
38 Laguna 1536: for his own experience, ff. 16v–17r, 28r, 29v, and for Tagault's, f. 24v. Guinter 1536; Nutton 2017a.
39 Stephanus 1545, 1546; Talvacchia 1999.
40 Nutton 2017a: 168; Guinter 1539: sig. 5v; for his religious views, later, p. 310.
41 Du Fail 1874: 2,145–6.
42 Sylvius 1555 (but written between 1536 and 1542); Kellett 1961.
43 Vesalius 1543. English translations by Richardson and Carman 1998–2009, and Garrison-Hast 2014 (which also translates the changes in the 1555 edition and the major corrections made by Vesalius in his notes to that edition).
44 Roth 1892: 128; Nutton 1998.
45 O'Malley 1964; Joffe 2014; Van Hee 2014, 2020, adding new biographical details: Nutton 2017a: 25.
46 Compier 2012.
47 Vesalius 1538; Singer and Rabin 1946: Kusukawa 2012: 185–90; Nutton 2018b.
48 Guinter and Vesalius 1538; Nutton 2017a: 167–75 transcribes the notes.
49 Zwinger 1577: 309 ('The doctor is to explain, the surgeon to cut'). Leonardo Fioravanti (1517–c. 1588) devoted Book II of his popular text on surgery (1582) to instructing the surgeon exactly how to cut at a public anatomy. Cf. also Findlen 1996: 212–13, for Bologna.
50 Eriksson 1959.
51 O'Malley 1964: 188–98. Panizza 1561: 76r; Soulier 2020a: 43–8.
52 Vesalius 1546; 2015.
53 O'Malley 1964: 270, 284–9; Steeno *et al.* 2020.
54 Nutton 2012a.
55 Vesalius 1564. For his mission to the Holy Land, see Dirix 2014: 112.
56 Nutton 2017a: 25. For Da Monte's attendance at a Vesalian dissection of a spleen, Da Monte 1558b: 642.
57 O'Malley 1964: 226.
58 Vesalius 1543: 538; for other examples, Vesalius 1546: 140–1; 2015: 166.
59 O'Malley 1964 remains the most detailed account in English. Recent books, in addition to those listed in note 45, include Vons 2016; Canalis and Ciavolella 2018; Gielen and Goyens 2018; Van Hee and Biesbrouck 2018; Van Hee 2020; Soulier 2020b.
60 Margócsy *et al.* 2018: 40–55.
61 Steinmann 1967: 36–7, 113–14. Vesalius himself paid for the paper for the second edition and seems also to have loaned Oporinus a considerable sum.

62 The 1555 printing may simply be a reissue with a new title page.
63 Note 43. A French translation has also been begun.
64 The most substantial and accessible survey of Vesalius's anatomical work in 1543 is given by Carman in the prefaces to the individual volumes of Carman-Richardson 1998–2009. See also Catani and Sandrone 2015.
65 Nutton 2012a: 435; Baker 2016: 62. Vesalius's original error was noted by Falloppia (Soulier 2020b: 426); Valverde 1556: 63, fig. 1; and by Colombo 1559: 220.
66 O'Malley 1964: 170 optic chiasmus; 115 oarsman.
67 Vesalius 1543: 589, 2014: 1192; Vesalius 1555: 734/746, 1543: 642 (rete), 2014: 1299–300, 1555: 797.
68 Guinter and Vesalius 1538: fol. 51v; Nutton 2017a: 171.
69 Eriksson 1959: 234–5, 238–9.
70 Vesalius 1543: 584–6; cf. Jasolino 1576, supporting Vesalius, a reference I owe to David Soulier.
71 Vesalius 1555: 585, 2014: 1183–4.
72 Massa 1550: fol. 58r.
73 Vesalius 1543: iii–iv. The conjunction of these names shows the ahistoricity of Vesalius's claims. For rhetoric, see Salas 2020: 270–83.
74 For the significance of the anatomy of a woman, see Park 2006; and for the hand and arm, Rowe 1997; Siraisi 2001: 257–62; Maurette 2018.
75 Galen 1541–2; Caius 1570c: fol. 6r–v; Nutton 2018a: 58.
76 Carlino 2012; Cornarius 1556: 69–70, a letter of April 1543. For his later reactions, see p. 238. Similar praise of Vesalius as a Galenist comes from Julius Alexandrinus 1548: 171.
77 Massa 1536; Lind 1975: 174–253; Palmer 1981b; Ross 2016: 79–110.
78 Massa 1550: fol. 58r., written originally in 1544 in response to the *Fabrica*.
79 Nutton 2017a: 31–2, 125, 172.
80 Vesalius 1544: 42–7; 2015: 47–53. Sylvius's claim would have seemed more credible to scholars brought up on the forgeries of Annius of Viterbo who claimed that there had been giants before the flood, Stephens 1979.
81 Nutton 2018a: 13–14.
82 London, British Library, classmark 9065–9 (2).
83 Ingrassia 1552: 156–7; Colombo 1559; Falloppia 1561; Canalis 2018b. For post-Vesalian teaching in Padua and Bologna, Klestinec 2011; Stolberg 2018a, 2018b.
84 Dryander, apud Vesalius 1555: 178; Vesalius 2015: 209–10; Soulier 2020b.
85 Vesalius 1543: 661.
86 Eustachi 1563–4; Kusukawa 2012: 237–41.
87 Barcia Goyanes 1994; Salas 2020.
88 Canalis 2018a.
89 O'Malley 1964: 275. One doubts whether Vesalius would have been pleased to be the dedicatee of the 1549 Basle edition of Benedetti, Hieronymus 2005: 190, despite its fulsome praise.
90 Roth 1895: 477–8; mistranslated in O'Malley 1964: 405.
91 Stolberg 2018b: 74.
92 Margócsy *et al.* 2018: 8; 164, a copy owned by Johann Friedrich, Elector of Saxony from 1543 to 1547, and in the Jena University Library in 1549; 165 a copy bought in 1545 by the Nuremberg physician Erasmus Flock (1514–68).
93 *Ibid.*, 242–5.
94 Nutton 1993: Helm 2001; Margócsy *et al.* 2018: 18, 72–3.
95 Carlino 1999b: cat. 30,2, 34,2, 35,1, 36–7.
96 Geminus 1545; Donaldson 2010; Lo 2018; Nutton 2020b; Valverde 1556; Skaarup 2015b. Vesalius's brother wrongly assumed that John Caius was behind Geminus's work.

97 Skaarup 2015a; Soulier 2020b.

98 Geminus 1545: pref.; Nutton 2020b.

99 Nutton 2018a: 28–9. He is more critical of Colombo, at least one of whose dissections he attended, Colombo 1559: 266.

100 Langton 1547: sig. D.4r.

101 Jones PM 1988; Margócsy *et al.* 2018: 388–9.

102 Lewis 1986: 217–8, with the qualifications on pp. 244–7.

103 Matthioli 1561: 151–2; *Epistolae medicinales* IV, 1; Thaddeus Hagecius in Gryllus 1566a: sig. D ii r: Adam Landau, *ibid.*: sig. Bii v; Zwinger 1577: 33 ("Vesalius, to whom we owe the recovery of anatomy").

104 Triebs 1995: 45; Semenzato 1995: 70–7. The new wooden theatre at Ferrara, built in 1567 at the expense of Faculty and students, was intended to last for several years, see Muratori 1969: 317–21.

105 See the poem copied into a 1555 edition of the *Fabrica*, Margócsy *et al.* 2018: 309.

106 Canano 1925; Van Glabbeek and Biesbrouck 2020; Botallo 1565 (which despite its title contains some of his anatomical writings; cf. Taccari 1971). For Paduan anatomy after Vesalius, Klestinec 2011; Stolberg 2018a, 2018b.

107 Colombo 1559: 177; Baldo 2014: xliii–xlvii, lxxii–lxxix.

108 Baldo 2014: lxxxv–xciii; Mudry 2013; Purkircher 1988: 154.

109 Adelmann 1966: 85–8; Grendler 2002: 337–40, noting also other universities.

110 Platter 1583; Bauhin 1590; Burckhardt 1917: 86–7, 100–7; Hieronymus 2005: 2664–708, 3034–52, adds many new details, reproducing, 3036, a poem by Peter Monau comparing Platter to Vesalius, Falloppia and Colombo.

111 Nutton 1993: 14–15.

112 Wallis 2018: 62.

113 Hobson 1999: 81.

114 Sawday 1995; Hillman and Mazzio 1997; Sugg 2012; Margócsy *et al.* 2018: 32–7.

115 Caius 1570c: 17v; Nutton 2018a: 69–70, 97.

116 Crato 1611: 95, 1619: 431–2; Ongaro 1971: 36–8; Celati 2015.

117 Ferrari 1987.

118 Daston and Park 1998; Ogilvie 2006.

119 Soulier 2021.

120 Eriksson 1959. He also showed the skull of one or two sheep and the larynx of an ox.

121 Park 1994: 16–21; Carlino 1999a.

122 Joffe 2014: 144.

123 Vesalius 1543: 539; cf. also 126, 538.

124 Nutton 1993: 14–15.

125 Murphy 2019: 81.

126 Murphy 2019: 81; Adelmann 1966: 753–9; Findlen 1996: 213.

127 Cunningham 1985; for a critique of this interpretation, Stolberg 2018b: 390–4.

128 French 1999: 59–67.

129 Klestinec 2011: xvi; Murphy 2019: 95.

130 Purkircher 1988: 150. For Landi (c. 1515–62), who published a short textbook of anatomy in 1542, see Ferretto 2012.

131 For later student reports of attending private autopsies, Zampieri 2021: 55; Soulier 2020b: 404n1, discusses a Paduan decree of 1549 forbidding digging for bones in cemeteries to put them on sale.

132 Purkircher 1988: 154.

133 For the real reason, earlier, p. 143.

134 Fioravanti 1567: 42v–6v, 1582: 117v–20r, 143r–v; Ferrari 2008: 361. For Fioravanti, see earlier, pp. 170–2.

135 Fioravanti 1582: 131v.
136 Vesalian anatomy had also been taught at the Portuguese and later Spanish University of Coimbra.
137 Skaarup 2015a: 98–105, 109–11. Cf. Granjel 1980: 156–72, and for similar statements at Bologna a century later, Adelmann 1966: 86–7.
138 O'Malley 1970: 94; Sticker 1927: 66; Giese and Von Hagen 1958: 17–18.
139 Coiter 1572: t.p.; Murphy 2019: 68–84.
140 Earlier, pp. 169–71.
141 Langton 1547: sig. D 4r. Cf. Ashley-Montagu 1953; Soulier 2020b.
142 For Fuchs and Isingrin, see earlier, pp. 16–7. For Vesalius's assistance with Oporinus's wayward son Jacob, Steinmann 1967: 108.
143 Janssen 2005: 10.
144 Vesalius 1538; Kornell 2018: Caiati *et al.* 2020.
145 Eriksson 1959.
146 Steeno *et al.* 2020: 119.
147 Jones PM 1984; Kusukawa 2012.
148 Berengario 1521; Canano 1929; Van Glabbeek and Biesbrouck 2020.
149 Dryander 1536; Vesalius 1538; Singer and Rabin 1946.
150 Schultz 1985; Kornell 1993; Laurenza 2003, 2011, 2012a; Guest 2014.
151 Cazort *et al.* 1996: 106–7, 15–38.
152 Literature on Leonardo is enormous. The fundamental study is Keele and Pedretti 1980–1985, with Roberts 1990: 53–6; Clayton and Philo 2012. For this division into periods, see Baur *et al.* 1984: 19–36; Laurenza 2003: 34–72; Nicholl 2004: 240–5, 418–23, 443–9.
153 Vasari 1984: 284; Giacomelli 2021.
154 Laurenza 2011; Nutton and Bos 2011: 110–12.
155 Clayton and Philo 2012: 19–21; Laurenza 2003: 54–67.
156 Nicholl 2005: 444.
157 De Beatis A 1979: 132; Roberts 1990: 60. The latter may have been Ms A, but that is not systematically organised.
158 Baur *et al.* 1984. For his work on the heart, Wells 2013.
159 One who did at the end of the century was Ambrogio Figino (1546/1553–1608), Laurenza 2012a: 36–9.
160 Kornell 2000.
161 Kornell 2000: 108–10; Jacobs 2002: 439–41.
162 Van Glabbeek and Biesbrouck 2020: 116–17; Colombo 1559, although some were planned and a contemporary knew of some copper plates, Kornell 2022: 126.
163 Milanesi 1875: 554.
164 Talvacchia 1999: 161–87; Kornell 2022: 97; for the possible involvement of the artist Rosso Fiorentino, at least at one remove, see Kornell 1989.
165 Kornell 2018; Caiati *et al.* 2020; Simons and Kornell 2008.
166 De Ferrari 1978.
167 Kornell 2000: 109.
168 Céard *et al.* 1990: 115–86.
169 Jacobs 2002; for the interaction of artists and anatomist at Bologna, Pigozzi 2012.
170 Jacobs 2002: 435. Stradanus was responsible with Allori for organising the dissection of 1573–4.
171 Fioravanti 1567: 42v–6v. For this dispute in late sixteenth-century Spain, Portmann 2018.
172 Vesalius 1543: 170–211; Cavanagh 1983.
173 Roberts and Tomlinson 1992: 168–87; Talvacchia 1999; Cazes and Carlino 2003, "a book for friends rather than students".

174 Nutton 2012a: 426–8.
175 For the substantial extra cost of printing images, see earlier, p. 70; for debates on the reliability of images, Kusukawa 2012: 124–36.
176 Piccolomini 1586.
177 Vesalius 1552, 1568; Elaut 1974.
178 Colombo 1559; Eustachi 1728.
179 Geminus 1545; Donaldson 2010; Lo 2018; Nutton 2020b; Valverde 1556; Skaarup 2015b. Geminus's images were later reused by Jacques Grévin (1538–70) for his 1569 *Portraits anatomiques* and its Latin version.
180 Saunders and O'Malley 1982; Van Hee 2020: 149.
181 The Lyons printer Clément Baudin included artists and architects among his projected audience for his selection of images from Vesalius, Baudin 1560; Kornell 2022: 30–1. The Paris (incomplete) copy, Bibliothèque Nationale de France, classmark Ta 12.64, was owned by an apothecary; a unique complete copy, sold at Christie's in London, Sale Catalogue, December 9, 2020, by a French aristocrat.
182 Earlier, note 103.

10 Paracelsus and Paracelsianism

From the 1550s onwards traditional Galenist medicine was challenged by a revolutionary new theory, Paracelsianism. It was revolutionary in that it broke down many of the hierarchies of knowledge upheld by the Church, the universities and the medical profession to such an extent that mere possession of Paracelsian books became a reason for investigation by the Inquisition, occasionally leading to execution.[1] Originally confined largely to German-speaking Europe, the publication of many Paracelsian writings in Latin for the first time in 1575 enabled it to spread more widely. It was based on the teachings of a doctor who had died in 1541, and whose published writings were confined to small almanacs of predictions for the coming year (a common side-line for doctors), a book on syphilis, another on a local spring and, the most successful, his *Great Book of Surgery*. His reputation increased after his death as stories of the almost miraculous cures of this great and wrongly despised healer proliferated and encouraged others to seek out and publish whatever of his writings they could still uncover. That many of the medical ideas contained within them fitted with the religious ideas of some Evangelicals was a further incentive for their publication, and the high level of literacy among the German-speaking inhabitants of Northern Europe ensured a profitable market for Paracelsian writings.[2] But as the great medical historian Owsei Temkin remarked over 70 years ago, Paracelsus remains elusive, and although subsequent scholarship has done much to pin him down, many difficulties stand in the way of understanding who he was, what he believed and how his ideas were interpreted and developed by his followers.[3] It is not only, as another great historian, Walter Pagel, insisted over and over again, that notions that were easily intelligible, if not commonplace, in the learned world of the late Renaissance are now likely to be dismissed as strange and unscientific, but also that their historical context has become even less familiar now than when Temkin and Pagel were writing 70 years ago.[4] The German-speaking world of today is a fraction of what it was then, and bitter religious struggles are a thing of the past in many parts of modern secular European society. This chapter aims to restore some of this lost context as a way of understanding the man and his work, while acknowledging that Paracelsus's own liking

DOI: 10.4324/9781003223184-14

for a quarrel and the relative lack of others' testimony from his lifetime still leave much that is uncertain.

The Life of Paracelsus

Philippus Aureolus Theophrastus Bombastus von Hohenheim, to give him his full name, was born in 1493/4, the son of a doctor at Einsielden in Switzerland, who shortly after moved to the mining centre of Villach in modern Austria.[5] He learned much about mineralogy from his father, but the belief that he studied philosophy and theology with various clerics, probably including the reformist mystic Abbot Trithemius of Sponheim, rests on a modern misunderstanding.[6] Where he gained his education remains unclear. He mentions a variety of universities, almost always critically, but he may have studied at Vienna before travelling to Italy to learn medicine, probably at Ferrara.[7] He seems then to have a made a peregrination around Europe, to Spain and England and as far as Turkey and Muscovy (if his claims can be believed), including periods as a military surgeon in the service of Venice and Denmark. In this, he differed from some of the wandering students we have met earlier only in his combative nature and, when practising in Salzburg and Strasbourg, in his support for poor citizens in their at times bitter struggles with the authorities.[8]

By early 1527 he was in Basle where a successful cure of the publisher Froben, who was in danger of having his leg amputated, gained him the approval of Erasmus and other humanists there and led to his appointment as a town physician with the right to lecture at the university. Although the plague had temporarily halted teaching, Paracelsus challenged the university by refusing to take its oath and by publishing a manifesto in which he promised to teach practical and theoretical medicine, not from Galen and Hippocrates, but from his own experience with nature and disease. In a further show of independence, he burnt a copy of Avicenna's *Canon* in a student bonfire on St John's Day (June 24th). Although the medical Faculty reacted by refusing to allow him the use of a lecture room and forbidding him to sponsor doctorands, he continued lecturing, but in German, not Latin, another innovation. Froben's death later that year robbed him of a protector, and after losing a lawsuit to a patient who complained of maltreatment and financial chicanery, he hurriedly left town, handing his possessions over to his pupil and assistant, Oporinus, the later publisher of Vesalius.[9] It is about this time that he began to call himself Paracelsus, possibly a Latinised form of 'from Hohenheim'. But the *Para-* prefix, meaning 'super', was also a favourite of his, in titles like *Paragranum* and *Paramirum*, and those who met or heard of him may have understood it to mean 'Greater than Celsus', the Roman doctor.[10] From Basle he headed for Colmar and then Nuremberg, causing controversy wherever he went, before arriving in 1531 in St Gallen, where he wrote his *Paramirum, The Wonderful Book*, dedicating it to the physician Vadianus, who was now the town's Mayor. In 1533

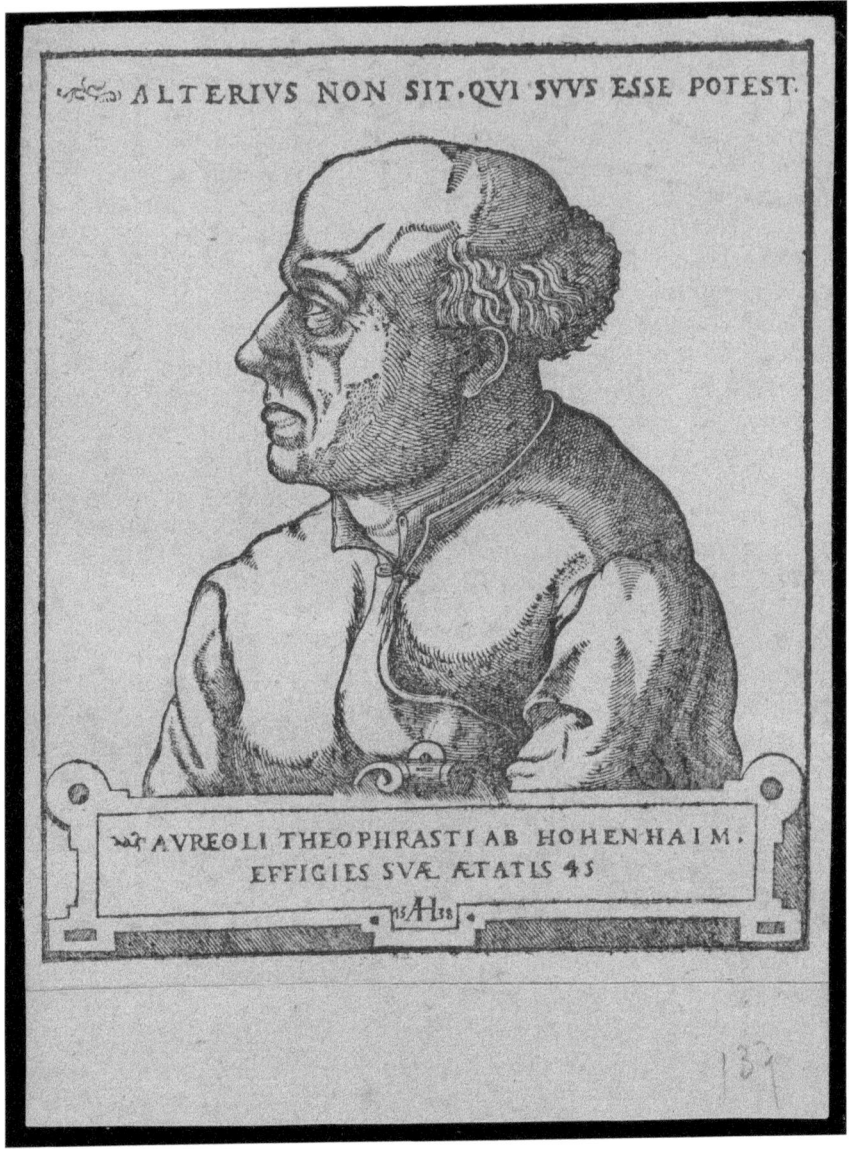

Figure 10.1 Paracelsus, aged 45. Woodcut by Augustin Hirschvogel, 1538. Paracelsus's motto, above, declares that "No one who can be his own man
should be bound to another".

he moved deeper into Switzerland as an itinerant preacher and surgeon and
then onwards into South Germany and the Tyrol, including Villach again,
before being summoned to Salzburg in 1541 to treat its Archbishop. Here he
died suddenly, bequeathing his few belongings to the poor.

His writings are filled with accounts of cases in which his use of chemical drugs or surgery had succeeded against all the odds and the opposition of medical and town authorities. Oporinus in a much later hostile note for Johann Weyer confirmed his master's deep interest in experiments with minerals and his disdain for, if not ignorance of, academic learning, as well as his strange behaviour – constantly drinking and rarely sleeping, always appearing to have money and constantly disposing of his old smelly clothes to the poor, who rejected them. He frequently railed against both the Pope and Luther for being unable to penetrate to what he saw as the kernel of the Christian gospel.[11] Oporinus's sketch confirms the evidence of Paracelsus's own writings that he attracted patients wherever he went who continued to pay him well, and that he performed several cures on the sick who had been given up for lost by others. But, leaving aside his time in Basle, it was his social and religious views, including his sympathy for outsiders, always vigorously expressed, that caused him greatest trouble with the authorities. One can see from Oporinus and other contemporary comments how after his death the story became established in the popular mind of Paracelsus as a great, almost miraculous, Christian healer, rejected by the upholders of official medicine in both church and state, and why, a decade or more after his death, some who shared his religious and political outlook should have sought to publish a corpus of Paracelsian writings, including some that had been left behind in Basle with Oporinus.[12]

Paracelsus the German

In the first half of the sixteenth century, native speakers of German could be found across Europe from the Vosges mountains in Alsace to Transylvania in the East and from Riga on the Baltic to the Tyrol and Carniola in the south. They spoke a variety of dialects, but Luther's translation of the Bible and the power of the printing press had begun to make his Saxon dialect of Central Germany commonly understood everywhere. German migrations in the Later Middle Ages had pushed German colonists yet further east and north, where they frequently constituted the majority of the population in the many small towns. They were often traders, hence at least functionally literate, and the many small courts of local magnates provided employment for administrators and doctors as well as being centres of literate culture. The Reformation, in origin largely a phenomenon of German towns, further stimulated a growth in education because of its insistence on a universal acquaintance with the word of God as expressed in the Bible. In short, the German-speaking community was larger and had access to more written material in the vernacular than any other European group, and, although not as universal as Latin among scholars and clergy across Europe, German penetrated extremely widely and more deeply into the urban communities of Northern Europe. Politically, the Holy Roman Empire (the additional words 'of the German nation' came into use much later) covered a multitude of states both great and small extending from modern Belgium,

Eastern France and Switzerland far to the east, where it faced the Ottoman Empire. Within its boundaries, and under the theoretical overlordship of the Emperor, travellers and traders, including doctors, moved easily across a network of towns that provided opportunities for lucrative employment. Towns like Strasbourg, Nuremberg, Augsburg and Prague were among the wealthiest in Europe, and even smaller communities such as Colmar and St Gallen contained potentially wealthy patients and employed their own civic physicians to look after their sick poor.[13] There were also many universities as well as courts to attract men of learning, and town regulations required doctors, surgeons and midwives to be appointed to treat the community, and, among other things, to investigate cases of leprosy and plague, both of which were described at length by Paracelsus. There was an abundance of opportunities for healers of all kinds, matched only in the richer areas of Italy or in a megalopolis like London.

Already in the Middle Ages there had been a flourishing medical literature of all kinds in German that circulated widely.[14] It included translations of Latin works as well as advice on plague and books of domestic medicine. Learned works on surgery, like those of the thirteenth-century surgeon Ortolf of Bavaria or of Peter of Ulm (fl. 1430–40), were often excerpted and their advice and remedies (and sometimes illustrations) were copied into other manuscripts and commonplace books across dialect boundaries.[15] University teachers of medicine like Heinrich Münsinger (fl. 1440) at Heidelberg wrote treatises in both Latin and German on human as well as on veterinary medicine.[16] Medicine at courts like that of Sigmund of the Tyrol (1427–96) at Innsbruck was likewise conducted in both languages, and some of the largest manuscripts and recipe collections were put together for the benefit of rulers and their households.[17] Elector Ludwig V of the Palatinate (ruled 1508–44) collected and himself copied out an enormous number of medical tracts, which he had bound in 13 volumes: his contemporary, the Elector John of Saxony contented himself with a mere four.[18] By deliberately choosing to write in German, Paracelsus was not cutting himself off from learned society, but aiming for as wide an audience as possible within a German-speaking world that had long been accustomed to reading printed books by other doctors on similar themes.

It was an audience already familiar with the genres in which Paracelsus published during his lifetime. Calendars of one sort or another had been common since medieval times, and printed almanacs containing predictions for the year were sure-fire sellers, often written by doctors who had been trained in medical astrology.[19] Plague texts were also ubiquitous in German as were short self-help handbooks of healing, some under such titles as *A Little Book of Medicine for the Poor Man Who Has No Physician* or *The Treasury of Health*.[20] This domestic medicine, or *Hausvatermedizin*, was especially encouraged by Evangelicals who held a high conception of the importance of family life. Particularly significant for Paracelsus's reputation in his last years was his big book on surgery, which drew on a long tradition of substantial and detailed writings on surgery, not least those of Hierony-mus Brunschwig and Hans von Gersdorff (Figure 6.2).[21] His own book, first published in Augsburg in 1536, was a great success: it was followed imme-diately by an unauthorised edition at Ulm and was among the first of his writings to be published or republished after his death.[22] That edition, the first of his books to appear from the Frankfurt press of Christian Egenolff, had as an appendix a description of the healing power of the 'quintessence', the distilled essence of all natural substances.[23] He himself mentioned his surgical cures at various points in his writings, but his book has relatively little to say about amputations and the treatment of fractures compared with wound management, relying particularly on a range of salves, oint-ments and powders, many of them mineral in origin. Typically, it combines wonderfully modern insights with others that appear extremely strange.[24] The body can heal itself through an innate 'balm' that it produces, and the duty of the surgeon is to allow this natural healing to take place. The vigor-ous interventions of medieval surgeons like Guy de Chauliac are rejected along with those of Galen as they prevent the wound receiving its natural nourishment from this balm. Paracelsus opposes notions of laudable pus and of sewing up the wound or encasing it in white of egg, for these procedures only assist harmful putrefaction. But his view that wounds are in some way infected as the result of poison is very different from that of surgeons like Vigo (earlier, p. 157) who treated gunshot wounds as if they were poisoned. Paracelsus's poison comes from outside and does not depend on the weapon that caused the wound, which merely opened up the body. Sometimes it is the stars that impress plague into the wound and an unpropitious heaven makes healing almost impossible; sometimes the poison is sent to the wound by the poisonous looks of (usually) jealous, hateful and perfidious women; sometimes the individual's own anger poisons the wound with bile.[25]

There are other parallels between the first published writings of Para-celsus and those of the earlier surgeon Hieronymus Brunschwig. Both wrote a *Practica*, a brief guide to domestic medicine, Brunschwig's *Thesaurus pau-perum*, *Treasury of the Poor*, or *Hausapotheke*, going through many edi-tions under a variety of titles from 1512, and appearing in English in 1561 as *A Most Excellent and Perfect Homish Apothecareye or Homely Physick Booke*. He too wrote a short book on surgery, again published in several editions, including an English version in 1525, *The Noble Experyence of the Vertuous Handy Warke of Surgerie*. His third best-seller, translated into English in 1527 as *The Vertuose Boke of Distyllacyon of the Waters of all Maner of Herbes*, continued a long tradition of writing in German on distillation. One of the earliest books on the subject was ascribed to a pro-fessor of medicine at Vienna, Michael Puff von Schrick (c. 1400–73), and was printed from 1473 onwards more often (at least 27 times) and in the company of a greater and more varied combination of other tracts on distil-lation than almost any other medical text, as well as circulating widely in manuscript form.[26]

This interest in distillation and what might be termed protochemistry was shared and extended by Paracelsus. From his early upbringing with his father at Villach and his later experiences in other mining areas Paracelsus gained a deep familiarity with mineralogy and mining techniques that sets him apart from many of his medical contemporaries. Whether in the Harz region, the Iron-ore mountains of Saxony and Bohemia, in Styria, Carniola or further east in the Carpathians and Transylvania, Germans had exploited the varied ores that provided them with sources of wealth surpassed in this period only by the silver mines of the New World. The first major book on mineralogy was written by a German physician, Georg Agricola's *De re metallica, Metallurgy*, and a variety of smaller writings in German described the properties of minerals that could be used in therapy.[27] Paracelsus's acquaintance with mining is most obvious in the three books on *Miners' Diseases, Von der Bergsucht oder Bergkranckheiten*, in which he distinguished the types of disease encountered by miners according to the substances mined, an observation already enunciated in 1473 by Ulrich Ellenbog (1435–99) in a *Consilium* for the goldsmiths of Augsburg, although not printed until 1524.[28] The previous year, 1523, another doctor in a mining town, Wenzeslaus Bayer, a town doctor at Joachimsthal in Saxony, had published a short health guide for the poor workmen whom he saw suffering from breathing problems caused by bad air in the mines.[29] Paracelsus was thus not alone in observing the problems of miners, but an understanding of the principles behind mining, smelting and distillation permeates his entire medicine from the very start. His universe is one of processes, constantly changing and developing, with close links and correspondences between the natural world, the macrocosm and the human microcosm. He laid great stress on fire as an active agent, and, although he mentions other substances, for him the universe is primarily based on three chemical (or alchemical) principles, salt, sulphur and mercury. But he saw them not so much as material substances, but rather as representing the qualities of solidity, flammability and spirituousness respectively. They were active, spirit-like and 'male' compared with the traditional 'female' and passive Aristotelian elements.

Paracelsus devoted much attention to the essences of things, including diseases, which he viewed as a sort of spiritual specificity, akin to the quintessence produced by distillation and sublimation. Diseases were thus best combatted by reducing the herbs or minerals used in therapy to their quintessence, which contained their properties in the most concentrated and hence most powerful form. His notion of anatomy similarly developed in an idiosyncratic direction. He rejected the anatomy of the medical school in favour of a true, living anatomy that revealed the body's processes not only, for example, by inspecting urine but also by 'dissecting' it chemically, seeing how it changed under the action of heat. Paracelsus similarly investigated the formation of 'tartar', progressively accumulated coagulations of salt from 'hellish' unwanted substances which took on different forms depending on their site, for example in the stomach, the heart or the mouth.[30] His view of dropsy was that it was caused by fluid generated by the liquid dissolution of tissues which causes the body to swell from the feet upwards until the "spirit of life is drowned in it like a man in a flood that overtakes him". Conditions like this could best be cured not by diet or traditional herbal drugs but by quicker-acting mineral ones, for their speed of healing action counteracted the swiftly developing poison of the disease. Dropsy, for instance, had first to be removed by 'mercurial essences', then sulphur and finally a metallic 'crocus' (or oxide). Sulphur acted in curing dropsy like the sun dispelling rain in the macrocosm, while the 'crocus' dried and firmed up the body.[31] Many of these ideas were not unique to Paracelsus, but the words he used to describe them were often his own and hence added to the impression that he possessed a secret or arcane wisdom, the mark to his followers of a remarkable physician, but to his detractors of a charlatan.

The Religion of Paracelsus

For many years, historians of medicine concentrated upon Paracelsus's ideas as they derived from other medical and philosophical writers, and it was not until the work of Kurt Goldammer in the 1950s that his writings on ethics, politics and, above all, religion were published in a modern edition, many of them for the very first time. Indeed, it was not until 2008 that a biography of Paracelsus was published that placed his religious and ethical views at the centre of his activities.[32] Arguably none of his writings and few of his actions, to say nothing of the opposition they aroused, can be understood without a reference to his religious beliefs in the context of the tumultuous final decades of his life.

As will be explained further in the next chapter, this was a period of great religious upheaval, and it was only to be expected that his demands for a more open and less authoritarian Christian medicine should be compared with what Martin Luther had achieved in his religious reforms. It was a comparison that he resented strongly, not least because he objected to both organised medicine and religion for their exclusivity.[33] Both of them he scathingly termed 'Scheinkirche', mere ecclesiastical mirages, or 'Mauerkirche', churches confined by walls, in which only a select few, defined by their academic and theoretical learning, could exercise authority.[34] For Paracelsus, like other radical reformers such as Caspar Schwenckfeld (1489–1561) and Sebastian Franck, (1499–1543), true Christianity was the result of a direct individual, personal revelation from God, mediated also through the Bible and the Light of Nature. It did not require participation in the Mass, let alone the mitre, staff, vestments and silk trousers of priests and bishops, in order to live a Christian life in preparation for the ultimate battle with the forces of the Antichrist – the devils, elves and demons that populate the universe.[35] Similarly, healing did not depend on a degree from a university or membership of a guild, but on any individual's understanding of and ability to bring about healing. It derived not from theological books, but from reading the Book of Nature, prayer and contemplation. Through God alone, the true doctor could now see like God into the very heart of creation and grasp the secrets of every individual living thing in a universe where heaven and earth were bound closely together.

This reversal of traditional epistemology, from book-learning to an inner intuition, is matched by a change from a Hippocratic to a Christian ethic. It is not the patient's trust in the Hippocratic doctor that will bring about healing, the message of the opening section in the Hippocratic *Prognostics*, but the belief of both doctor and patient in the Christian God. Christian love, not book-learning, must lie at the basis of all healing.[36] Sometimes Paracelsus departs almost completely from the ideas of Galen and Aristotle, at others he gives them only a slight twist. His discussion of madness, for example, combines humoralism with chemical analogies. Melancholic madness is the result of an excess of melancholic humour, and, like Galen, Paracelsus accepts that mania and epilepsy both arise from a physical cause. But in his view the former is the result of the distillation and sublimation of harmful vapours in the body, whereas epilepsy, a sort of earthquake in the brain, is provoked by a 'spirit of life' arising in the body, rising to the brain, and causing the body to shake and tremble, just as the action of sodium causes vinegar to boil when it is dropped into it. Both processes could be successfully counteracted by chemical drugs that reversed them. By contrast, the truly mad are difficult, if not impossible to cure. Some, the lunatics, have been affected by the influence of the Moon while still in the womb. Although the madness of the truly insane also often originates in the womb, here it results from a weakness in the seed that formed the foetus, sometimes brought on by an excessive desire for coitus. But insanity can also result from the sinful behaviour of the two partners, the result of inebriation brought on by excessive food and drink that drove them to make love inappropriately. However, those who are born from such intercourse with a choleric disposition are likely to become ever more pugnacious and warlike, which is no insanity at all.[37]

Other standard Hippocratic and Galenic statements were reinterpreted within an Evangelical context.[38] The injunction in *Airs, Waters and Places* to travel in order to discover the different effects of environment becomes an encouragement to see the world as God created it. Only then will one understand Nature truly. "Whoever wishes to investigate things fully should walk in the Book [of Nature]. Books are revealed letter by letter, Nature land by land. One land, one page; one must turn over the pages in the book of Nature." Thus, in the Light of God and Nature one can come to understand, for example, something that only a pear knows: how to be a pear.[39] This intuition, the gaining of knowledge through contemplation and prayer, is vastly different from the book-learning of the schools. It is open to all Christians and leads directly to effective practice. Anyone can experiment and see, for example, the different colours left by urine on the inside of a glass, or watch iron change colour, shape, and even substance as it is heated in a furnace. These insights can then be made public in the certainty, familiar among Evangelicals, that these revelations from God cannot be gainsaid by any detractors.

The Mystical Paracelsus

The third strand in Paracelsus's thinking, which links him to other ideas that enjoyed a wide circulation in the early sixteenth century, can be loosely termed Neoplatonist or Gnostic. Although their ultimate origins lay in some of the ideas of the philosopher Plato in the fourth century BCE, they had been developed by both Christian and non-Christian thinkers in the Greek world of the second and third century CE. Bitterly resisted both by Aristotelians and orthodox Christians, they were promoted by a few Christians in the Western Middle Ages, most notably the Spaniard Ramon Lull (1234–1315), and they received a renewed impetus in the fifteenth century from the rediscovery in Greek of forgotten works of Plato and his Neoplatonist followers. Particularly influential on his contemporaries in Italy and beyond, and one of the very few doctors whom Paracelsus mentioned with approval, was Marsilio Ficino (1433–99), a Florentine philosopher, although the precise extent of Paracelsus's dependence is far from clear. Pagel, for example, suggested that Paracelsus derived his ideas on plague from Ficino, who had argued that plague was a pestilential poison that operated like the corrosive vapour found in mines. Webster, on the other hand, thought that the writings of another Renaissance Neoplatonist, Pico della Mirandola, (1463–94) may have been more relevant to Paracelsus's ideas.[40] Ficino believed that there was throughout the universe an immaterial soul-substance that gave life to corporeal beings: at the peak was a World Soul, followed by the souls in the celestial spheres, and finally those that animated all living things. The universe was full of souls, spirits and demons who interacted with humans for good and ill. This was an idea that Ficino and others believed could be found in all religions, including Christianity, whose truths could be further illuminated by exploring both Christian and Jewish mysticism, including the Jewish Cabala.[41] Only through possession of this true *gnosis* or knowledge, including a knowledge of the workings of the heavens, could one fully understand how the body worked. This knowledge was gained both by revelation and by observing the secrets of Nature, or, as some called it, *magia naturalis*, Nature's magic. The adept was both priest and physician, for medicine without heavenly grace was ineffective and even harmful.[42] Ficino's philosophy in many ways resembles that of Paracelsus, although the latter was more sceptical than Ficino of many aspects of astrology as well as being more deeply versed in the Bible.

For Paracelsus, the true doctor was guided throughout by God, who had placed clues in Nature that the adept could recognise and act upon. These so-called signatures indicated correspondences between diseases, processes within the body (and also outside it), and the appropriate therapy.

Knowing these connections explained why the colours, shapes or patterns of certain herbs and minerals indicated that they were to be used against certain conditions. The leaves of a thistle prick like needles; hence there is no better remedy against stitches and other sharp abdominal pains. Eyebright shows the image of eyes, hence it is led by sympathy towards and cures the eyes. Iris cures cancer for "its image locates itself in the body at the place to which it belongs by form".[43] This notion that like should be used to cure like ran counter, at least in theory, to the standard Galenic doctrine of allopathy, that the body should be brought back into balance by using remedies that opposed the disease, such as a cold therapy for a hot condition. At times, these correspondences are only visible to the adept. Atrophy, for instance, occurs when the sun in the body continually dries up its moisture, and hence requires to be fed with moist nourishment to prevent it drying the body further. This hot sun is not eliminated, as in Galenic medicine, but controlled: "the doctor must sow water that grows in man in the same way as grass grows in the field, so that heaven stands in our hand". The sympathy and antipathy between the ill part and the remedy are thus viewed in much wider terms than in the treatise of Fracastoro that bears that title.[44]

Separating out these three strands in Paracelsus's writings, the mystical, the religious and the German, shows that almost all his individual views were shared by someone or other at the time, whether it was a doctor, preacher or philosopher. But this dissection, as he would say, does not give life to his message, for what makes Paracelsus distinctive is their combination, for he can switch instantaneously from what opponents would judge to be one type of argument to another. That is also because he is not interested in Galenic logical analysis but only in what might be termed the logic of the Gospel, the intuition of the adept, the expert, whose acquisition and use of knowledge is derived directly from an acquaintance with God. But they also reveal that Paracelsus was a learned man, even as he claims to be writing for those less learned or close to illiterate. His writings are filled with punchy expressions, vivid analogies and caustic denunciations of his opponents, and his frequent support for the common people in their sufferings would undoubtedly have also gained him many followers.[45] But at the same time, his coinage of unusual words as well as the combination of at times apparently contradictory ideas within a single paragraph or even sentence hamper easy comprehension. In this he is writing for the adept, the physician who has gained access already to the true learning in and through the Christian light of Nature and who shares his Evangelical beliefs and can understand his message – and, one should not forget, knows German. This combination poses problems for all who seek to understand Paracelsus, whether as a religious radical, a proto-chemist, a practitioner of alternative medicine or a Ficinian philosopher. Structuring an account around one of Paracelsus's programmatic descriptions of his ideas, his *Seven Defences*, *Defensiones*, as Bruce Moran has recently done, provides welcome clarity, but it still fails fully to express the strangeness, or in Owsei Temkin's phrase, "the elusiveness of Paracelsus".[46]

Immediate Reactions

At his own request he was buried in 1541 in the chapel of the almshouse of St Sebastian in Salzburg, whither he had been summoned by its Prince-Bishop Ernest of Wittelsbach. He clearly still saw himself as a faithful Catholic whose zeal for reform and insistence on personal belief did not, at this stage, contradict any official rulings. Some of his early publications were reprinted in Augsburg and other German cities, and a Flemish translation of his *Secrets of the Philosophers*, an alchemical tract, appeared at Antwerp in 1556, but it was not until 1560 that the great majority of his non-theological writings began to appear in print.[47] Until then he was little more than a name, as Conrad Gessner discovered in 1545 when he wrote his entry on him in his *Universal Library*.[48] The catalyst was Adam Karlstadt von Bodenstein (1528–77), the son of Luther's colleague and later opponent, Andreas Karlstadt, who had left his position as a preacher in Wittenberg after an argument with Luther and the Elector of Saxony, eventually becoming Professor of Hebrew in Basle between 1534 and his death in 1541. His son studied first in Basle before embarking on travels to study medicine in Freiburg, Leipzig, Mainz and Ferrara, where he took his MD degree. After spending time in Venice and examining plants in a Swiss monastery, he returned to Basle where in 1557 he published a small tract on gout and the relevant medicinal herbs organised according to their zodiacal properties. He was also attached to the court of Elector Otthein-rich at Heidelberg, who looked favourably on alchemical physicians and who apparently encouraged him to read Paracelsus.[49] The following year he was elected to the Council of the Basle Medical Faculty, and in summer 1559 he edited another alchemical work, the *Rosarium Chymicum*, *The Chemical Rose-Garden*, by the medieval professor at Montpellier, Arnald of Villanova (c. 1240–1311). In neither of these two books is there any mention of Paracelsus, which suggests that Karlstadt had not yet come across any of his manuscripts, as opposed to printed books, and may not have known much about his alchemical writings.[50] This had changed by 1560 when he published an edition of the Paracelsian *De vita longa*, *Longevity*, that opens with a substantial preface explaining his new interest in Paracelsus and his knowledge of the secrets of Nature. Who put up the money for this publication is unclear, as is the manuscript source of this (possibly spurious) book, which in a revised version two years later Karlstadt admitted was incomplete and lacked the fifth section. By then he and others such as Gerard Dorn (fl. 1567) and Michael Toxites (1515–81) were collecting manuscripts of Paracelsus from his wealthy patrons such as Duke Heinrich of Pfalz-Neuburg, apothecaries like Melchior Dorss of Colmar, and his former assistant Oporinus. Copies of these first Paracelsian publications were dedicated to a variety of important figures in Basle and elsewhere, and some were presented to members of the university. From 1561 onwards, many were published by Pietro Perna (1519–82), who became the main printer of Paracelsian writings in Basle.[51] At this stage there is no indication that Karlstadt was acting unusually, or that he expected the hostile reactions that were soon to follow. But in 1564 he was expelled from the Physicians' Council, and there were undoubtedly others among the physicians who had experienced or knew about the conflict between Paracelsus and the physicians 30 years earlier and who disapproved of what they termed the "false doctrines" of Paracelsus. Exile from the Faculty did not, however, prevent Karlstadt from continuing to enjoy a successful practice as writer, editor and physician in the city or from gaining a wide range of influential contacts across Europe.[52]

Although it is not easy to determine the extent to which Paracelsus's ideas were known and discussed before 1560, the scale and the impact of the Basle printings of his writings is obvious. Karlstadt and his colleagues, assisted by Perna, created a propaganda storm akin to that produced by the Galenist translators 30 years earlier. As well as publishing in German, they translated many Paracelsian writings into Latin, which made them accessible to a wider learned audience across Europe. Perna's links with the community of Italian Evangelical exiles, of whom he was one, in Basle and elsewhere helped to spread his Paracelsian publications even within Italy, despite their inclusion on the Index and the severe penalties that possession of them might bring.[53] He also published other tracts by some of the followers of Paracelsus such as the Dane Petrus Severinus (1540–1602) and Georg Fedro of Nuremberg, and later Cologne, although his views were repudiated by Karlstadt.[54] Many of these books were in octavo format, cheap to obtain and easy to smuggle to areas where they were forbidden. Some were published in the original German, others in Latin, a few had been published previously, but most had not, and some may have been written by Paracelsians rather than by the master himself.[55] A glance at the prefaces to these Paracelsian books as translated by Frank Hieronymus, as well as his notes on the dedications and ownership, indicates a variety of reasons why they were bought.[56] Many of the early owners were Evangelicals, Protestant theologians or like-minded magnates, for whom the Christian message within some of the books was important. Many prefaces stress the superiority of this practical and accessible medicine over long-winded Galenic disputations, which would appeal to apothecaries and local physicians alike. Other buyers would have been already interested in astrology and alchemy and appreciated that this strand of medicine formed part of an ancient tradition of wisdom that went back to the Egyptians, the Babylonians and such Late Antiquity texts as the *Poimandres*.[57] Books on natural magic, such as those by Agrippa von Nettesheim, had been best sellers, and these new books fell squarely within that category. It was also particularly the young who were attracted to this new way of thinking, as

Gessner lamented when sending a copy of the first edition of the *De vita longa, Long Life,* to Crato.[58]

Reactions were not slow in coming, not least because many of Paracelsus's original claims threatened the authority of learned Galenist physicians. Karlstadt was expelled from the Basle Faculty in 1564 on the grounds that he had published some of his books before they had been approved by the Censor, and was propagating the false ideas of Paracelsus.[59] There were accusations of magic, Arianism, ignorance and charlatanry.[60] Arguments over the use of chemical drugs and the respective roles of apothecaries, surgeons and physicians could easily provoke public uproar, as at Cologne in 1565 when the physicians quarrelled with the Paracelsian Georg Fedro. Complaints about incompetent treatments by non-physicians and demands for further restrictions on those who were unqualified became louder. Oporinus's memories of his time with a drunken and boorish Paracelsus, sent to the Cologne physician Johannes Weyer, only added fuel to the flames, and opponents of Paracelsus were only too happy to discover that the spectacular cures that he had trumpeted so often were mere shams, for those he had treated all died within a year.[61] Thomas Erastus (1523–83), another of Crato's correspondents, who had been a court physician and professor at Heidelberg when Karlstadt was there, responded with a series of books denouncing the errors of Paracelsus. In his view Paracelsus was a Magus in league with the devil, a Gnostic heretic, who mistook the workings of natural forces for miracles. His ignorance of logic and learning was shown by his doctrine of three principles, which, far from being the basis of all matter, were themselves formed from the Galenic-Aristotelian elements. His doctrine of the correspondence between microcosm and macrocosm turned an allegory into a serious confusion, and his theories of disease were mere nonsense. Christian belief and the physician's own experience played no part in Erastus's critical and logical reasoning, which was vigorously employed in dissecting the many inconsistencies that could be found in his opponents' writings.[62]

Erastus's *Disputations* provided the template for many subsequent attacks on Paracelsian medicine, whether in England, France or the Crato circle around the Emperor. That Perna should have published the attacks of Erastus alongside all the Paracelsian material may occasion surprise, but Perna had to make money, and publishing both sides in the controversy was good for business.[63] Crato continued to worry about his reluctance to accept advice and his preference for testing the boundaries of the imperial patience, not least because he himself might lose both a contact at the heart of medical publishing and an outlet for his own and his friends' compositions. Others in his circle doubted Perna's wisdom in promoting Paracelsian literature, much of which did not sell, at the expense of 'good books', when he had had on occasions been so impoverished that he had to pay another Basle press, that of Heinrich Petri, to do the printing for him.[64]

This ambivalence towards Perna on the part of those who detested almost all that Paracelsus stood for is mirrored in the reaction of Conrad Gessner.

A sound Galenist, who strongly disliked the posturings of the Arian Paracelsians, and who encouraged his friend Crato to write a rebuttal of all that they professed, he nevertheless saw something valuable in their attention to distillation and their interest in mineral waters.[65] In 1554 he had published his *Thesaurus Euonymi, The Treasury of Euonymus*, which included several 'secret' chemical remedies among its recipes. A second edition in 1569 included many more remedies, some taken from Paracelsus, but also a warning about the dangers and limitations of this medicinal chemistry. Both books were translated quickly into German, French and English, and, in what Allen Debus called the "Elizabethan compromise", encouraged the introduction of some chemical drugs into the practice of orthodox Galenist physicians.[66]

More significant was the intellectual development of Theodor Zwinger from a vigorous defender of Aristotle and Galen in his student days at Padua to a sympathiser with some aspects of Paracelsianism and the sponsor in 1581 of two of the most devastating attacks on the Aristotelian-Galenic synthesis, Francesco Patrizi's *Discussiones Peripateticae, Peripatetic Discussions*, and the renegade doctor Agostino Doni's *De natura hominis, The Nature of Man*, both printed by Perna.[67] His early summaries of his lectures on Galen's *Art of Medicine* and *The Make-up of the Art of Medicine* reflect his Paduan education, after which he was immediately elected to the Basle Faculty and became a member of its Council in December 1559. From then on, until his death in 1588, he played the leading role in the Faculty, writing its new constitution and taking great care of its finances, although he did not hold a medical chair until 1580.[68] In 1564 he seems to have had little interest in Paracelsus's medical writings, refusing to comment on his personal morality, and noting only that many people treasured his religious writings as precious jewels, although he was universally believed to be an Arian.[69] But the more he read of his writings, the more he adopted a nuanced approach towards his chemical remedies and pharmacology, and sought ways to distinguish what Paracelsus himself, "the most important author of this type", had said from the fantastic speculations of followers like Karlstadt and Toxites.[70] In his lectures towards the end of his life he compared Paracelsus with Vesalius, praising him for bringing pharmacology out of the secret hiding places of the alchemists to become a public art, open to all, and thereby winning for himself a place of honour in Germany akin to that of Avicenna among the Arabs.[71]

Not only had he been convinced of the merits of Paracelsus's therapies and of those of another chemical doctor with Basle connections, Leonhard Thurneisser (1531–1596), both of whom in his view relied on the evidence of experiment and experience, but he also saw how much Paracelsus's ideas in fact owed to Hippocrates and to Dioscorides.[72] His chemical remedies were far from new, and his methods were not always precise, but he had understood the basic principles of healing correctly. In his Hippocratism Zwinger was sharing in a more widespread move away from strict Galenism

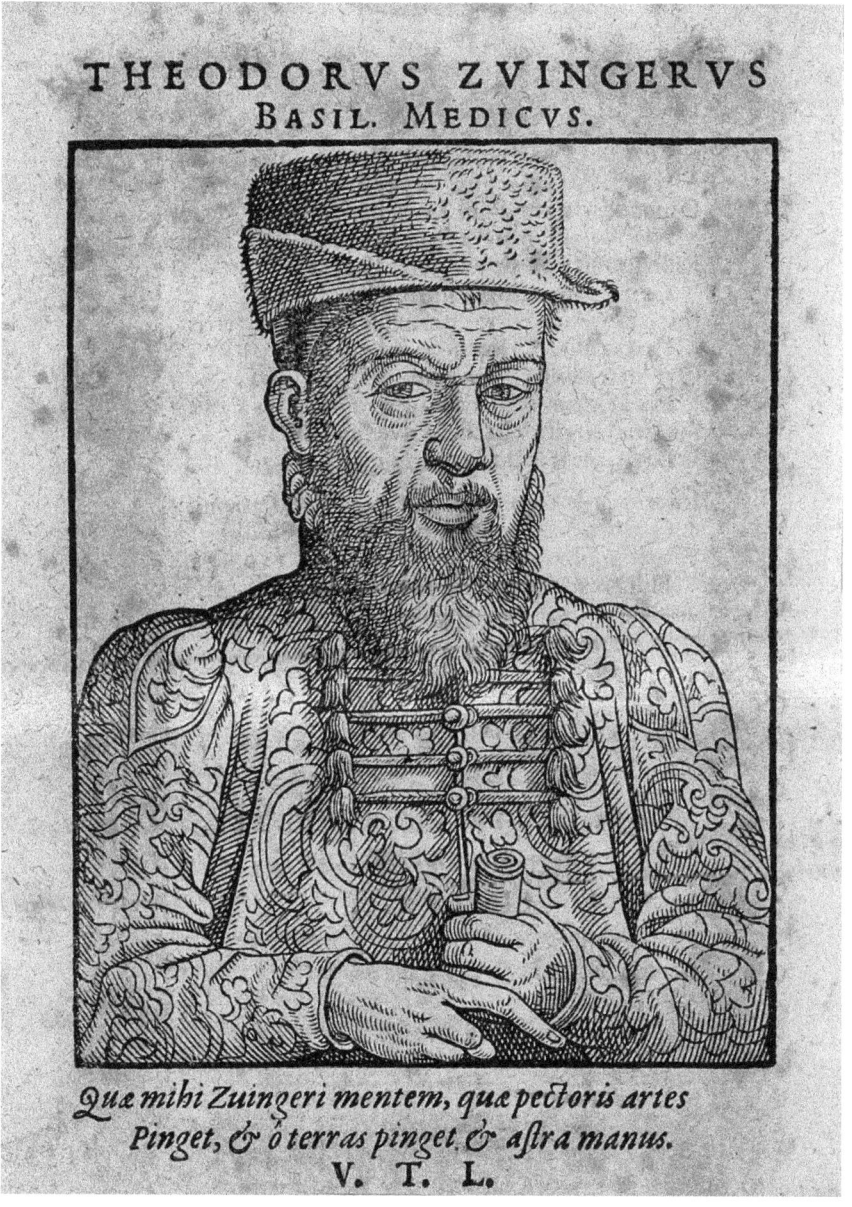

THEODORVS ZVINGERVS
BASIL. MEDICVS.

*Quæ mihi Zuingeri mentem, quæ pectoris artes
Pinget, & ò terras pinget & astra manus.*
V. T. L.

Figure 10.2 Theodor Zwinger (1533–88), a leading Basle professor, proponent of a modified Paracelsianism, and a pan-European correspondent. Woodcut, 1589. The lines below read: The hand that designed the mind of Zwinger and the skills in his breast will surely be the designer of the earth and stars.

to a greater interest in Hippocrates (earlier, pp. 293–4) and making use of the linguistic skills which had earned him the Basle chair of Greek in 1565. In 1579 he produced a major edition of Hippocrates with a commentary that won him the respect of Mercuriale, and provided his readers with a detailed breakdown of the contents and medical value of the Hippocratic texts.[73] This allowed him to introduce much Paracelsian doctrine into his university lectures, where he explained Paracelsian therapies in a clearer and more succinct way than their author had originally presented them.[74] In 1575 he sponsored Joseph Duchesne, Quercetanus (1544–1609), "famous for his chemical skill", and later a controversial Paracelsian in France, for a doctorate, even though he had never technically matriculated. The fact that the degree was conferred privately in Zwinger's house suggests a certain unease about the procedure. A similar secrecy enveloped the grant of the MD in 1591 to another French Paracelsian, Bernard Penot (c. 1525–c. 1615), perhaps with even better reason, for he never matriculated at all, and is described as trained more in chemistry than in real medicine, "but not entirely a stranger to Hippocratic medicine". At his degree ceremony, in the house of Felix Platter, he was also told to brush up on his Hippocrates and Galen and promise to say nothing against their teachings.[75] Other students of Zwinger, such as the Englishman Thomas Moffet (1553–1604), openly argued for the compatibility of Hippocratic doctrine with that of Paracelsus.[76]

Paracelsianism Beyond Basle

Zwinger's position within the Basle establishment and his European-wide fame as the author of the multi-volume encyclopaedia, *Theatrum humanae vitae*, *The Theatre of Human Life*, helped to establish the respectability of Paracelsianism as a system of therapy taught in other universities in some Protestant regions, such as Montpellier, Marburg or Copenhagen. Even if the majority of Galenists remained unreconciled, several others tried to find a middle way between the two systems. One who did was Vesalius's old teacher, Guinter von Andernach, who after leaving Paris during the Wars of Religion moved to Strasbourg where he wrote a large volume *De medicina veteri et nova facienda*, *Creating a Medicine Both Old and New*, that was published by Perna in 1571. Its preface sets out its aim. Medicine has developed by constant additions of new material, from biblical times onwards, and it would be foolish to disregard the enormous strides made recently in pharmacology, especially by Paracelsus, who has added more mineral drugs to those already obtained by distillation. But he drew the line at the Cabala, demonology and spirits, which he regarded as a perversion of the truth that all medicines were created by God. As a good Protestant, he approved of the Christian ethic that pervaded Paracelsus's writings, and did not concern himself with the complicated theories that underlay them, except to argue for the compatibility of the three Paracelsian principles with the four Aristotelian elements.[77]

A similar reconciliation was published five years later by Johann Jacob Wecker (1528–86), who had served as Dean of the Basle Faculty in 1565, before leaving the next year to become civic physician at Colmar. His published writings were largely derivative, including two popular collections of recipes as well as an edition of the *Book of Secrets* attributed to Alexis of Piedmont.[78] In his Colmar period he was a Paracelsian chemist, who illustrated his books with drawings of distillation apparatus and furnaces. His argument coincides with that of Guinter, although beginning from the Paracelsian end. He too traced the descent of medicine from God via Hippocrates and Galen, who employed both logic and experience, to the present day, and in the huge *Book of Secrets* of 1582 he took over several recipes from Paracelsus. But in 1576 he also accepted that there were Paracelsians who trumpeted their miraculous cures and employed what could only be described as a methodology based on fantasy, and he wished to reassure his readers that he was not one of them.[79] To make his synthesis more accessible to students, he divided it up with Ramist tree-like diagrams that showed visually how his statements related to one another. His book went through two further editions in Basle and one in Lyons and large sections of it appeared in London in 1585 in a translation by the surgeon John Banister. Banister, however, was not entirely satisfied with Wecker, for he found too many errors in his therapeutics, although not in his recipes, which he attributed to an excessive reliance on classical texts.[80]

Zwinger, Guinter and Wecker are all good examples of the way in which physicians on both sides of the Paracelsian divide tried to produce a synthesis of chemical and Galenical medicine, believing that it was possible to reconcile both their respective underlying theories of matter. But there were others in Northern Europe who adhered more consistently to all the medical theories of Paracelsus despite their initial education in Galenic medicine. One of the most influential exponents of Paracelsianism was the Dane Petrus Severinus (1542–1602), who had spent time at Padua in 1566 alongside another Danish student Jason Pratensis (1543–76). Both became firm adherents of the new medicine, and on their return to Denmark were rewarded with important positions, Pratensis as professor of medicine at Copenhagen, Severinus as a royal physician. Severinus wrote his *Idea medicinae philosophicae, A Sketch of Philosophical Medicine*, in 1570, having studied also in Wittenberg, Heidelberg, Rostock, Paris and Basle, where he had made friends with Zwinger. His book quickly became a standard work among the new Paracelsians, and Severinus gained an enormous reputation, not least among court physicians. Thomas Moffet, who visited Denmark in 1582 on royal business, two years later dedicated to him his treatise defending Paracelsian chemical medicine, *De jure et praestantia chymicorum medicamentorum, The Legality and Superiority of Chemical Drugs*.[81]

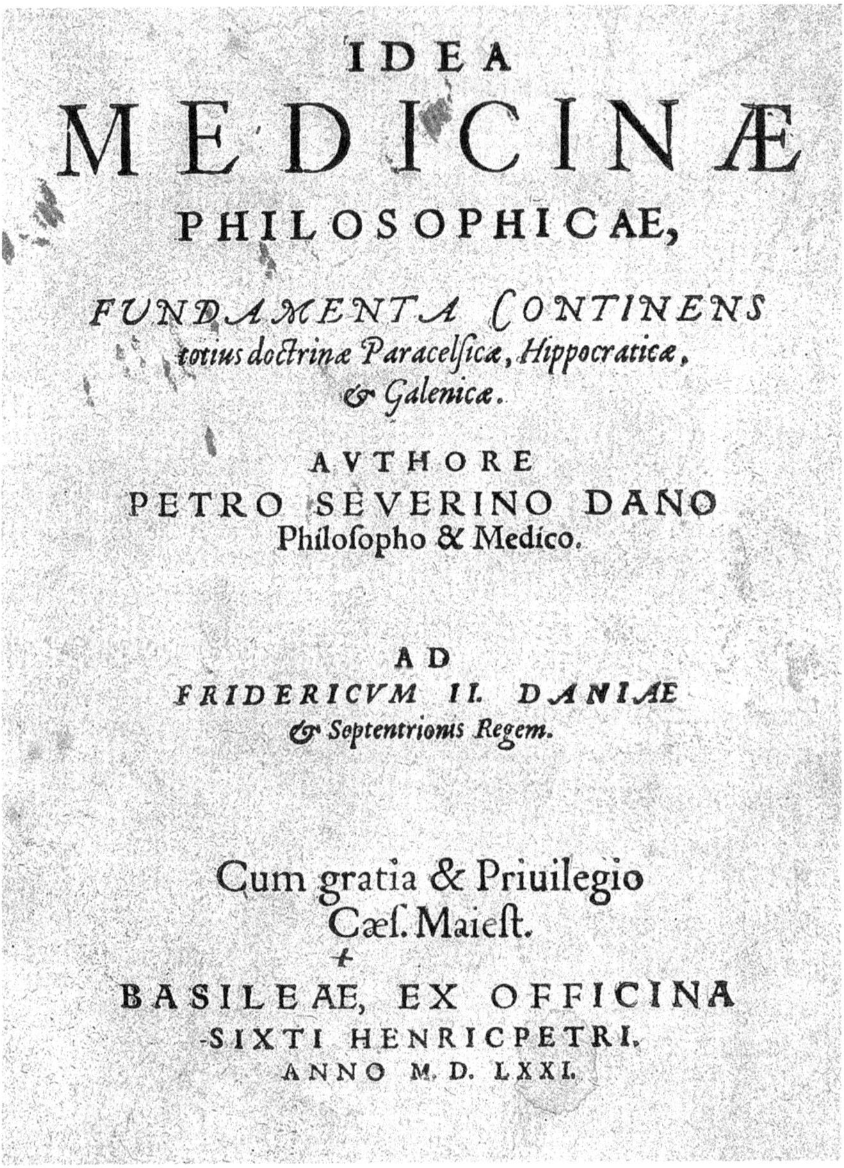

IDEA
MEDICINÆ
PHILOSOPHICAE,

FUNDAMENTA CONTINENS
totius doctrinæ Paracelsicæ, Hippocraticæ,
& Galenicæ.

AVTHORE
PETRO SEVERINO DANO
Philofopho & Medico.

AD
FRIDERICVM II. DANIÆ
& Septentrionis Regem.

Cum gratia & Priuilegio
Cæf. Maieft.
✝
BASILEAE, EX OFFICINA
SIXTI HENRICPETRI,
ANNO M. D. LXXI.

Figure 10.3 Petrus Severinus, *Idea medicinae philosophicae, fundamenta continens totius doctrinae Paracelsicae, Hippocraticae et Galenicae*, Basle, S. Henricpetri, 1571, the most significant attempt to reconcile Paracelsian and Galenic medicine.

Precisely when Severinus adopted Paracelsianism is not entirely clear, but the title of a treatise preserved in manuscript in the British Library, Ms Sloane 3005, ff. 1–37, and dated from Paris in 1567, *A Book of Essays on Questions of Philosophy, Astronomy, Medicine and Cabalistic*, shows that his ideas were already taking shape then. His book repeats in clearer terms Paracelsus's objections to academic anatomy and the Aristotelian theory of elements in favour of an emphasis on vital spirits (going far beyond what Fernel had argued) and the role of 'seeds' of disease, in causing illness. He emphasises the role of spagyric, alchemical remedies, as well as the importance of fire in governing and correcting the processes of the body. Like Paracelsus he traces all these ideas back to Hippocrates and Plato, who had understood the links between the macrocosm and the microcosm, but he insists that mere theoretical learning is not enough. One needs to know about farming and mining, and constantly experiment in the laboratory.[82]

The list of topics in his 1567 essays, philosophy, medicine, astronomy and cabalistic, shows why he, and Paracelsians like him, quickly found supporters among monarchs and magnates. Together they show his claim to secret wisdom, deriving from philosophy (a common description of alchemy), a knowledge of the stars, and access to the long and hidden tradition of Jewish magic and mysticism. All these were commonly pursued by kings and the wealthy eager to seek out ways to extend their lives, foretell the future, and make money by transmuting base metals to gold by means of the philosopher's stone. Many treatises on these themes had been written in Antiquity and the Middle Ages (and ascribed to Ramon Lull, Arnald of Villanova and other reputed magicians), and they proliferated in the world of print. Paracelsus drew on this literature, as did Severinus. Even in Britain, as Charles Webster has shown, books on these themes circulated widely, preparing the ground for the introduction of Paracelsian ideas from the 1560s onwards. Courts had long employed astrologers, many of them reputable physicians, and others who claimed magical abilities or an understanding of natural magic, and it was no large step from this for a Paracelsian patron to set up a chemical laboratory. Several rulers in Germany indulged personally in these activities, while the court of the Holy Roman Emperor under Rudolf II was filled with such adepts of secret wisdom.[83] The fact that many of these Paracelsians were also Evangelical Christians both recommended them to Protestant rulers and guaranteed the moral legitimacy of their activities.

Their religious affiliations and their positions at the very centre of political power played a major role in the two most famous confrontations in Paris between Paracelsians and orthodox Galenists, many of whom remained loyal Catholics at a time of great political and religious turmoil. Roch le Baillif, sieur de la Riviere (1540–98), a gentleman from Normandy who had published in 1578 a summary of Paracelsian doctrine, was soon after appointed one of the doctors to Henri III. Catholics were already alarmed by what they saw as a growing Huguenot domination in all aspects of court life and politics, and here was another example of a pugnacious Huguenot

on the make. The Paris medical Faculty, which had earlier in 1567 condemned the use of antimony as a remedy, banned him from practising and
from lecturing.[84] There followed a trial before the Parlement of Paris, which
ended in the victory of the medical establishment and in Le Bailliff's return
to Rennes, where he continued to practise.[85] Two years later he published a
tract on plague, defending the three principles of Paracelsus, and another on
anatomy, rejecting traditional anatomy in favour of investigations into the
macrocosm and microcosm.

The verdict of the court produced only a short lull in the hostilities
between Galenists and Paracelsians. This ended in 1593 with the accession
to the throne of Henri of Navarre, who abjured his Huguenot beliefs to
reign as Henri IV. Henri may have changed his religion, but he remained
loyal to his Huguenot physicians, all immigrants from Calvinist Geneva and
all committed followers of Paracelsus, albeit to slightly different degrees. In
1594 Jean Ribit (confusingly, also titled sieur de la Rivière, c. 1546–1605),
was appointed first physician and soon after secured the appointments of
the prolific Quercetanus and, in 1597, of the younger Theodore Turquet de
Mayerne, who began a series of lectures on chemical medicine for surgeons.
There followed a decade of controversy, in which both the Faculty and
their opponents issued equally vigorous denunciations, ending with another
apparent victory for the Faculty. Henceforth the royal doctors had to be
Catholic, only drugs approved by the Faculty were to be used, and antimony
and other chemical drugs were forbidden. By then both Ribit and Quercetanus were dead, and in 1610, after the assassination of Henri IV, Mayerne
moved to England as one of the doctors of James I.[86] But the Faculty's writ
did not extend to the whole of France, Paracelsian books continued to circulate and Paracelsian doctrines were still taught at Montpellier. Nor could
it prevent individuals from employing Paracelsians as private doctors or
outsiders such as Andreas Libavius (1546–1616), a great chemical experimenter but no friend of Paracelsian mysticism, from condemning what they
saw as outdated and unreasonable behaviour by the Faculty.[87]

The position of the London College of Physician when Mayerne came to
London was different from that of the Paris Faculty. As we have seen (earlier,
p. 136), it had difficulty enforcing its authority in the megalopolis of London, and it had already elected doctors like Moffet who openly espoused the
new chemical medicine. However, compared with Germany, which Zwinger
considered eminently sympathetic to Paracelsian doctrines, few such treatises were published or circulated in London. The earliest would appear to
be Richard Bostock's *The Difference between the Auncient Physicke . . . and
the Later Physicke Proceeding from Idolaters, Ethnickes and Heathens*, of
1585, whose appeal to a tradition of healing as taught by the "godly forefathers" condemned both Galen, "a dealer in dualitie, discorde and contrari-
etie", and Aristotle whose departure "from the truth of God's words" was
"injurious to Christianitie and sounde doctrine".[88] Bostock was a lawyer
and a friend of the magus John Dee, who left for Europe in 1583 taking

his Paracelsian books with him, and, although many works on alchemy were circulating at the time, the arguments in England over Paracelsian medicines had a more mundane focus. London surgeons such as George Baker (1540–1600) and the always controversial John Hester (d. 1593), as Deborah Harkness has shown, were publicising Paracelsus's chemical writings as part of their campaign to strengthen their own position against the College in their use of antimony and similar metallic drugs against syphilis and skin diseases.[89] Another surgeon, William Clowes, confessed his inability to understand what Paracelsus was talking about, but had tried out many of his recommendations for surgery and found them "singularly good and worthy". Although he was aware that there was "much strife between the Galenists and the Paracelsians, as was in times past between Ajax and Ulysses for Achilles' armour", he trusted to reason and experience, whether it was found in Galen, Paracelsus, Turk, Jew or infidel.[90] But that did not stop him from devoting some of his most scintillating pages to denouncing a Paracelsian exile from Cologne, Valentin Rasworme of Schmalkalden, as a "marvellous monster, captain cozener and quacksalver" "who had abused many of the Queen's good subjects under the habit of honesty and title or names of *Medicus, Spagiricus, Chirurgus, Lithotomus* and *Ophthalmista,* . . . this great Bugbear, stinging gnat, venomous wasp and counterfeit crocodile". In 1574 Rasworme was put on trial at the London Guildhall for his malpractice but fearing that he would be convicted and put in the pillory, he absconded.[91]

Clowes's wonderful rhetoric disguises the fact that, far from being among "the bungling botchers, ignorant makeshifts, caterpillars in a commonwealth", Rasworme was an experienced surgeon and lithotomist, who had made a respectable name for himself in the Rhineland despite several brushes with the authorities. While there he had come to use some Paracelsian remedies, which he introduced to London and employed, apparently successfully, to treat acquaintances of Lord Burghley himself.[92] The length and acerbity of Clowes's denunciation of him reflects the increasingly vigorous debate in London between older surgeons such as George Baker, Clowes and John Banister on the one hand and younger ones such as John Hester who saw these new drugs as a way of increasing their reputation and (as Burghley's informant noted) making a lot of money.[93] Clowes was deriding foreign competition far more than he was attacking the new chemical remedies.

Supporters like Lord Burghley ensured a certain place for Paracelsian remedies, and the growing membership of the London College of Physicians with an interest in chemical remedies helped to promote a cautious acceptance of chemical remedies alongside Galenicals in English medicine. How cautious is obvious from the publication of the *Pharmacopaea Londinensis* in 1618, often seen as a major step towards a new chemical philosophy. But it is better viewed as a reluctant acknowledgement of the importance of the new drugs. It permitted only those that had already appeared in books and it showed little sign of involvement with new chemical experiments.[94] It was only with the Helmontians and the importing of the ideas of the Rosicrucians and others more than a decade later that Paracelsian theories played a large part in English medicine, albeit greatly modified from their original form.

Paracelsus was always a controversial figure, well suited to an age of major changes in religion and society. In his lifetime he constantly supported the poor against the rich and objected to authority wherever he found it. It was this reputation that after his death made him and his ideas appear so controversial. In his writings he drew on established traditions, whether in Germany or in learned medicine, but combined, and perhaps more importantly, expressed, them in ways that baffled and frightened many of his readers. Reactions to the flood of Paracelsian publications that appeared from the 1570s covered the whole spectrum from wholesale acceptance of even the strangest of notions to a complete rejection and, in Italy, involved the imposition of the death penalty for those caught with a Paracelsian volume.[95] But from then on, particularly through the activities of Zwinger in Basle, Paracelsian practical medicine and the uses of experiment and chemical drugs became more and more acceptable to physicians and learned surgeons. The publication of the two volumes of Latin translations in 1575 and, still more, of the ten (later 11) volumes of Huser's edition of the collected works of Paracelsus in German in 1603 confirmed his importance both within and outside Germany.[96] But by then the notion of chemical experimenting was well established, and its practitioners, such as Libavius, did not always see the need to immerse themselves in Paracelsian mysticism to carry out and explain their discoveries.

Notes

1 Later, pp. 316–7.
2 Brady 2009: 1–68, provides a good overview of German economic and social life.
3 Temkin 1977: 225–38 (originally 1952). Grell 1998 calls him an enigma.
4 Pagel 1982.
5 Pagel 1982: 5–31; Webster 2008: 5–29; Moran 2019.
6 Webster 2008: 254.
7 In a lawsuit at Basle he claimed to hold a medical degree; the records of Ferrara for the relevant period 1513–17 are lost.
8 Earlier, pp. 129–33.
9 Pagel 1982: 19–22.
10 Webster 2008: 39–43, 259–60.
11 Pagel 1982: 30–1; Webster 2008: 20–4; Moran 2019: 4–17.
12 Gilly 1998: 151.
13 In general, Brady 2009: 11–28; for civic doctors, earlier, pp. 46–50.
14 Useful introductions are Assion 1973; Crossgrove 1994; Keil 1993.
15 Keil 1993; Crossgrove 1994: 74–6.
16 Assion 1973: 124, 146.
17 Assion 1981.

18 Assion 1973: 150; Hagenmeyer 1981; Crossgrove 1994: 77.
19 Zinner 1964; Welker 1988.
20 Assion 1973: 150; Zimmermann 1986; Keil 1995; Webster 2008: 47–50.
21 For the German surgical tradition: Panse 2012: 143–214, has valuable comments about distribution.
22 Vollmuth 2001.
23 Paracelsus 1549.
24 Pagel 1982: 148.
25 Paracelsus 1923–33: 10, 36, 41–2.
26 Welker 1988: 85–98, 226–48.
27 Agricola 1556, with Hieronymus 2005: 897–945; Assion 1973: 149; Crossgrove 1994: 140–1.
28 Paracelsus 1567; 1941 (trans, Sigerist); Ellenbog 1524; Crossgrove 1994: 140–1.
29 Clemen 1905: 293–4.
30 Pagel 1982: 153–61.
31 Temkin 1977: 230–2; Wear 1995: 313–15.
32 Webster 2008; cf. Webster 1993; Nutton 1995.
33 Nutton 1995. For the background, later, pp. 308–9.
34 Paracelsus 1922–33: 13, 373, 4, 38, 43–5; Gilly 1998: 153–4.
35 Paracelsus 1955–86: 2,140–50.
36 Moran 2019: 119–21.
37 Moran 2019: 145–7.
38 Benzenhöfer and Triebs 1992.
39 Pagel 1982: 50–8; Moran 2019: 96, 38–40.
40 Pagel 1982: 174–7, 218–23; Webster 2008: 110–13.
41 Ruderman 1988.
42 Pagel 1982: 322.
43 Paracelsus 1922–33: 13,378; Pagel 1982: 149, noting the compatibility of this doctrine with that of the quintessence.
44 Pagel 1982: 68–9, 149. For Fracastoro, earlier, p. 225.
45 Webster 1993, 2008.
46 Moran 2019; Temkin 1977.
47 For the development of Paracelsianism in general see Grell 1998; Telle 1998; Sudhoff 1894–99 pioneered the modern study of Paracelsian writings.
48 Gessner 1545: 614v.
49 Telle 2008.
50 Karlstadt 1557, 1559: much information on Karlstadt and his Basle editions is given by Hieronymus 2005: I, 422–36. The whole section, 1,375–703, is a mine of information on Basle printings, editors and owners of Paracelsian works, along with many illustrations of pages and annotations.
51 Paracelsus 1560; Rotondò 1974: 274–391; Perini 2002; Hieronymus 2005: I, 431–50.
52 Burckhardt 1917: 57; Telle 2008.
53 Later, pp. 316–7.
54 Severinus 1571; Paracelsus 1571.
55 Kahn and Hirai 2019.
56 For Perna's view of his Paracelsian publications, see his preface to Paracelsus 1577a; translated in Hieronymus 2005: 1,630–6.
57 Paracelsus 1577b; Walker 1972; Hieronymus 2005: 1,637.
58 Gessner 1577: 10r.
59 Burckhardt 1917: 57 n. 1 gives the text of the Faculty decision.
60 Erastus 1571–3: I, 24.
61 Pagel 1982: 29–31, 327; Webster 2008: 19–21.
62 Erastus 1571–3; Pagel 1982: 311–33.

63 Something on which both Erastus and Perna came to agree. Information from Dr Tilmann Walter, who is working on the unpublished correspondence between the two men.

64 Rotondò 1974: 366–71, with similar comments from others about Perna's unreliability.

65 Gessner 1577: 5v, 11v.

66 Gessner 1554, 1569; Debus 1965: 52–7.

67 Rotondò 1974: 371 (Padua), 370, 372, 408–21.

68 Burckhardt 1917: 89–95; Benkert 2020: 41–64.

69 Gilly 1998: 157.

70 Zwinger 1577: 120; Gilly 1977. For his relations with Severinus, later, pp. 295–7.

71 Zwinger 1610: 56–7.

72 For Thurneisser, Morys 1982; Eikermann and Kaiser 2012.

73 Zwinger 1579; Siraisi 2008.

74 Zwinger 1610: 56, 79–90.

75 Burckhardt 1917: 158–9.

76 Moffet 1588; Dawbarn 2003.

77 Guinter 1571: pref.; Debus 1987: II, 190–1, 1991: 19–21, citing the similar views of Johannes Wimpenaeus in 1569; Hieronymus 2005: 2,2480–5, no. 56.

78 Wecker 1576, a much enlarged version of a book of 1562; Eamon 1994: 276–8; Burckhardt 1917: 54–5; Hieronymus 2005: 21,608–64, quoting his prefaces and giving examples of his pictures of apparatus.

79 Wecker 1576: sig. 3r; for drugs, Wecker 1582: sig. 6v.

80 Wecker 1585: pref.

81 Biographical details in Severinus 1979: 1–15; very brief English summary, 64–5. Danish translations of letters to Zwinger, *ibid.*: 45–58; Shackelford 2004.

82 Severinus 1571, 1979, with English summary 67–73; Grell 1998: 245–68; Shackelford 2004.

83 Evans 1984a; Trevor-Roper 1985, 1990; Moran 1991; Zemla 2016. See also earlier, p. 142.

84 The earlier opposition has been led by Jacques Grévin, earlier, p. 277.

85 Trevor-Roper 1990: 84–5; Debus 1991: 38–41; Kahn 2007.

86 Nance 2001; Trevor-Roper 2006: 30–100.

87 Trevor-Roper 1990: 85–6; Debus 1991: 46–73; Brockliss and Jones 1997: 122–4.

88 Bostock 1585; Debus 1965: 24; Harley 2000.

89 Harkness 2007: 80–96; Pelling 2003.

90 Clowes 1602: pref.; 1948: 48–9.

91 Clowes 1585: 10r–12v (modernised): 1948: 80–3. The 1579 edition devoted a single paragraph to him. The expanded version owed much to the argument among surgeons about the use of chemical remedies.

92 For a French Huguenot and Basle graduate in 1591 who was "more inclined to chemical medicine than the true art" and "an exile for his religion", Burckhardt 1917: 159.

93 Jütte 1993; Harkness 2007: 57–96 (although misspelling his name as Russwurin).

94 Clark 1964: 227–30.

95 See later, pp. 316–7. Paracelsus was similarly condemned in Spain.

96 Paracelsus 1575, 1603. For a typical Paracelsian circle in Germany, Paulus 1994; for an early English owner, Thomas Langley, buying the Latin edition immediately after publication, see London, Wellcome Collection, EPB 4791.

11 Religion and Medicine

In the sixteenth century, more than at any time since the fourth century CE, religion interacted significantly with medicine in new ways and with unexpected and at times undesirable consequences. In 1500, an apparently triumphant Christian Europe, emboldened by the recent conquest of the Muslim kingdom of Granada, was opposed by an increasingly aggressive Ottoman Empire in the Balkans and Eastern Mediterranean. The subjugation of mainly Greek Orthodox Christians there was more than balanced in the eyes of Catholic theologians by the conversions of hundreds of thousands of natives in the Americas. The papacy, united again after the ending of a century of Antipopes, faced calls for reform following the blatant worldly behaviour of its incumbents. Martin Luther's ideas, far from novel theologically, and his subsequent defiance of papal injunctions attracted increasing numbers of supporters, firstly in Germany and then throughout most of Europe, leading to major breakaways from the Catholic Church. These Evangelicals, later called Protestants, continued to splinter into a variety of groupings, both large and small, along a wide spectrum of belief and church organisation, distinguished at least as much by the ferocity with which they defended their doctrinal standpoints, often marked by bloodshed, as by their equally fierce unity in denouncing the errors of their Catholic opponents. In their turn, from the 1540s and, particularly with a series of ascetic and uncompromising Popes during the second half of the century, the Catholics fought back hard, sometimes literally, to regain control and to eliminate dissent particularly in Iberia, Italy, France and Southern Germany. It was difficult, if not impossible, to stand aside from these conflicts, for, except for small numbers of Jews and Muslims, always in danger of persecution as non-Christians, belief in a Christian God and a Christian world was universal in Europe. Doctors might thunder about their medical adversaries as Epicureans, followers of an ancient Greek sect who denied any place for gods in their world view, and non-medics might joke that two out of every three doctors were atheists, but these were largely rhetorical formulations without much foundation in reality, although still potentially dangerous for any one so accused.[1] Europe in the sixteenth century was not as starkly polarised between Catholic and Evangelical as it was to become

DOI: 10.4324/9781003223184-15

in the next, but religious divisions were beginning to coalesce and to harden into political ones as well. Religious belief mattered, and healers of all types had to take account of that belief, for better or worse.

Christianity had from its very outset proclaimed its concern for the sick and needy.[2] Throughout the Middle Ages, the accounts in the *Gospels* and *Acts* of healing miracles performed by Christ and his Apostles were supplemented by myriad stories of saints who healed the sick and even brought the dead back to life. Paintings, mosaics, stained glass windows, votive tablets and sculpture reinforced visually the message that the unlettered could also hear in readings and sermons in churches everywhere.[3] In towns and even villages, hospitals housing under the aegis of a religious community those suffering from disease, old age or simply "the misfortunes of life" as they were termed, were imposing sights, often surpassing in size and area nearby churches and demonstrating to all the world the charitable concern and the saving power of the Christian religion.[4] A morality play published in Paris in 1533 used long familiar analogies to show how Christ, the heavenly healer, could, like the earthly physician, diagnose and cure all ills, both physical and social.[5] There was a shared understanding of what it meant to live in a Christian world. All believers accepted that they were living in a universe that had been created by a purposeful God, a message easily reconciled with Galenism, and that He had the power to alter the natural world for good or ill. Even though changes in the heavens that brought about 'bad air' and its consequent epidemics were regarded as part of the natural order of things, this still left space for a religious explanation for plague as a divine punishment for the sins of the world. Individual sickness could also be explained similarly as a consequence either of the body's physical condition or of some personal sin (an accusation far more often directed at those with whom one disagreed than a conclusion reached about oneself after examining one's conscience and past behaviour). The two explanations overlapped rather than opposing one another. The writers of plague tracts regularly began with an acknowledgement of God's involvement before going on to discuss individual prophylaxis and treatment, for He might have intended the illness as a warning to repent rather than a way of dispatching a sinner quickly to Hell. Theologians approached the question from the other end. John Calvin stood in a long line of preachers who asserted that if it was the will of the Almighty, death was inevitable, and no medicine could avert it. A good death was not simply one that occurred peacefully in the fulness of years and allowed time for the sick person to organise his or her affairs on earth. It mattered, above all, to confess one's sins and enter into an appropriate relationship with God and the church that would, as far as was humanly possible, permit access to the heavenly life everlasting. In England the Elizabethan prayerbook reiterated that whatever form an illness took, the clergyman should remind the sick person that it was a visitation from God. One might follow the advice of the doctor, but all remedies should be employed cautiously and in the knowledge that they worked only if God allowed them to, and all medical practitioners, whether doctors or surgeons, should pray from the very outset of treatment that their interventions would be successful. But where to draw the line was always a matter of choice, for few medics rejected completely the possibility of divine aid, and few Christian believers put their trust solely in the hands of God and His saints.[6]

The church also had its own institutions and methods that could be deployed to deal with illness. In many areas, a clergyman was one of the few who were literate and was often expected to provide physical as well as spiritual healing from whatever book of practical therapy he might have to hand. Not every cleric was as well qualified as William Bullein, a Suffolk vicar and a Fellow of the London College of Physicians, nor were all their patients as fortunate as the girl whose friend persuaded the vicar of Yalding in Kent, who practised both medicine and surgery, to abandon his unsuccessful therapy and take her to London to see William Clowes.[7] Guilds or confraternities, groups of Christians who banded together for religious and charitable purposes, were ubiquitous, looking after their members in poverty and sickness, and, after their deaths, praying for the repose of their souls. In large cities holding office in a major confraternity might convey prestige and even simple membership was expensive. In the countryside, however, contributions were much smaller, often a mere twopence, easily eclipsed by those of the ostentatious and well-to-do who might donate a whole flock of sheep.[8] These associations often bore the name of a saint, acknowledged as a mediator between heaven and earth who might be called on for assistance at any time. Some saints were universal or national, others like St Thomas of Cantelupe or St Radegund were very local. Some were attached to a specific trade like St Blaise, the patron saint of woolcombers, who was held to have a special power to cure diseases of the throat. Through the name given them at baptism everyone had their own patron saint who might offer life-long protection. Processions and festivals on their annual holy day and individual chapels and altars within a church made the saving activities of individual saints visible in the community. Pilgrimages to holy sites near and far confirmed to those who made them (and recovered) their power over illness.[9] But it was not necessary for the sick to travel in order to invoke heavenly aid, for in moments of great peril there were always at hand saints whose own lives and experiences had given them special expertise in treating illness: St Roch against the plague, St Erasmus (St Elmo) against intestinal disorders (doubly helpful if one happened also to be a seafarer, whose patron he also was), St Petronilla against the ague. One did not require a large volume, almost a telephone directory of heavenly healers, such as appeared in the nineteenth century, or even the popular book of stories of saints by Jacopo di Voragine, the *Golden Legend*, in order to identify an appropriate intercessor, for one could see their images on screens and windows in parish churches, attend plays in their honour, or hear sermons or simply the readings of poetry detailing their miraculous interventions.[10] Intercessory prayers, anointing with holy oil (the sacrament of unction) or simply the touch of a monarch, one of God's representatives on earth, could all contribute to the cure of patients who had repented of their sins and placed their faith in divine assistance.[11] Alongside these officially approved religious healings must be set the many ways in which other aspects of church teaching and practice were reinterpreted by the laity in less orthodox ways. The water poured over a child at baptism, to take one example, was eagerly sought after as a remedy for the ills of both humans and animals. Such types of healing were strongly opposed by medical practitioners as useless and by theologians as illicit magic, but, as Keith Thomas has shown, they were equally strongly defended by those who believed they had been cured by them.[12]

But if there was disagreement over the boundaries between religious and magical healing, there was universal agreement that this world was also peopled by devils, demons and evil spirits who were responsible for both mental and physical ailments. The truth of the Gospel stories of Christ's healing by casting out demons was further confirmed in the sixteenth century by popular broadsheets telling of new instances of monstrous births and demonic apparitions, often illustrated with a striking woodcut. Johannes Weyer (1515–88), the German physician who in 1563 published a thick volume, *De praestigiis daemonum et incantationibus ac veneficiis*, *The Tricks of Demons, Incantations and Poisonings*, accepted the existence of demons and witches, even though he then went on to argue that those who were accused of being witches or possessed by demons were in fact suffering from some form of mental illness, especially melancholia, arising out of a "corrupted imagination", and thus did not deserve the punishments inflicted upon them.[13] Nonetheless, he agreed that, with God's permission, demons could act upon humans, an opinion he supported with many learned references to both medical and theological authorities. He was equally vigorous in his denunciation of poisoners and especially magicians, a reminder that the boundary between what was thought to be dangerous magic and what was not rested at least as much on perceptions of what was being done, by whom and to what end as on any formal legal or theological distinction between licit and illicit.[14]

During the fifteenth century this essentially sacramental view of religion was supplemented by the "strivings of lay people to invent, promote and protect ways to live a spiritual life in the world" in such movements as the so-called *Devotio moderna*.[15] The development of printing at the end of the century further encouraged a move towards an emphasis on the word of God as something that could be read and heard directly. Reformers such as Trithemius of Sponheim and Erasmus contrasted the simplicity of the Christian message of the Gospels with the elaborate and expensive rituals they saw in the contemporary church. Many of its leaders behaved as monarchs, not least the Pope, who in the Renaissance period often conducted himself in an imperial style with a large and elaborate court, even waging war on his enemies, not all of them non-Christians. It was the excesses of

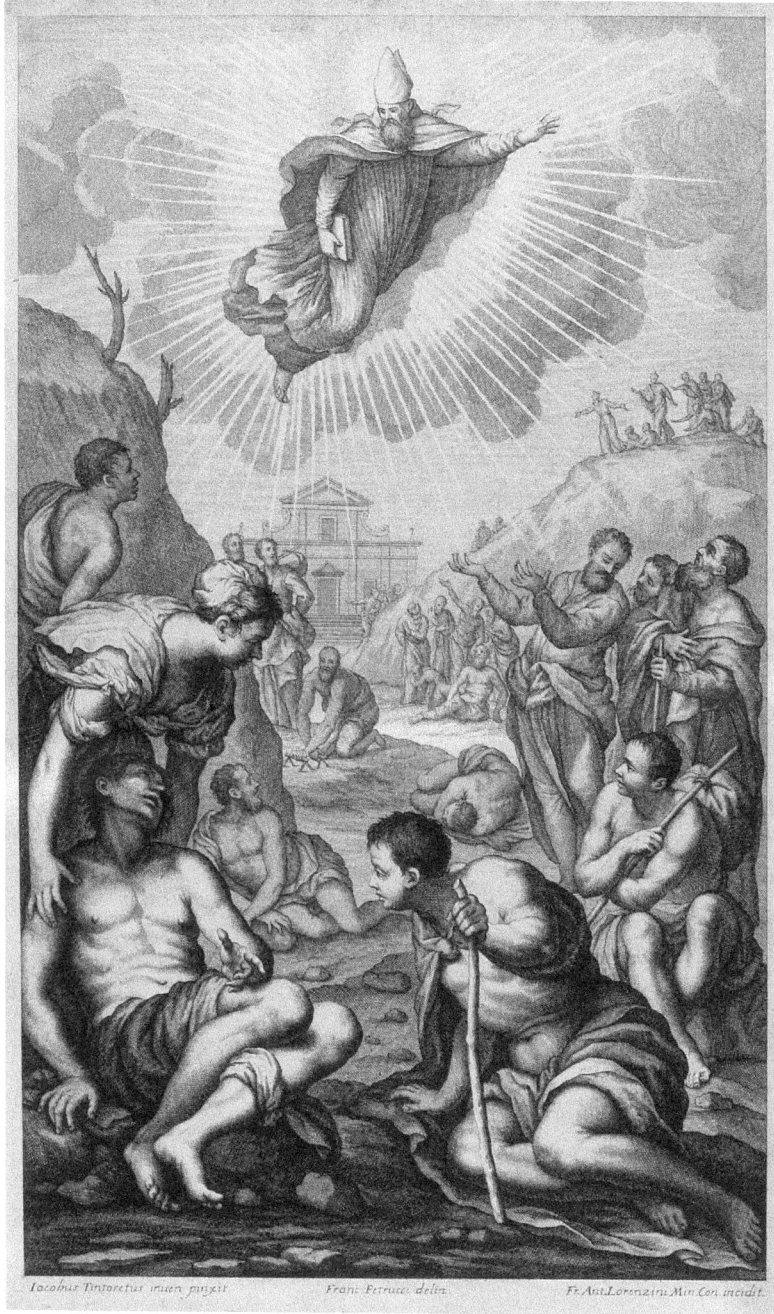

Figure 11.1 St Augustine of Hippo healing the sick. Large altarpieces of saintly
healings are typical of Counter-Reformation Catholicism. Engraving by
G. A. Lorenzini after Tintoretto (1518–94).

the Popes and their scandalous behaviour that aroused the anger of those in France, Germany and beyond who looked for a reformed church, simpler in style and more biblical in orientation, and who in Italy in the 1530s and 1540s came to be nicknamed the *Spirituali*. Many of their complaints were widely shared, not least by those who had contributed to the Pope's coffers to pay for these secular extravagances. In 1517 a relatively unknown German monk, Martin Luther, a member of the Augustinian Order, one of the most ascetic of monastic groupings, promulgated a series of theses for discussion in public, a typical procedure at his university of Wittenberg, which led first to major arguments and, within a few years, to a variety of splits and conflicts within the Western Church as a whole. Such theological debates were nothing new. Theologians had long argued over the precise weight to be given to individual interpretations of the New Testament contrasted with the decisions of the Church going back to the fourth century, and monarchs had had an equally long series of disputes with the Pope over their right to run the Church in their own countries. It was the combination of doctrinal, social and particularly political unrest that led first to the formation of an Evangelical alliance against the Pope, and then to further splits within the alliance itself. Luther's insistence on faith alone as the route to eternal salvation, and his rejection of the notion of the efficacy of good works, allied to the humanist discovery that the Greek New Testament did not always say what generations brought up on Jerome's Latin translation had believed, produced an intellectual crisis that challenged the very basis of Christian belief as it had been taught and practised for centuries. If faith in Christ was the sole way to heaven, what use were elaborate ceremonies or the countless masses paid for at chantry altars to secure the salvation of the soul of the donor? If Christ alone had the power to save, there was no need for intermediaries such as saints or even the Blessed Virgin Mary to plead with Him on behalf of the sinner. In her play, *Le mallade, The Patient*, the reformist-minded Marguerite de Navarre (1492–1549), poked fun at both the learned medicine of the physician and the appeal of the man's wife to amulets, herbs and the Mass. It is the successful plea of the young servant girl for him to place all his hope in Christ that brings about a cure, a position that she defends in the subsequent colloquy with the others.[16]

The Medical Consequences of the Reformation

As we have seen (earlier, p. 58, 61), rulers and town councils had long cast eager eyes on the wealth of medieval hospitals, and the complaints about the wealth of monastic orders only encouraged a trend towards the municipalisation of hospitals and charitable care, but few went so far as the reformers in the British Isles in abolishing many of them completely. Elsewhere pilgrimages to healing shrines were neglected and officially frowned upon, and many healing shrines were actually destroyed. Lutherans accepted that miracles were possible but thought them extremely unlikely at best, whereas

Calvin rejected the notion of miracle entirely in favour of some form of natural explanation.[17] For William Perkins (1558–1602), the most influential English Calvinist writer at the end of the century, the miraculous gift of healing given to the apostles had now ceased, and the anointing carried out by the Catholic Church was a worthless charade: all those anointed by the apostles had recovered, but most of those anointed in his own day died almost immediately. All that was left for the reformed church was "but a ministry of reconciliation", reconciling the sick person to God, who alone could decide whether one lived or died.[18] Prayer might supplement secular healing and, at the very least, would ensure a Christian death.[19] Nonetheless, popular belief in miracles and the efficacy of the saints was hard to stamp out and revived afresh in South Germany and the Habsburg Empire during the Counter-Reformation at the end of the century.[20] The Counter-Reformation insistence on the authority of tradition as vouchsafed to and in the Church led to the renewed beautification of its buildings with artistic representations of healing by Christ, the Apostles and the saints. By contrast, Evangelical stress on individual belief within a family group led to a greater insistence on the moral values of those concerned with the care and upbringing of children from birth onwards and a concomitant dislike, and in some groupings, abandonment of the religious ceremonies around birth such as the churching of women.[21]

Medical practitioners were caught up in these ecclesiastical convulsions in a variety of ways. Their fabled rapacity and their apparent reluctance to leave a space for God in healing had long been the stuff of polemic or satire. The well-worn tag that Galen guaranteed wealth and Justinian honours was given an added twist by the German poet Caspar Brusch (1518–59) in a series of poems circulated on a single printed sheet. In them he derided physicians and lawyers as hypocrites, ostensibly engaged in the valuable service of treating the sick and protecting the innocent, but in reality greedy snakes, denying the saving word of God. Flatterers in the courts of kings and pontiffs, they hid their black wickedness under a cloak of kindness. Only if they repented and, believing in the true gospel, joined the tiny number of true Christian physicians that still existed in Germany, would they avoid the pains of Hell and attain the place in heaven reserved for true believers.[22] This is splendid rhetoric, a series of riffs on a very traditional theme, but its message was potentially dangerous in an era of religious strife.

Doctors might find themselves in difficulties with the authorities for their adherence to Galen, since some of his arguments, as newly revealed in his Greek texts, challenged Christian theology. Although personally remarkably interested in Jews and Christians, particularly for their high morality, he drew the line at the notion of miracles, rejecting the ability of the Creator to change at random the organisation of the world he had created so purposefully.[23] Some doctors in the sixteenth century still repeated the legend that he had died on a pilgrimage to Jerusalem, debating whether he was a Catholic or an Evangelical, but there was a major obstacle to identifying him with any branch of Christianity: he rejected the notion of a Aristotelian unitary soul located in the heart in favour of Plato's tripartite soul with three separate locations in the liver, heart and brain.[24] Christian Aristotelians, not least in Padua, naturally took issue with their medical colleagues, who defended Galen on the grounds that his three separate 'souls' were simply three faculties of a unitary soul operating through the three systems of the Galenic body.[25] Lutheran theologians, encouraged by Melanchthon and with a strong belief in the resurrection of the soul and body together, were more sympathetic to Galen, and the medical teachers at Wittenberg participated fully, if not always happily, in wider discussions on ethics. Their message of the close relationship between body and the Christian soul, and of the duty of all Christians to know about the workings of both of them, was passed on in lectures to all Wittenberg students and, in a suitably simplified form, even in Lutheran high schools.[26] Others, particularly in the second half of the century, interpreted what Galen had said in a small tract *Quod animi mores, The Soul's Behaviour Depends on the Body's Mixtures*, to mean that he held a materialist view of the soul, although in reality he had refused to commit himself to any position on the nature or immortality of the human soul, save that it was universally accepted that human behaviour could be influenced by bodily changes, for instance, by a lack of sleep or an excess of drink. This was enough for Juan Huarte (1529–88) to assert bluntly that "Galen, dying went to hell . . . this Physition had Knowledge of the Evangelicall [i.e. Gospel] doctrine, and could not receive it".[27]

Suspicions of the doctor's less than whole-hearted belief in church doctrine were not confined to philosophers. The cleric and doctor William Bullein acknowledged this when, in a dialogue in his book on plague, he made his character Medicus, a doctor, openly prefer Aristotle to the Bible and claim to have no specific faith, "like many of our secte".[28] Although Bullein makes it clear that he does not share the opinion of Medicus, who in the end is condemned by Death, not all his readers will have followed closely his somewhat tortuous rhetoric. But if unbelief laid one open to punishment, for much of the century it was even more dangerous to believe in the wrong brand of Christianity. Nicodemism, disguising one's true beliefs for as long as one could and keeping a low profile, offered some protection, for an overt expression of one's religious beliefs was more likely to lead to imprisonment and even death if it was uttered in the wrong place or at the wrong time. Had the Spanish anatomist Miguel Servet in 1553 not stopped in Geneva on his flight from imprisonment by the French Inquisition in Vienne and even attended a sermon by Calvin, with whom he had earlier engaged in an argumentative correspondence, he would not have given his enemies a renewed chance to imprison him, and ultimately for Calvin to allow him to be burnt on a pyre of his own books for denying both the Trinity and infant baptism. In his recently published book, the *Restoration of Christianity*, he had used his discovery of the circulation of the blood from one side of the heart to the other via the lungs as one of his arguments to support the idea he found in *Leviticus* and *Deuteronomy* that the soul was to be found in blood, not in the heart, the brain and the liver, as Galen had taught. His belief in the inerrancy of the Bible may have further blinded him to the extent to which Calvin, a biblical scholar of distinction, was strongly opposed to this and many other of his theories.[29]

Religious Persecution and Exile: England

Servet aside, most historians have concentrated upon Catholic persecution of non-Catholics, whether Evangelicals, Jews or converts from Islam, to which we shall return in a moment, but the British Isles also saw persecution directed against Catholics in the later years of Henry VIII, and the reigns of Edward VI and Elizabeth. The most notable of the Catholic medical exiles was John Clement, the former servant of the Chancellor Thomas More and the husband of More's ward, Margaret Giggs. Their proximity to the More family after More's execution in 1535, and the outspokenness of Margaret Clement in defence of her fellow Catholics, caused them serious difficulties in the years immediately following.[30] Henry VIII's change of policy on religion after the execution of More's successor as Chancellor, Thomas Cromwell, in 1540 allowed Clement to return to public life. He became President of the London College in 1544 and a member of its Council in 1547, a period which Caius, a close friend of Clement, looked back on almost as a golden age. It ended abruptly with the accession of the Evangelical Edward VI in 1547, causing Clement and his family to flee in July 1549 to Louvain "for the sake of religion", as Caius delicately put it in the *Annals* of the College.[31] He returned in 1553 on the accession of Queen Mary, who was determined to restore her kingdom to the old faith, only to find that his London house had been taken over by another Fellow of the College, Alban Hill, and he had to go to law to regain possession. Although he was later given permission to absent himself on grounds of health from meetings of the College, he remained active in it as an Elector and occasionally a member of the Council until 1562 when he wisely returned to Flanders. His family suffered further in the Spanish sack of Malines (Mechelen) in 1572, when almost all of what remained of his magnificent library was destroyed or dispersed around Northern Europe, and his son Thomas was reduced to begging the Pope for financial assistance.[32]

Clement was only the most distinguished of the several members of the London College who were punished or fled abroad because of their adherence to the Catholic Faith. George Smith went into exile, John Friar was imprisoned and Thomas Vavasour, a medical graduate of Venice and the most celebrated recusant in the north of England, spent years in gaol after being on the run for more than two years.[33] His fellow northerner, Dr Lee, so the authorities alleged, meanwhile passed unhindered from Papist family to Papist family encouraging the faithful among the gentry.[34] Balthasar Guersey (d. 1556) was specifically excluded from the Act of Pardon under

Edward VI because of his part in earlier machinations against archbishop Cranmer. Under Elizabeth I, Dr Atslowe was twice tortured on the rack, and Dr Good imprisoned for treacherous correspondence with Mary Queen of Scots.[35] By contrast, only two Evangelical physicians were forced into exile for a while, Andrew Boorde, whose *Breviary of Helthe*, first published in 1547, became an English best-seller, and the fiery cleric, William Turner, later Dean of Wells, who took the opportunity of his European exile to study medicine and to pursue his botanical researches in Germany.[36]

The consequences for English medicine were two-fold. Firstly, the direct link between England and Italy was effectively severed for half a century. Between John Caius in 1541 and Edward Jordan in 1591 only a tiny handful of medical students studied at Venice and Padua, almost all Catholics, who went there "out of an abundant zeal for religion", and the sole exception, Samuel Foxe in 1585–6, did not persevere with his medical studies and may indeed have been sent there to spy on other Englishmen.[37] Even at the end of the century, those who attended were likely to be Catholic sympathisers like William Harvey, the reference on whose degree certificate to the fact that he had sworn the standard oath of loyalty to the Catholic faith was omitted by the scribe of his personal copy on the instructions of the university authorities.[38] Secondly, the authority of the London College was seriously weakened by the popular belief, not entirely unfounded, that many of its members remained attached to the old beliefs. Many of those who had studied at Padua had known Cardinal Pole well, and, even if, like Edward Wotton, they managed to free themselves of suspicion, the energetic action of the College against outsiders while the Cardinal was Queen Mary's chief adviser hardly endeared them to those of an Evangelical persuasion.[39] In 1572, a memorandum was sent to the authorities, naming names, and complaining of the ease with which recusants like John Friar of Godmanchester (a recent Paduan student) and George Turner (who had a degree from Venice) were admitted when "any whom they think to be well affected towards the true religion now renewed" were rejected.[40] Matters came to a head a dozen years later when Thomas Moffet (or Muffet) wrote a vigorous letter of protest to the College complaining that he had been passed over unfairly for a Fellowship. Moffet, a Basle graduate and an expert on spiders (whose daughter's discomfiture is familiar to every small English child), was a supporter of Paracelsian therapies. A protégé of the Sidney family, the Earls of Pembroke, he was a convinced Evangelical and the dedicatee of the *Antidicsonus* by the Cambridge pillar of Calvinism, William Perkins.[41] In his letter he protested that he was being excluded from the Fellows' "musick and jollyty" on the grounds that he was not a Papist. His complaint did not fall on deaf ears for within months he attained his ambition and was elected a Fellow.

Religion undoubtedly played a part in the hostility of the College towards those more evangelically inclined, but its members were even more annoyed by the fact that many of the Protestant refugees from mainland Catholic

Europe were being employed or recommended by members of the aristocracy or wealthy Londoners, thus depriving them of the rich patients to which they thought themselves entitled. Initially, numbers of such immigrants were small and a royal physician such as Cesare Adelmare could easily be accommodated within the College.[42] But as the sixteenth century wore on, more and more exiles flocked to London in the hope of finding lucrative patronage. Some, like Guillaume de Laune, who had studied medicine at Paris and Montpellier, Daniel Celerius, a German protégé of the Earl of Huntingdon, or Raphael Thorey, a Leiden graduate, seem to have confined their practice largely to the foreign religious communities and were not troubled unless they took on English patients, and, even then, might in the end be given a licence.[43] Gerard Gossen, an MD of Louvain, claimed he had left his degree certificates behind when he was compelled to flee from Flanders, and promised to return home as soon as possible, but he never did, dying in London in 1603, having obtained an archbishop's licence to practise medicine as long before as 1582.[44] Others brought before the College were harder to deal with. Bartolo Sylva, a surgeon from Turin, first appeared in 1569, accused of bad practice that killed one patient and caused an abortion in another, but little could be done as he had to go and attend to surgical business at the behest of his master, the Earl of Bedford. He was back six months or so later, failing in his application for a licence because he was judged to be utterly ignorant of medicine and philosophy, and was fined £20 for causing enormous harm to the community. Undeterred, he continued to practise, was briefly thrown into the College's own jail and only just escaped being sent to the Fleet prison through the intervention of the two most powerful members of the government, Lord Burghley and Lord Leicester.[45]

Persecution and Exile: Northern Italy

England was not the only northern country to welcome Evangelical exiles from Italy. The eastern end of the Po valley, in particular, had a long tradition of independent religious thought, especially before the papal conquest of Bologna in 1506, and the first decades of the sixteenth century there saw several initiatives for religious reform along Erasmian lines, with which the future Cardinal Pole was in sympathy. There was also considerable support for many of Luther's ideas, particularly among a group of so-called '*spirituali*', but from the 1530s onwards they were forced to hide their beliefs or to face exile (or worse). After the marriage of the future Ercole II to Renée of France in 1527, Ferrara became suspect as the home of many such thinkers. Some of them came to Ferrara with the future Duchess, who was sympathetic to Evangelicals like Calvin, while others were more local, like the poet Marco Antonio Flaminio or the theologian Bernardino Ochino.[46] The medical Faculty was regarded as a hotbed of heresy. Brasavola, although opposed to Luther, was in favour of a Catholic reform, writing in his *Vita di Jesú Cristo*, *Life of Jesus*, of 1538 that religion must be a matter of individual conviction if one was to seek to live like Christ, the motto of the *spiritu-ali*.[47] Johannes Sinapius (1505–60), who was influenced by the Strasbourg Reformers, taught at Ferrara from 1534 to 1539 before becoming doctor to the Queen and he remained in frequent contact with Calvinists in Germany, Switzerland and France.[48] A third member of the Faculty with strong Evangelical leanings was Francesco Severi (c. 1508–70), originally from Argenta in the Po delta, who taught logic, natural philosophy and medicine in a career that lasted from 1543 until 1568, as well as acquiring considerable fame as a poet and humanist.[49] He was associated around 1548 with Nascimbene Nascimbeni and Giorgio Siculo, both of whom were arraigned before the Inquisition, and although Severi claimed to have tried to persuade Siculo to remain loyal to the Catholic church, he instead fell under his influence. Brought before the Inquisition himself in 1567, imprisoned and accused of reading Siculo's *Libro grande* and other heretical books, as well as of denying the Trinity and other errors, Severi was found guilty, but, after abjuring his errors, he was freed to continue treating the Ducal family and to resume his teaching for a year in 1568. His punishment was only delayed. He was brought back when it was alleged that this was not the first time he had made a similar recantation, and that he had continued nonetheless to hold his heretical beliefs, a much graver crime, for which he was executed and his body burnt in 1570.

But many of the Italian doctors who were suspected or even imprisoned for their religious views managed to escape north of the Alps, firstly to Basle and then to such Calvinist citadels as Geneva and Heidelberg. Many of them, like Guglielmo Massari (c. 1483–1564) and Guglielmo Gratarolo (1510–68), participated vigorously in both the medical and the religious life of their new homes, often on different sides of the theological arguments that developed as these religious communities began to fracture. Following the execution of Servet, Massari moved towards advocating religious tolerance, while Gratarolo, who had exchanged letters with Servet about his opinions, strongly supported the Calvinist line.[50] Others, like Niccolò Buccella (1520–99), Marcello Squarcialupi (1538–99) and Giorgio Biandrata (1515–88), migrated yet further east, where as doctors to the rulers of Poland and Transylvania or to great magnates they could help fellow religious exiles and make these regions a welcome home for anti-trinitarians as well as Calvinists.[51] Many of them were associated with the court of Emperor Rudolf II and were frequent correspondents of Crato von Crafftheim and Andreas Dudith.[52] They were not easy companions wherever they went and they changed their places of work and their religious adherences frequently. Fabio Nifo (fl. 1565–99), for example, had been a valued Dominican monk before becoming attracted to Calvinism while serving on the staff of a clerical diplomat in Paris. He left his order to study medicine in Padua in 1575 but was denounced to the Inquisition. He managed to escape from the bishop's prison and reach Vienna, where he was befriended by Crato, who helped him obtain a post as court doctor in Cracow with a salary of 600 florins. Disagreements with his colleague Buccella led quickly to his move in 1578 to Transylvania, but he did not stay long there either. In 1580/81 he turned up in London and was enrolled as a member of the Italian Church there, but a series of arguments and lawsuits with other members of the congregation saw him leave for the Spanish Netherlands, where he became a Catholic once again.[53]

Equally quarrelsome, although a far more significant academic figure, was Simone Simoni of Lucca, who initially returned home after taking his medical degree at Padua in 1562. When and where he became attracted to Calvinist ideas is unclear, but he was soon afterwards forced to flee on horseback from Lucca to Geneva, where he earned his living by giving private lessons to his fellow exiles. He quickly became a citizen of Geneva and was promoted to the chair of philosophy at its Academy, a remarkably swift recognition of his undoubted talents. But it was not long before he fell out with the pastor of the Italian church and, deprived of his post, was forced to move with his young family to Paris, where in 1567 he was giving lectures on philosophy at the Collège Royal with great success, or so he claimed. Shortly afterwards, an edict of Charles IX banned Calvinists from lecturing there, and he moved on to Zurich and Basle, where he was employed as a proof-corrector by Pietro Perna, another Italian exile who was engaged in publishing books on theology as well as the new Paracelsian medicine.[54] Following the death of his wife, Simoni left Basle for the Palatine court at Heidelberg, but his religious views displeased the Lutherans there, and, after a brief return to Basle, he made his way back to Germany, furnished with a letter of recommendation by Caspar Peucer, professor at Wittenberg and Melanchthon's son-in-law. His attempt to find a position at the university of Marburg failed, but in 1569 he managed to secure a chair in medicine at Leipzig as well as a post at the Saxon court.[55] Quarrels with his professorial colleagues led him to withdraw from the university, but his court position gave him power and influence beyond its walls. He was behind the reforms planned by the Elector of Saxony for the university, and his account of the plague at Leipzig in 1575 shows some of his ambitions and abilities, even if, at the crucial moment, he had already left town for the distant mountain town of Annaberg and, as he acknowledged, any success against the plague was owed to the efforts of the Leipzig Mayor, Hieronymus Rauscher.[56] Complaints about his religious belief, and his own quixotic, some said contentious, temperament led him to resign his post and leave Saxony in 1581 for Prague, where he converted back to Catholicism in 1582 before a crowd of imperial dignitaries.[57] He quickly moved on yet again, to the Polish Court, where he joined (and soon fell out with) Buccella. The death of the Polish king in late 1586 led to further accusations against him, and to a further pamphlet war. He lost his court position and had to rely for financial assistance on his aristocratic friends in the region, such as the Bishop of Olmouc. Despite appealing to the Pope for permission to return to Italy, he seems never to have done so, and died in Cracow in 1602. His tombstone records his wanderings in search of appropriate outlets for his "heroic" learning as well as his services to monarchs, but others found it difficult to understand all his changes of professed belief and his inability to remain for long in one place.[58] As Peter Monau put it in 1581,

> From a supporter of the pope he has become a Calvinist, from a Calvinist an antitrinitarian, from an antitrinitarian a Lutheran, and now he's a papist again; he says he will go off to Poland or Transylvania to join the antitrinitarians. But I will never stop thinking of him as a Galenist.[59]

His former employer, Pietro Perna, played a crucial role in linking the Italian exiles in Switzerland and Germany with like-minded groups in their home towns, and his role as a publisher of Paracelsian medicine will have strengthened, even if it did not occasion, the perceived link that developed from the 1560s onwards between Paracelsianism as a medical and as a theological heresy.[60] The development of censorship by the Inquisition had been formalised in 1559 by the publication of the first Papal Index of prohibited books, following on previous local Indexes issued in Paris (1544), Louvain, Venice, Spain and Portugal, and was extended throughout the century. It prohibited the ownership and reading of books by non-Catholic authors, especially by those who had written or commented on theological matters, such as Gessner and Fuchs. But its net was wide, and it included not only medieval medical authors like Arnald of Villanova and Pietro d'Abano but also modern editors of ancient medical texts such as Cornarius and Georg Agricola (who remained a Catholic). Even the name of Giambattista Da Monte was carefully excised from a book on distillation written by one of the censors himself, Girolamo Rossi, the historian of Ravenna. This produced an outcry, especially as many of the banned medical authors were regarded as essential for a proper medical education, and some were subsequently allowed back, albeit with excisions and corrections.[61] But banned books continued to be read, and communication was maintained between leading scholars across the confessional divide, but it required considerable caution, even from so well-connected and internationally famous scholar as Mercuriale, to avoid falling under suspicion.[62] Pietro Longo, who had acted as courier for books from Frankfurt and Basel to Venice, was imprisoned and then drowned by the Venetian authorities in 1588, having been caught smuggling in prohibited books, including a copy of Gessner's *Bibliotheca Universalis* destined for Mercuriale.[63]

The previous year had seen the similar trial and execution of one of the leading doctors in Venice, Girolamo Donzellini (c. 1513–87) who had corresponded with Zwinger and the Elder Camerarius and had long maintained contacts north of the Alps.[64] A student of Da Monte, he arranged for the publication of some of his writings in Basle with Isingrin and later with Perna. He was first named by the Inquisition in 1544, which occasioned his flight from Rome to Venice, where he helped in the import and distribution of large quantities of books from Perna. Implicated again in a heresy trial of a fellow humanist from Brescia in 1553, he fled at midnight to Ferrara and thence, to Germany, where he spent the next six years. In 1560, furnished with a safe conduct from the Emperor Ferdinand, he returned to Venice, appearing voluntarily before the Inquisition to abjure his former behaviour. He admitted reading some of the forbidden books but claimed that he had read Averroes through the lens of Thomas Aquinas, and Avicenna through that of Galen, being uniquely trained to separate the useful contents of these books from their mistaken contexts. Given a mild sentence of a year's confinement in a Venetian monastery, he became a Venetian citizen, joining the College of Physicians and even becoming its Prior. But during a controversy between 1570 and 1573 on the properties of theriac, he annoyed his opponent by emphasising his travels in Germany, and, having survived an attempt on his life, he was again brought before the Inquisition in 1574. This time more evidence was produced, and he was charged again, tortured, convicted and imprisoned for life. The outbreak of the great plague in Venice in 1576 gave him a new opportunity. Having written his own plague tract while in prison, he was freed again in 1577. But within a year he was back before the Inquisition, condemned to a period of house arrest for his involvement in the escape of another medical heretic Nascimbene Nascimbeni, whom he had been allowed to treat in his house.[65] By now he was sufficiently frightened to approach the ubiquitous Crato for assistance in finding a post at the Imperial court, something Crato had earlier promised him, but the opportunity had now passed. He continued to work and study in his large library, arranging for books to be conveyed to him from Basle either by students or concealed in bales of cloth or other merchandise. It was one of these books that brought about his final trial. He had managed to reach Padua on his flight north when bad weather prevented him going further, he was re-arrested, and brought back to Venice where, as a lapsed heretic, he was soon afterwards drowned in the lagoon.

The case of Donzellini illustrates neatly some of the consequences of the religious splits caused by the Reformation. The years after 1550 hardened the divisions, disrupting, although they did not entirely prevent, communication between the Evangelicals and the Catholics, and imposing constraints on what could be read or done. Belief in the stars, as Cardano found out to his cost, or the use of chemical remedies, and, still more, adherence to the Paracelsian theories behind them, risked imprisonment and even death in Spain and Italy, unless one had a powerful patron, such as Llorenç Coçar (1540–92) found in Philip II, and hampered the movement of students from England and other parts of the North to Italy.[66] At the same time, the Protestant networks, whether Lutheran, Calvinist or Unitarian in outlook, provided learned exiles from Italy with employment with publishers, academic posts and, in particular, high positions at court where they could introduce many up-to-the-minute ideas on therapy and medical organisation. Wherever they went, they continued to debate and write on theological as well as medical and philosophical themes, and to quarrel constantly with any-one with whom they might disagree. Many of them shared the same broad humanist outlook, brought up on Aristotle and Galen, and trained to com-pare and criticise texts, something that came up against officially approved limits when commenting on Holy Scripture, whether as interpreted by Luther, Calvin or the Council of Trent.

But these were constraints on individuals and, England apart, the hos-pitals and similar healing institutions did not change much and may even have prospered because of the increased emphasis on works of charity and, among Protestants, on the importance of looking after the welfare of the whole community of God. At Groningen in North-East Holland in 1594, following the incorporation of this previously multi-faith com-munity into the Calvinist Dutch Republic, the new political and religious elite gave increased powers and obligations to its surgeons within a much expanded social construction of charity, partly from theological reasons but also to emphasise its superiority to the Spanish administration that had preceded it.[67]

Persecution and Exile: Iberia

During the sixteenth century this renewed sense of the Christian commu-nity (whether as the Church universal or as the gathered faithful) and an increased hostility and suspicion to any outsiders who might reside in its midst badly affected two other religious groups, Jews and Muslims. Both had shared in the flourishing medical Galenic tradition of the Middle Ages, often co-operating with Christian translators, and contributing, in Latin translation, some of the seminal writings studied by European medical faculties down to the sixteenth century and, in the case of Avicenna, even beyond.[68] There were substantial Jewish communities in Venice and Rome, served by their own doctors, who were often called in to assist Christian colleagues and even to treat Popes.[69] Many of them were extremely learned. Vesalius describes co-operating in translating Arabic and Hebrew anatomi-cal terms with Lazarus de Frigeis, "a distinguished Hebrew physician", who may or may not be the same as Lazarus Friscus, a Jew who attended Brasavola's lectures on the *Aphorisms* at Ferrara in 1540–1.[70] The long-lived Jacopo Mantino (d. 1549) was given permission by the Doge to hear lectures at Padua, and his Latin translations, via the Hebrew, of the two most familiar parts of Avicenna's *Canon*, *Fens* I, 1 and 4, were several times reprinted and their accuracy widely discussed.[71] He later lived in Bologna, Florence, Venice and finally Rome, where he treated many members of the papal court, and even the Pope himself. His authority as a scholar was such that both sides sought his aid in deciding whether the marriage of Henry VIII to his deceased brother's wife was valid or not according to church law. His refusal to abandon the rules in the book of *Deuteronomy* that declared it invalid in favour of the later ones in *Leviticus* that allowed such a marriage in very special circumstances was gratefully welcomed by Pope Clement V, whose patron, the Emperor Charles V, was the nephew of the unfortunate Catherine of Aragon.[72] In 1593, Abraham ben Hananiah Yagel (about 1530–1623) was given the right to treat both Christian and Jews at Rubiera in the Po valley in the absence of a Christian doctor: his appointment document describes him as a doctor in both arts and medicine, which suggests that he had attended a university.[73] His printed works show a blend of Galenism, astral medicine (in therapy as well as in prediction) and Jewish religious ideas, "supported by the secrets of the Torah".[74]

Like Abraham in his earlier career, Jewish doctors were largely confined to their own community and were always living on the verge of disaster.[75] One of their most eminent, Amatus Lusitanus, moved from Portugal to Antwerp, to Ferrara (where he assisted Canano in some of his dissections) and then in 1547 to Ancona, a port with a Jewish community of over 100 families. Benefitting from a papal dispensation of 1547 allowing these Portuguese refugees to practise their own religion, he enjoyed a successful practice there and elsewhere in Italy for a while. But the bull of Paul IV in 1555 withdrawing this permission and confining Jews to a ghetto, led almost immediately to confiscations and arrests, including that of his uncle, and within months to the complete dispersal of the *conversos*. Amatus himself fled hurriedly to Pesaro, Ragusa and ultimately Salonica, leaving behind his belongings and his books.[76] Another Portuguese *converso*, Manuel Brudus, the son of a Portuguese royal physician, tried his luck in England in the 1540s. He travelled as far as Scotland for information he included in his book on *Diet in Fever*, praising haggis and the English preference for red meat and bear as appropriate for their climates, but despite support from noblemen and courtiers, he failed to find permanent position, and left for the Jewish community in Antwerp.[77]

The doctors who had converted in Spain from Islam fared even worse than the Jewish *conversos*. Although very many of the Islamic population of Granada chose to go into exile, a large number remained behind, forming a majority in some southern areas and constituting a continuing threat in the eyes of their conquerors. Unlike the Jews, Muslim doctors had previously confined their practice mainly to their own co-religionists, whose social and economic standing suffered substantially as more and more wealthy members preferred to leave for North Africa. Some clerics, most notably Archbishop Cisneros of Granada and Archbishop Juan de Ribera of Valencia, sought to assimilate the learned new Christians within a college or university, so that they could continue to serve their own community, but their numbers were always small and they faced great pressure to abandon all traces of their old faith.[78] Besides, at least for the first half of the century, Morisco physicians continued to be trained in the old *ijaza* system, studying certain books with a master in a form of apprenticeship in a madrasa like that of Saragossa; only a few obtained a university degree or permission to practise from one of the royal regional tribunals.[79] Morisco midwives were still allowed to function, but only under the strictest of Christian supervision, for fear that they might carry out illicit circumcisions or repeat traditional Muslim prayers. But, increasingly, the investigators of the Inquisition insisted that they should not treat 'old Christians', and tax records confirm that by mid-century it was extremely rare for a Morisco to call himself a doctor. In Valencia in 1552, only one of the 35 doctors and licentiates in the city, Gomis Fajardo, was a Morisco, who had resided there for at least five years.[80] As García Ballester puts it, if there was any degree of assimilation, it was timid and quickly abandoned.[81]

By the 1570s, coexistence between the two groups had broken down. Morisco healers might be occasionally called on for their empirical skills, as when a Morisco healer, Pinterete, was called in to apply efficacious ointment to Don Carlos, the son of Philip II, much to the annoyance of the royal surgeon Daza Chacon, but they were also forbidden to practise even among their own community.[82] Local conditions and a certain reputation might for a while protect a popular healer such as Jeronimo Jover in Valencia in 1577, but even he was in the end brought before the Inquisition and forced to flee to North Africa. The dispersal around Spain of 80,000 Moriscos after the Morisco revolt of 1568–71 further diminished any standing that these healers might have had. Some of them had a few books in Latin or Spanish, but they had lost any acquaintance with the medieval authors in the original Arabic, which was easily interpreted by the Inquisition as a series of magical symbols. Possession of an Arabic book, and even a prescription in Arabic, was likely to lead to imprisonment or, very occasionally, burning as a heretic.[83] Accusations of magic, witchcraft and belief in demons are common in trials of Morisco healers, but not in those of Jews, a further indication of the different status of the two communities.[84] In 1609 the King issued the first of a series of orders expelling the Moriscos from the various parts of Spain. Possibly as many as 300,000 left for North Africa, and a similar number may have remained behind, too poor or insignificant to be worth the effort of pursuing them. It was a sad end to a learned tradition of medicine, paradoxically coming at a time when the older pre-humanist Galenism as represented by Luis Mercado, the royal *Protomedico*, was gaining a tighter grip on university medicine.

These expulsions, whether of *conversos*, Moriscos, *spirituali* or Protestants and Catholics who found themselves living on the wrong side of a religious divide, are a feature of the growing religious tensions in Western Europe. Except for the Moriscos, whose whole culture was destroyed, most doctors managed to make a living in their new homes, even if they were often suspected of heretical beliefs or, like Queen Elizabeth's doctor, the *converso* Rodrigo Lopez, of conspiring with enemies of the state.[85] Others, particularly Jews, found themselves unable to settle down in one place, a constant source of turmoil for themselves and their families. At the same time, their mobility helped to spread new ideas around Europe among learned physicians. Compared with their impact on individuals, the religious changes during the sixteenth century affected the institutions of healing relatively little. Even among Protestants, many continued to practise as before or maintained their old beliefs surreptitiously, and the 'sacred magic' of the old Church still had its power, despite official attempts to replace it.[86] Only in England and Scotland, where the religious Reformation was tied closely to a political one, were many of the earlier charitable institutions abolished rather than handed over to the new religion or to secular lords. Elsewhere, the same emphasis on the Christian community engaged in caring for its members physically as well as spiritually, is found in both Calvinist Geneva and the Counter-Reformation Milan of Cardinal Borromeo. Christian belief and practice intersected, and usually harmonised, with the professional ethics of physicians and other healers, but, as the fates of Servet and Donzellini show, there were also limits to what might be publicly expressed. There was, as yet, no *Religio Medici*.[87]

Notes

1 For the joke, Kocher 1947; cf. also Gilly 1991.
2 In general, Porterfield 2005; MacCulloch 2003.
3 Henderson 2006: 113–33, 339; for votive tablets, Laven 2016.
4 Earlier, pp. 57–61.
5 Malingre 1533.
6 Brief account in the classic Thomas 1973: 98-9. Some medical prayers from books of surgery are given in Kocher 1947: 447; for some Catholic prayers against plague, Cyrus 2021, and earlier, p. 91, n. 43.
7 Clowes 1602: 41–2, 1948: 56–8. For clerics in the Netherlands, De Waardt 1996.
8 For Italy, Pullan 1971: 33–238; Henderson 1994; for England, Duffy 1992: 132–54 (noting that charity was only the third most important activity of most guilds).
9 Duffy 1992: 190–205; for France, Brockliss and Jones 1997: 73–5.
10 Du Broc de Segange and Morel 1887; Thomas 1973: 29–30; Duffy 1992: 177–83, a good selection of English examples.
11 Thomas 1973: 44–9, 146–8, 227–35.
12 For some German examples, Karant-Nunn 1997: 62, cf. 54; Thomas 1973, *passim*.
13 Weyer 1563, 1991; for a Jewish physician rejecting demons as a primary cause of illness, Ruderman 1988: 51–2; for the German context, Brady 2009: 336–46.
14 Weyer 1991; Thomas 1973 remains a classic; Ankarloo *et al.* 2002 is a useful overall survey.
15 Brady 2009: 61–5, 132–44 (survey of different approaches to reform in the years before Luther).
16 Marguerite de Navarre 1946; Broomhall 2004: 139–42.
17 Porterfield 2005: 24–5.
18 Wear 1985: 60–1.
19 Mann 2020, summarises seventeenth-century attitudes.
20 Evans 1984b: 224, 390; MacCulloch 2003: 329, 361, 454.
21 Karant-Nunn 1997: 72–90; Flügge 1998: 332–42, 369–71.
22 Clemen 1911, probably published around 1550.
23 Nutton 2020a: 82.

24 Nutton 2009: 216–24.
25 Nutton 1990b; Bigotti 2019.
26 Nutton 1990b; Helm 2001.
27 Bigotti 2019: 130, n. 46. *Ibid.*, 107–36, 150–66 discusses Renaissance uses of this treatise.
28 Bullein 1564: sigs. B2v–4v; Kocher 1947: 230–2.
29 Servetus 1553: 170; Bainton 1960; Ongaro 1971: 4–10; MacCulloch 2003: 244–6.
30 Brigden 2012: 406.
31 Caius *Annals*: Roberts 1912: 17.
32 Wenkebach 1925: 17–29: for the lawsuit with Hill over the house and library, Reed 1925–6; for his son and the remains of his library after the sack, Guilday 1914: 183–9.
33 Caius, *Annals*: Roberts 1912: 17; Palmer 1983, 137, 177; Rex 1990–91.
34 Bastow 2007: 202–3.
35 Clark 1964: 127–8; Nutton 2011: 173.
36 Jones W 1988.
37 Woolfson 1998: 249; Nutton 2011: 169–70.
38 Rossetti 2006.
39 Brigden 2012: 180–1.
40 Nutton 2011: 173.
41 Clark 1964: 133–5; Yates 1992: 265, 275; Dawbarn 2003.
42 For Adelmare, earlier, p. 53.
43 Clark 1964: 142.
44 Pelling and Webster 1979: 185. For an Archbishop's licence, earlier, p. 135.
45 Roberts 1912: 64–9.
46 Flood and Shaw 1997: 86–9.
47 Horne 1958; Firpo 1984; Marcantonio Doni, unpaginated pref. to Brasavola 1551.
48 Food and Shaw 1997: 89–90.
49 Raffaelli 1983, 1984; Quaranta 2018.
50 Celati 2018c; Hieronymus 2005: 884–96 adds useful material on Gratarolo's publications and his writings.
51 Caccamo 1970: 109–52; Palmer 1993.
52 For the significance of Crato in supporting these networks, Evans 1984a: 98–105; Louthan 1994, 1997.
53 Caccamo 1970: 55–6.
54 Earlier, p. 43; Rotondò 1974 remains fundamental for his career and publication of unorthodox writings; Perini 2002.
55 Ludwig 1909; Verdigi 1997: 62–81; Madonia 1980.
56 Nutton 2008b.
57 Firpo 1984; Madonia 1980: 171; Verdigi 1997: 95–108.
58 Verdigi 1997: 16; Nutton 2008b: 5.
59 Gillet 1860: 2,340.
60 Perini 2002; Hieronymus 2005.
61 Donzellini's name was removed from his authorship of Galenic translations in the 1556 Giunta edition of Galen, whose editor, Gadaldino, also fell foul of the Inquisition.
62 Siraisi 2008; Agasse and Pennuto 2016.
63 Donato 2019; Marcus 2020; for Rossi, 80–95.
64 Palmer 1993; Celati 2014; Marcus 2020: 43–5.
65 Ginzburg 1970 gives the wider context of this relationship.

66 Siraisi 1997; for the expurgation of his books, Marcus 2020: 121–2. For Coçar, López Terrada 2009: 21–5.
67 Huisman 1996: 73–9.
68 Siraisi 1987; García-Ballester 1993.
69 Esposito 2013.
70 Vesalius 1543: 166; O'Malley 1964: 120, 438; Nutton 1990c: 243.
71 Siraisi 1987: 135–6.
72 Kaufman 1893.
73 Ruderman 1988: 26.
74 Ruderman 1988: 25–42: quotation on p. 31.
75 For Portuguese Jewish physicians, Maclean 2009: 397.
76 Andreoni and Fortuna 2019; I have not seen Gutwirth 2004, which puts his career in a wider context.
77 Nutton 1999: 280.
78 García Ballester 1984: 51–3, 60–3.
79 García Ballester 1985: 249–50, 262.
80 García Ballester 1993: 172–6.
81 García Ballester 1984: 62–3.
82 García Ballester 1985: 252, 1993: 169–73.
83 García Ballester 1985: 265–8, 1993: 161–2, pointing out that Moriscos were burnt far less frequently than Jews.
84 García Ballester 1984: 158–210, 1993: 185.
85 Earlier, p. 145.
86 Only Paracelsus appears in Waddell 2021, who says little about theological differences.
87 For Renaissance medical ethics, Gadebusch-Bondio 2014. For the medical background to Sir Thomas Browne (b. 1605), Barbour 2013.

12 Conclusion

The main characteristics of medicine during the sixteenth century are best grasped by a comparison with those of the preceding and succeeding centuries, as well as by a consideration of their relationship to two familiar historical constructs, the Renaissance and the Scientific Revolution. Both terms have been strongly debated in recent years, but with little concern for medicine, and much Anglo-American scholarship has subsumed the whole period under the vague denomination of 'Early Modern', a catch-all that can cover almost anything between the Black Death in the late 1340s and the nineteenth century. Inevitably, perhaps, in such a periodisation, the sixteenth century fares badly by comparison with the better and more accessibly documented later centuries. Even such excellent surveys of early-modern medicine as those by Andrew Wear and Mary Lindemann focus more on the period after 1600 than before it.[1] The decline of Latin, once universal in British schools and understood by most of the medical profession, and the increasing remoteness of the cultural presuppositions of a classical heritage that accompanied it, have meant that many Anglophone writers on this period confine themselves to works written in or translated into English, and neglect the European dimension. This book, it is hoped, will help to restore that balance.

Two major developments mark off the medicine of the sixteenth century from its predecessor: the opening up of the world via exploration and the effects of printing. The medical changes that followed the European discovery of the Americas and the expansion of Europeans into India and further east were not immediate, with the possible exception of the major epidemic of the French Disease, or syphilis, which some physicians came to associate, rightly or wrongly, with Columbus's discoveries. While drugs continued to come in from the East, those from the Americas did not figure prominently in lists of recipes or in pharmacists' shops until the last third of the century. The few exceptions were those, like guaiac, that were thought to be particularly appropriate for this foreign disease, syphilis. It should not be forgotten too that the transfer of peoples, whether as conquerors or slaves, from one hemisphere to the other also brought European diseases to the Americas,

DOI: 10.4324/9781003223184-16

with disastrous consequences for many of their original inhabitants. The Columbian exchange was not an equal one.

But it was the world closer to home that was revealed in greater detail than ever before to readers in the sixteenth century. Local histories and geographies were supplemented by the expeditions of naturalists to discover and classify the native flora and fauna of their regions. Botanists had a template for this in the treatise on materia medica by the Greek Dioscorides, and many of the early discoveries and debates were made public in the form of commentaries or notes on his book. But by mid-century the abundance of new material, whether from Italy, Britain, Germany or further afield, had largely outgrown this model and independent herbals, many of them illustrated, began to be produced in quantity. At the same time, communities of naturalists, sharing information and sometimes objects, brought a new sense of a joint intellectual endeavour that could transcend political and religious boundaries. Besides, as new plants and herbs were discovered, the more likely it became that even more still remained to be found, thus encouraging expeditions to local mountains or to Mediterranean islands and beyond. At the same time, local pride and practical utility encouraged the development of medicinal spas and a more detailed study of their medical effects, which could then be communicated to a wider audience by means of print. 'New' local diseases, like the English Sweat, the Moravian Pestilence or land scurvy also attracted attention and led Fracastoro and his followers to more extensive investigations into contagious diseases.

This new learning was spread throughout Europe and to the Spanish Empire through the power of print. Although medical books had been printed as early as the 1470s, numbers were small, and the range of titles was restricted to a few university staples, plague tracts and home medicine. Most were in Latin, and hence inaccessible because of language and, probably, cost to all but male members of the upper classes. Most were also printed in Italy, and although networks of booksellers were beginning, medicine at the end of the fifteenth century was still to a large extent a manuscript culture. This changed dramatically in the first quarter of the sixteenth century, with the development of more publishing centres, not least Paris and Basle, and with the publication of a much wider range of subjects in a variety of formats and, increasingly, languages. The success of Paracelsian medicine from the 1560s onwards was dependent on the existence of a market for learned medicine in German. The growth of literacy across Europe, even if confined to a small percentage of the male population and an even smaller one of the female, also stimulated the production of new types of books aimed at filling the gap between the academic learning of a university-trained physician and a basic home help manual. Some of these authors, like Leonardo Fioravanti or the German Walther Hermann Ryff (c. 1500–48), were extremely prolific, transmitting, some would say plagiarising, the ideas of others to produce popular summaries on a variety of subjects, including medicine.[2] Such authors, although they are relatively unfamiliar today, contributed substantially to the spread of new discoveries and new ideas in medicine.

The format of books also changed. Stately folios containing the complete works of an author or combining many tracts on a single theme were still produced in numbers, although, like the later Giuntine editions of Galen, some were little more than reissues with a new frontispiece. But alongside them came many shorter texts on specific themes such as bloodletting or diet, almost always in a much smaller format. Printing also made possible the production of works on botany and anatomy with more illustrations than had been possible in an age of manuscript. Some of them, like Fuchs's *Herbal* or Vesalius's *Fabrica*, were extremely expensive. Students, however, were able to make use of the shorter *Epitome* of Vesalius and the compilations of images put out by Valverde, Jacques Grévin or Thomas Geminus, or content themselves with a set of anatomical fugitive sheets that they could take to lectures or study at home. It would be wrong to think of this as the democratisation of medicine, for most of these students came from the upper bourgeoisie or gentry and expected to become wealthy themselves. But as the evidence of medical libraries shows, it allowed the publication of a greater range of authors with a correspondingly variety of ideas, even if they were working within the same Galenist medical tradition. A comparison between the library of Giovanni di Marco, a learned Paduan-trained doctor from Rimini (d. 1474) and those a century later of Thomas Lorkyn in Cambridge and Georg Palma in Nuremberg is telling. The first is entirely manuscript, with far fewer volumes, and concentrates on a small number of authors in Latin from Antiquity and the Middle Ages, only a handful of them Giovanni's contemporaries. Those of Lorkyn and Palma have only a very few manuscripts, but very many printed books covering a wide range of topics, most written by authors who lived in the sixteenth century. Most are still in Latin, but many are not, and they show many marginal annotations that confirm that these were working libraries contrasted with the untouched beauty of many of Giovanni's codices, few of which contain his notes. In short, printing brought about not only an increase in accessibility and range, but also different kinds of use.[3]

In the conclusion to her study of medicine before 1500, Nancy Siraisi sketched very briefly some of the continuities between that period and the sixteenth century, concentrating largely on the intellectual milieu rather than social and structural developments. She rightly pointed to the continued importance of Galenic medicine in some form or another as the basis of the understanding of medicine among the laity as well as learned physicians. Only Paracelsus and his more extreme followers from 1560 onwards rejected Galenism entirely, and several physicians sought to reconcile the two at least in practice, and occasionally in theory. But there is a major shift of emphasis in attitudes towards Galen, beginning among a small group of North Italians around 1490 who decried the errors of earlier translators and medieval doctors and demanded a return to his original Greek, or at least to more accurate Latin versions of it. They could also point to newly accessible ancient texts, mainly by Galen but also by Dioscorides, 'Hippocrates' and some less familiar names. Basing themselves on the newly printed Greek texts of Galen (1525) and Hippocrates (1526) and even more on the subsequent flood of translations, physicians could rightly claim that they were both engaging with something new and retaining the cachet of centuries of success. Like those of Dioscorides in botany, the newly discovered books by Galen brought about major changes in medicine, not least in the understanding and role of human anatomy. Intellectually, by the 1550s Vesalius had equalled, if not surpassed, Galen as an authority on the anatomy of the human body, although he and his successors were still hampered by a shortage of suitable bodies to dissect. At the same time in Padua, basing himself on a wider range of genuinely Galenic treatises than his medieval Latin predecessors, Da Monte was advocating a range of methods that might be used in diagnosis to supplement a more cautious use of pulse and urines. Astrological medicine continued, despite attacks on it, although its practitioners became increasingly suspect, especially after it was shown that a work on astrology ascribed to Galen was not by him. This revived Galenism of the so-called neoterics continued to be the mainstay of university medicine down to the middle of the seventeenth century and, in some respects, down to the nineteenth.

It was accompanied by a greater emphasis on experience, whether in the publication of observations and case histories (although the latter genre was already familiar in the Middle Ages), or in such more empirical subjects as anatomy and medical botany. If learned medicine in the first quarter of the sixteenth century can still be characterised as medieval and that in the second as revived classical, the third saw the institutionalising of this empiricism through the creation of botanical gardens and anatomy theatres, some temporary but others permanent, for the annual dissections that were now conducted on a much more regular basis. But while anatomists like Vesalius, Falloppia and Colombo made many new discoveries about the structures of the human body, acquiring bodies for dissection, especially those of women, presented problems, for cutting up a human body still carried with it a taint of desecration or at least of something disgusting. More and more in the last quarter of the century anatomists, led by Coiter and Fabricius, were content to investigate the workings of the human body and the purposes of its structures by a careful comparison with those of animals, a reversion to the procedures of Aristotle's and, still more, Galen.

The sixteenth century also differs considerably from the preceding centuries in the spread of medical institutions of all kinds. The number of universities expanded and with them the number of academically qualified doctors and, at least in Italy, academically trained surgeons. At the same time, growing competition from others less qualified led to an increase in public supervision and in institutions such as medical colleges approved by the authorities as a way of improving standards and of exercising control over those considered less knowledgeable. This corporatisation of medicine was a process begun in Italy that spread across Europe, sometimes causing legal battles between groups of healers fearful that they would be excluded from access to wealthy patients and disadvantaging women who lacked the social and, as was often alleged, the intellectual capabilities to compete. Even midwives and so-called charlatans came under forms of regulation. Similarly, complex social provisions against plague that had been made in only a few Italian cities before 1500 became more widespread and more onerous with the growth of Health Boards and the imposition of quarantines. Samuel Cohn also argues that the Italian plagues of the 1570s led to new genres of medical writing as well as serving as a template for how a community should respond to plague.[4] Simple cleaning of the streets and a minimal local response were no longer considered adequate. Hospitals also grew larger and more numerous (except in the British Isles where many were destroyed in Henry VIII's Reformation), and both Evangelicals and, in the second half of the century, Catholics developed a new social conscience, although their ideals were somewhat different. Evangelicals stressed the importance of the family, Counter-Reformation Catholics the role of the church and its saints. Christian religion mattered, but now it was divided into ever more hostile camps.

Developments in the first quarter of the seventeenth century did not differ greatly from what had gone before, except in the greater abundance of documentation and in the beginnings of a shift away from Italy, although Padua and Bologna still remained important, towards northern universities such as Basle, later Leiden, and even Helmstedt, which enjoyed a boom in this period. Although Paracelsianism continued to win converts and there was a much greater interest in alchemy and medicinal chemistry among its adherents, most universities continued to teach a modified Galenism. William Harvey, a Paduan graduate, developed his anatomical studies along the lines taught him by Fabricius, using a variety of animals to determine the different movements of the heart and, partly reverting to an experiment of Galen, to posit the circulation of blood around the whole body. The circulation from heart to lungs and back to the heart, discovered by Colombo, had been accepted by all younger anatomists by 1600, and some had argued for a greater transfer of blood from arteries to veins but only in unusual circumstances.[5] But for Harvey this discovery of something normal and universal did not entail the abandonment of Galenic medicine, rather the reverse, for it explained better both the value of bloodletting and the action elsewhere in the body of a drug taken by mouth. But increasingly, experimental investigations, whether in Oxford or Leiden, took a physiological turn, which together with iatrophysics and iatrochemistry, as well as new ideas on measurement and instrumentation, meant that learned medicine, particularly in Northern Europe, evolved a very different approach from that of the sixteenth century. Latin was also gradually losing its place as the universal language of medicine as treatises in the vernacular, even on academic themes, became more popular. Some diseases seem to have become less virulent or even disappeared, like the English Sweat or plague in most of England after 1665. Notions of quarantine were almost universal, and cities and governments developed stronger means to control infectious disease, even if they could not cure it. Surgery, and particularly military surgery, also developed substantially as a result of new conflicts and civil wars, notably the Thirty Years War and the British Civil War. As more and more Europeans settled in the Americas, the traffic in substances from there increased greatly, and was accompanied by further studies of the environment of these distant places. All these developments took place over time and at different speeds, but while it is hard to see major changes in the first quarter of the seventeenth century, 50 years later the overall picture differs considerably.

Medicine, the Renaissance and the Scientific Revolution

Compared with the Scientific Revolution the Renaissance was both more extended in time and more extensive in scope, including art, architecture, music as well as literature and medicine. There are obvious continuities between Renaissance Italy in 1400 and Shakespeare's England in 1600. Principally among them was the belief that Classical Antiquity, and principally to begin with the Latin world of Cicero, Virgil and Livy, provided a model for contemporaries to follow in different areas, whether in art, morals, literature or even language. Latin had long been the universal language of Europe, but now it was a revived or reborn (hence Renaissance) Latin that avoided the allegedly barbarous constructions of the medieval scholastics. It served as a marker of gentility, for even after the expansion in the sixteenth century of humanist grammar schools only the reasonably wealthy or the sons of the urban bourgeoisie could afford to attend. Physicians displayed their adherence to this so-called humanist movement not only by composing their treatises in elegant Latin but also by displaying their talents in the verses they composed either for the wider public, like Eobanus Hessus or Fracastoro, or, more often, in the Latin odes and epigrams printed at the front of publications by friends and colleagues. These talents made them welcome in the societies of poets and literati that met in places like Rome, Florence or Erfurt, where one can still sit and debate in the surviving part of the Engelsberg complex that once contained the *Museum*, the Hall of the Muses, owned by the poet and physician Georg Sturtz (d. 1548).[6]

By contrast with many other Renaissance activities, the new medicine depended far more on a Greek renaissance than on a Latin, for the simple reason that the most significant and most extensive medical writings that survived from Antiquity were in Greek, a language that was not commonly studied until the sixteenth century, and, even then, proficiency in it was confined to a relatively small number of experts. But the publication of the Greek Galen in 1525 followed by the Greek Hippocrates the next year stimulated a huge wave of translations into the new, modern Latin that were more extensive and more accurately rendered than earlier versions. By contrast with the humanist movement a century earlier which spread only slowly from Italy, these new Latin versions were produced all over Europe and quickly became the staple source of information on the medicine of Antiquity. They provided models to emulate as well as a basis for adding new information or criticising the interpretations of others. Only Paracelsus and his followers deliberately wrote learned treatises in the vernacular, and arguably it was not until the publication of major syntheses in Latin in 1571 by Guinter and Severinus or the appearance of a body of Latin translations in 1575, that his doctrines penetrated the non-German world to any significant extent.[7] Certainly their readers felt themselves to be part of a culturally unified world that can justly be termed the Renaissance.

The relationship of medicine to what is often termed the Scientific Revolution is more problematic, largely because what is meant by the term is far from clear both in its chronology and in its specifics. Science, in the modern English sense of the word, is an invention of the nineteenth century. Before then '*scientia*' applied to all kinds of knowledge from law and theology to medicine, mathematics and astronomy: its modern German equivalent, '*Wissenschaft*', still requires to be qualified by the area of expertise that is being discussed, such as *Naturwissenschaft*, 'natural science' or *Medizinwissenschaft*, 'medical science'. In the sixteenth century there were many crossovers between disciplines. Medical information fed into debates between philosophers, and an interest in plants and herbs was shared by medics, diplomats, lawyers and aristocrats. In turn, many medical practitioners took a very close interest in astronomy, natural history and the workings of drugs, whether herbal or, as with the Paracelsians at the end of the century, chemical. But late nineteenth-century presuppositions about what constituted science left medicine in an ambiguous position, neither fully scientific nor entirely remote from the laboratory. The twenty-first century emphasis on the biomedical sciences has in turn emphasised only one part of the activities of medical practitioners, while also relegating its earlier history to an antiquarian study of centuries of failure.

Equally misleading is the term 'Revolution', for it implies a relatively short and decisive period rather than one stretching over a century and a half that links a variety of different periods, individuals and achievements. This is not to say that contemporaries in the sixteenth century did not quickly recognise major departures from what had gone before. Giovanni Manardi recognised almost at once the significance of the new voyages for views on climate and Aristotelian cosmology (earlier, p. 11), while the doctor-astrologer at the Habsburg court, Thaddeus Hagecius, had no hesitation in 1566 in linking Vesalius and Copernicus together as marking a major break with the past.[8] But to think of this period as one of frequent and revolutionary change, let alone one leading inexorably towards modernity is a major misunderstanding. Nor is it easy to find a Kuhnian revolution in which an abundance of small discoveries leads to a sudden overthrow of the old paradigm and its replacement by another. This argument may seem to work well for Vesalian anatomy or medical botany with Fuchs and Mattioli, but these breakthroughs are then followed by decades of consolidation before this new paradigm is itself changed. Indeed, the Vesalian credo that the structures of the human body should only be investigated from themselves, not from animals, faced enormous barriers and was substantially modified, and at times rejected, by many of his successors. It was an ideal that was realised at best sporadically.

But it is not just the different rhythm of change and consolidation that distinguishes the sixteenth-century investigators from those of the mid to late seventeenth, but their relationship to experience and experiment. The downgrading, rephrasing or supplementation of many ideas of their ancient predecessors by scholars such as Da Monte, Fernel and Mattioli was the result of their confrontation of what they had read or been taught with the data of their own experience. It was descriptive more than experimental, and they expected to find new information simply by observing the natural world or the human body. Paracelsus also fitted his own experiences in distillation or in mining into a new cosmology, but it was his followers at the end of the century who embarked on actual experiments that tried to go beyond what was naturally observable. They had predecessors in medieval alchemists and in some Renaissance Platonists, and their search was aimed more at producing practical benefits than new theoretical insights. Harvey's researches into the circulation and later into generation gained from his association with Fabricius and his dissection of animals, but were based on a programme of experiment that went far beyond that of his teacher. Experimentation involving precision and measurement, a major characteristic of the seventeenth century, is a long way from the qualitative reasoning of sixteenth-century physicians.

But medicine is more than biomedical science. It involves human beings whether as individuals in the patient-healer relationship or in the institutions and beliefs of the society around them. New ideas did make their way into wider public consciousness, but most people continued to believe in a modified Galenic and Aristotelian system, and, until the last third of the sixteenth century, they were treated in traditional ways with mainly herbal remedies, the so-called Galenicals. Indeed, the effect of the Renaissance was to give greater authority to this remoter past, simply because the Middle Ages could be shown to have misinterpreted many aspects of earlier medicine. The growing power of the state also encouraged the development of institutions such as hospitals, plague precautions and medical colleges at least in towns, thereby giving physicians, surgeons and apothecaries greater confidence in their own abilities and in their superiority to those who did not possess what they deemed to be appropriate knowledge. Patients could still choose how best to manage their ailments and who first to consult, but their choices were becoming more and more constrained by expectations and regulations within society at large.

In this book I have deliberately used the word kaleidoscope to emphasise the variety within medicine in the sixteenth century. But a kaleidoscope also imposes boundaries that apply to all of its pieces. By using examples drawn from across Europe, often from places that few except for locals can easily locate on a map, I have tried to give a sense of what was shared across Christian Europe and the links that might explain why, for example, a French-educated Scot could successfully agitate for the foundation of a medical college in Glasgow. Learned men could travel around Europe and make the acquaintance of famous names, and the availability of books and improved postal communications together allowed those who remained at home to have access to some of the new ideas and debates. These shared experiences were not always positive. A doctor might find himself among unwilling patients, a wife suddenly drop dead because of plague, a lady of the manor be obliged to minister to sick villagers, or a surgeon be faced with the horrid miseries of war. Adherents of Paracelsus faced a very different future in Italy and Spain compared with Northern, Protestant Europe, one of the fault lines opened up by the Reformation and Counter-Reformation. Today's Covid pandemic has also given us a limited acquaintance with what it must have once been like to face killer diseases such as plague, small-pox or the Sweat and to be subject to the harsh realities of lockdown and quarantine that, once again, have impacted most severely on those already disadvantaged.

This survey has depended on the work of many scholars who have delved into the archives and studied in the rare book rooms of libraries, yet much still remains to be done. But it will not be easy, as few today have the same fluency in humanist Latin as their predecessors or the same familiarity with European history and culture possessed by historians two or three genera-tions ago. The outlines of medicine in this period are clear, and some of the famous names have stimulated almost a scholarly industry in themselves. But beneath these generalities and highpoints, relatively little is known, and names once familiar around Europe, such as Simone Simoni, Van Foreest or Girolamo Mercuriale, are no longer remembered outside their homeland. For much of our information we are still indebted to indefatigable local historians of a century or more ago whose researches into local libraries and archives still provide a valuable base for modern historians. To balance that we may also expect more studies based on local archives, better statistics, and more investigations into the impact of medicine on literature, low as well as high. If this book encourages others to venture into this Renaissance medical jungle, its author will have succeeded in his ambition.

Notes

1 Lindemann 2010; Wear 1995, 2000.
2 Earlier, p. 172; for Ryff, Eamon 1994: 96–102.
3 Manfron 1998; Jones PM 1988, 1995; Murphy 2019: 96–121.

4 Cohn 2010.
5 French 1994, discusses this in detail.
6 Clemen 1907a; Nutton 1997a: 168–9.
7 Paracelsus 1575; Guinter 1571; Severinus 1571.
8 Thaddeus Hagecius in Gryllus 1566b: sig. D ii r; Evans 1984a: 203–4, 278–9.

Chronological Table

Date Medical Events	Date Contemporary Events
1490 Galen's *Opera Omnia* published in Latin	
	1492 Columbus's first voyage
1493 Leoniceno's *De erroribus*	
	1495 French capture of Naples
1497 Brunschwig's *De chirurgia*	
	1498 Vasco da Gama reaches India
1499 Dioscorides published in Greek	
1519 Death of Leonardo da Vinci	
1521 Berengario da Carpi's *Commentary On Mondino's Anatomy*	
	Manardi's first collection of *Medical Letters*
1525 Galen published in Greek	
	Hippocrates published in Latin
1526 Hippocrates published in Greek	
1527 Marburg University founded	
1528 London College of Physicians founded	
1530 Fracastoro's *Syphilis*	
1531 Guinter's translation of Galen's *Anatomical Procedures*	
	1536 Death of Erasmus
1540 Company of Barber-Surgeons of London founded	
1541 Death of Paracelsus	
1542 Fuchs's *De historia stirpium*	
1543 Vesalius's *De humani corporis fabrica*	
	1543 Copernicus's *De revolutionibus*
1544 Matthioli's *Commentary on Dioscorides*	
1544–5 Botanical gardens founded at Pisa and Padua	
	1545 Council of Trent begins

Date Medical Events	Date Contemporary Events
1546 Fracastoro's *De morbis contagiosis*	
	1547 Death of Henry VIII
1551 Death of Giambattista Da Monte	
	Last outbreak of the English Sweat
1552 Caius's *A counseill against the Sweate*	
1553 Servet burned at the stake in Geneva	
	1555 Pope Paul V's legislation against Jews
1557 Van Foreest becomes town physician at Delft	
	1558 Elizabeth I becomes Queen
	Death of Emperor Charles V
1559 Colombo's *De re anatomica*	Death of Henri II
1560 Fernel's *De abditis rerum causis*	
1560–81 Crato von Crafftheim imperial physician	
1561 Garcia D'Orta's *Coloquios*	
1562 Death of Falloppia	
1565 First part of Monardes's *Dos Libros*	
	Death of Conrad Gessner
	Fabricius becomes professor at Padua
	1568–71 Revolt of the Moriscos in Spain
1569 Mercuriale's *De arte gymnastica*	
1571 Severinus's *Idea medicinae philosophicae*	
	Guinter's *De medicina veteri et nova*
	1572 St Bartholomew's Day massacre in Paris
1575 Paracelsus *Opera* in Latin	
	Leiden University founded
1575–6 Great plague in Venice and Italy	
1577 The *lues Morava* in Brno	
1578 Joubert's *Erreurs populaires*	
1582 Fioravanti's *La cirurgia*	
1585 Clowes's *A briefe and necessarie practise*	
1587 Execution of Donzellini	
	1588 Defeat of the Spanish Armada
1590 Death of Paré	
1597 Tagliacozzi's *De curtorum chirurgia*	
1628 Harvey's *De motu cordis*	

Bibliography

Abbreviations

Allen: Allen PS, Allen HM and Garrod HW (1906–1947) *Opus epistolarum De. Erasmi Roterodami*. Oxford: Clarendon Press.
DBI: *Dizionario biografico degli italiani* (1960–). Rome: Treccani.
ODNB: *Oxford Dictionary of National Biography* (2004–). Oxford: Oxford University Press; online edition, consulted November 30, 2021.

Primary Sources

aa.vv. (1533) *Novae Academiae Florentinae opuscula adversus Avicennam et medicos neotericos, qui Galeni disciplina neglecta. barbaros colunt*. Venice: L. A.Giunta.
aa.vv. (1552) *Opuscules de divers autheurs médecins*. Lyons: J. de Tournes.
aa.vv. (1553) *De balneis*. Venice: Tommaso Giunta.
aa.vv. (1556) *Epistolae medicinales diversorum authorum*. Lyons: Heirs of Giacomo Giunta.
aa.vv. (1566) *Gynaeciorum: Hoc est, de mulierum tum aliis tum gravidarum, parientium et puerperarum affectibus et morbis, libri veterum et recentiorum aliquot*. Basle: T. Guarinus.
aa.vv. (1597) *Gynaeciorum sive de mulierum tum aliis tum gravidarum, parientium et puerperarum affectibus et morbis, libri Graecorum, Araborum, Latinorum veterum et recentiorum quotquot extant*. Strasbourg: L. Zetzner.
aa.vv. (1980) Epistolae academicae 1508–1596. In Mitchell WT (ed) *Oxford Historical Society*, n.s. 26. Oxford: Clarendon Press.
Achillini A (1521) *De humani corporis anatomia*. Venice: G. A. Di Sabio.
Agricola G (1550) *De precio metallorum et monetis*. Basle: H. Froben and N. Episcopius.
Agricola G (1556) *De re metallica*. Basle: H. Froben and N. Episcopius.
Alexandrinus J (1548) *Galeni enantiomaton aliquot libri*. Venice: Giunta.
Alexandrinus J (1575) *Salubrium sive de sanitate tuenda libri*. Cologne: G. Calenius.
Amatus Lusitanus JR (1551) *Curationum medicinalium centuria prima*. Florence: L. Torrentinus.
Aranzi B (1579) In *Hippocratis librum De vulneribus capitis....commentarius brevis*. Genva: J. Stoer.
Aubrey J (1962) *Brief Lives*, ed. Lawson Dick O. Harmondsworth: Penguin.
Bacci A (1572) *De thermis*. Venice: V. Valgrisi.

Baptista P (1534) *Epistolae tres*. n.p.

Bartisch G (1583) *ΟΦΘΑΘΜΟΔΟΥΛΕΙΑ. Das ist Augendienst*. Dresden: Matthes Stöckel.

Baudin C (1560) *Description et demonstration des membres interieurs de l'homme et de la femme . . . selon la vraye anatomie de André Wesal . . . Oeuvre utile & nécessaire non seulement aux Medecins & Chirurgiens, ains aussi aux Portrayeurs & Architeces*. Lyons: C. Baudin.

Bauhin C (1590) *De corporis humani fabrica: Libri IIII. Methodo anatomica in praelectionibus publicis proposita, ad Andreae Vesalii tabulas instituta: Sectionibusque publicis et privatis, comprobata*. Basle: S. Henricpetri.

Bauhin C (1602) *Introductio pulsuum synopsin continens*. Basle: L. König.

Benedetti A (1502) *Historia corporis sive Anatomice*. Venice: B. Guerraldo.

Benivieni A (1507) *De abditis nonnullis ac mirandis morborum et sanationum causis*. Florence: F. Giunta.

Bentivoglio E (1719) *Opere poetiche*. Paris: F. Furnier.

Bentivoglio E (1987) *Satire, a cura di Antonio Corsaro*. Ferrara: Deputazione provinciale Ferrarese di storia patria.

Berengario da Carpi J (1521) *Commentaria . . . super Anatomia Mundini*. Bologna: H. de Benedictis.

Berengario da Carpi J (1522) *Isagoge breves . . . in anatomiam humani corporis*. Bologna: H. de Benedictis.

Berengario da Carpi J (1529) *Galeni Pergameni libri anatomici*. Bologna: G.B. Phaelli.

Beroaldo P (1505) *De terraemotu et pestilentia*. Bologna: J. de Herberia.

Besti GF (1578) *Vera narratione del successo della peste, che afflisse l'inclita città di Milano l'anno 1576*. Milan: Paulo Gottardo & Pacifico Pontij Fratelli.

Bisciola P (1577) *Relatione verissima del progresso della peste di Milano*. Ancona and Bologna: Alessandro Benacci.

Boaistuau P (1570) *Le theatre du monde ou il est faict vn ample discours des miseres humaines*. Antwerp: C. Plantin.

Boorde A (1547) *The Breviary of Helthe, for All Manner of Syckenesses and Diseases the Whiche May Be in Man, or Woman Doth Folowe*. London: W. Middleton.

Borgarucci P (1565) *De peste*. Venice: M de Maria.

Borgarucci P (1566) *La fabrica de gli speziali*. Venice: V. Valgrisi.

Bostock R (1585) *The Difference Between the Auncient Physicke First Taught by the Godly Forefathers . . . and the Later Physicke Proceeding from Idolaters, Ethnickes and Heathens*. London: R. Walley.

Botallo L (1565) *Commentarioli duo: Alter de medico, alter de aegroti munere*. Lyons: A. Gryphius.

Bourgeois L (1626) *Observations diverses, sur la sterilité, perte de fruict, foecondité, accouchements, et maladies des femmes et enfants nouveaux-naiz*. Paris: M. Mondière.

Bourgeois L (2017) *Louise Bourgeois, Midwife to the Queen of France: Diverse Observations*, trans. O'Hara S and ed. Klairmont Lingo A. Toronto: Iter Press.

Brasavola AM (1536) *Examen omnium simplicium medicamentorum, quorum in officinis usus est*. Rome: A. Bladus de Asula.

Brasavola AM (1541) *In octo libros Aphorismorum Hippocratis et Galeni, commentaria & annotationes*. Basle: Froben.

Brasavola AM (1551) *Index refertissimus in omnes Galeni libros*. Venice: Giunta.

Brasavola AM (1561) *Examen omnium loch, id est linctuum, suffuf. Id est pulverum, aquarum, decoctionum, oleorum quorum apud Ferrariensese pharmacopolas usus est, ubi de morbo gallico . . . tractatur.* Lyons: P. Michael for S. Honoratus.

Bretonnayau R (1583) *La Generation de l'homme, et le Temple de l'âme avec Autres oeuures poëtiques extraittes de l'Esculape de René Bretonnayau.* Paris: A. L'Angelier.

Bright T (1580) *A Treatise: Wherein Is Declared the Sufficiencie of English Medicines, for Cure of All Diseases, Cured with Medicine.* London: Henrie Middleton for Thomas Man.

Brissot P (1525) *Apologetica disceptatio, qua docetur per quae loca sanguis mitti debeat in viscerum inflammationibus, praesertim in pleuritide.* Paris: S. de Colines.

Brissot P (1539) *De vena secanda . . . libellus apologeticus. Matthaei Curtii de eadem re libellus. Victoris Trincavellii . . . de eadem re rudimentum.* Venice: B. de Zanettis.

Brudus M (1544) *Liber de ratione victus in singulis febribus secundum Hippocratem . . . ad Anglos.* Venice: Heirs of P. Ravano.

Brunetto O (1548) *Lettere.* Venice: A. Arrivabene.

Brunfels O (1530) *Herbarum vivae ei coneb [sic, i.e. eicones] ad naturae imitationem, summa cum diligentia et artificio effigiatae, unà cum effectibus earundem.* Strasbourg: J. Schott.

Bullein W (1559) *A Newe Book of Physicke Called ye Government of Health. . . . Whereunto Is Annexed a Sufferain Regiment Against the Pestilence.* London: Jhon Day.

Bullein W (1564) *A Dialogue Against the Fever Pestilence.* London: Jhon Kingston.

Burton R (1624) *The Anatomy of Melancholy: What It Is.* Oxford: J. Lichfield and R. Short for H. Cripps.

Cagnati M (1581) *Variarum observationum liber.* Rome: G. Ferrarius for V. Accoltus.

Caius J (1544) *De medendi methodo libri duo, ex Cl. Galeni Pergameni & Jo. Baptistae Montani Veronensis, principum medicorum sententia.* Basle: H. Froben and G. Episcopius.

Caius J (1549) *Galeni De sanitate tuenda.* Basle: H. Froben.

Caius J (1552) *A Boke or Counseill Against the Disease Commonly Called the Sweate or Sweatyng Sicknesse.* London: R. Grafton.

Caius J (1556) *Opera aliquot et versiones, partim jam nata, partim recognita atque aucta.* Louvain: A.M. Bergagne.

Caius J (1568) *De antiquitate Cantebrigiensis academiæ libri duo, Londinensi authore: Adiunximus assertionem antiquitatis Oxoniensis academiæ, ab Oxoniensi quodam conscriptam.* London: H. Bynneman.

Caius J (1570a–c) *De canibus Britannicis, liber unus: De rariorum animalium et stirpium historia, liber unus: De libris propriis, liber unus.* London: W. Seres.

Caius J (1574a–d) *De antiquitate Cantebrigiensis academiæ libri duo, Londinensi authore: Adiunximus assertionem antiquitatis Oxoniensis academiæ, ab Oxoniensi quodam conscriptam. Historia Cantebrigiensis academiae ab urbe condita. De pronunciatione Graecae & Latinae linguae cum scriptione nova libellus.* London: J. Day [Printed together with separate paginations].

Caius J (1576) *Of Englishe Dogges, the Diuersities, the Names, the Natures and the Properties: A Short Treatise Written in Latine by Johannes Caius . . . and Newly Drawne into Englishe by Abraham Fleming.* London: Rychard Johnes.

Caius J (1904) *The Annals of Gonville and Caius College Cambridge*, ed. Venn J. Publications of the Cambridge Antiquarian Society 40. Cambridge: Cambridge Antiquarian Society.

Caius J (1912) *The Works of John Caius, M.D., Second Founder of Gonville and Caius College and Master of the College 1559–1573*, ed. Roberts ES. Cambridge: Cambridge University Press.

Canano GB (1925) *Musculorum humani corporis picturata dissectio (Ferrara 1541?)*, facsimile edition annotated. Cushing H and Streeter EC. Florence: Lier.

Canappe J (1552) *Opuscules de divers autheurs médecins, redigez ensemble pour le proufit et utilité de chirurgiens*. Lyons: J. de Tournes.

Cardano G (1555) *Geniturarum exemplar*. Lyons: T. Paganus.

Cardano G (1580) *Opus novum cunctis de sanitate tuenda, ac vita producenda studiosis apprime necessarium*. Rome: F. Zannettus.

Cardano G (1663) *Opera omnia*. Lyons: Jean Antoine Huguetan and Marc Antoine Ravaud.

Carrarius V (1581) *De medico et illius erga aegros officio*. Ravenna: Miseroccus.

Celsus (1971) *De Medicina*, with an English translation by W. G. Spencer. London: William Heinemann Ltd.

Cermisone A (1476) *Consilia medica contra omnes fere aegritudines a capite usque ad pedes*. Brescia: Henricus de Colonia.

Clowes W (1585) *A Briefe and Necessarie Treatise, Touching the Cure of the Disease called Morbus Gallicus*. London: T. East for T. Cadman.

Clowes W (1588) *A Prooued Practise for All Young Chirurgians*. London: Thomas Orwyn for Thomas Cadman.

Clowes W (1596) *A Profitable and Necessarie Booke of Observations*. London: Edm. Bollifant for Thomas Dawson.

Clowes W (1602) *A Right Frutefull and Approoved Treatise for the Artificiall Cure of That Malady Called in Latin Struma*. London: Edwarde Allde.

Clowes W (1948) *The Selected Writings of William Clowes*, ed. Poynter FNL. London: Harvey and Blythe Ltd.

Clusius C (1847) *Ad Thomam Redigerum et Carolum Clusium epistolae*, ed. Ram PFX. Brussels: M. Hayez.

Coiter V (1572) *Externarum et internarum principaliunm humani corporis partium tabulae, atque anatomicae exercitationes, observationesque variae, novis, diversis ac artificiossimis figuris illustratae*. Nuremberg: T. Gerlatzen.

Colombo R (1559) *De re anatomica*. Venice: N. Bevilacqua.

Condio L (1581) *Medicina filosofica contro la peste*. Lyons: Alessandro Marsilii.

Conte Da Monte (1591) *De morbis ex Galeni sententia*, ed. 2. Venice: G. Gueriglio.

Cornarius J (1531) *Parthenii Nicaensis De amatoriis affectionibus liber*. Basle: H. Froben and N. Episcopius.

Cornarius J (1536) *Galeni libri V jam primum in Latinam linguam conversi*. Basle: Froben.

Cornarius J (1556) *Medicina sive Medicus*. Basle: J. Oporinus.

Cortesi P (1510) *De cardinalatu*. Castel Cortesiano: S. N. Nardi.

Crassus JB (1581) *Medici antiqui graeci*. Basle: P. Perna.

Crato J (1555) *Methodus θεραπευτικη, ex sententia Galeni et Joannis Baptistae Montani*. Basle: J. Oporinus.

Crato J (1563) *In Cl. Galeni diuinos libros Methodi therapeutices Perioche methodica*. Basle: P. Perna.

Crato J (1591) *Consiliorum et epistolarum medicinalium liber ex collectaneis . . . Petri Monavii . . . selectus.* Frankfurt: Heirs of A. Wechel, C. Marnius and J. Aubrius.

Crato J (1592) *Consiliorum et epistolarum medicinalium libri II et III.* Frankfurt: Heirs of A. Wechel, C. Marnius and J. Aubrius.

Crato J (1593) *Consiliorum et epistolarum medicinalium libri IV et V.* Frankfurt: Heirs of A. Wechel, C. Marnius and J. Aubrius.

Crato J (1611) *Johannis Cratonis et aliorum medicorum consiliorum et epistularum libri VI et VII.* Hanau: Wechel.

Crato J (1619) *Johannis Cratonis et aliorum medicorum consiliorum et epistularum liber V.* Hanau: Wechel.

Curio J (1553) *Conservandae sanitatis praecepta saluberrima regi Angliae quondam a doctoribus scholae Salernitanae. . . . Per Joannem Curionem . . . recognita ac locupleta.* Frankfurt: Heirs of Chr. Egenolph.

Cuspinianus J (1553) *Austria . . . cum omnibus eiusdem marchionibus, ducibus, archiducibus, ac rebus praeclare ad haec usque tempora ab iisdem gestis.* Basle: J. Oporinus.

Daléchamps J (1569) *Les discours d'Hippocrate sur les fractures des os.* Lyons: G. Rouille.

Da Monte GB (1552) *Summaria declaratio eorum que ad urinarum cognitionem maxime faciunt, ex publicis . . . praelectionibus in Patavina schola a quodam auditore excerpta.* Vienna: Egidius Aquila.

Da Monte GB (1554a) *In libros Galeni De arte curandi ad Glauconem explanationes.* Venice: B. Constantino.

Da Monte GB (1554b) *Consultationum medicinalium centuria prima.* Venice: V. Valgrisi.

Da Monte GB (1554c) *In nonum librum Rhasis ad Mansorem exposition.* Venice: B. Constantino.

Da Monte GB (1558a) *Opuscula varia ac praeclara.* Basle: M. Isingrin for P. Perna.

Da Monte GB (1558b) *In primi libri Canonis Avicenna primam Fen, profundissima commentaria.* Venice: V. Valgrisi and B. Constantino.

Da Monte GB (1583) *Consultationes medicae . . . olim quidem Joannis Cratonis . . . opera atque studio correctae, ampliataeque, nunc vero post secundae editionem appendicem et additiones, insigni novorum consiliorum auctario ex Ludovici Demoulini . . . exornatae.* Basle: H. Petri and P. Perna.

Da Monte (1587) *Medicina Universa.* Frankfurt. Heirs of A. Wechel, C. Marnius and J. Aubrius.

De Baillou G (2021) *Les deux livres des épidémies et éphémérides de Guillaume de Baillou: Édition critique, traduction et notes par Joël Coste.* Paris: Les Belles Lettres.

De Beatis A (1979) *The Travel Journal of Antonio de Beatis. . . . 1517–1518.* London: The Hakluyt Society.

Della Porta GB (1586) *De humana physiognomia.* Vico di Sorrento: J. Cacchi.

De Rojas F (1958) *Celestina: A Play in Twenty-One Acts.* Madison: University of Wisconsin Press.

De Rojas F (1970) *Celestina.* New York: The Hispanic Society of America.

Di Montagnana B (1476) *Consilia medica.* Padua: L. Canozius.

Di Montagnana B (1497) *Consilia medica.* Venice: B. Locatellus for O. Scotus.

D'Orta G (1563) *Coloquios dos simples e drogas he cousas medicinais da India*. Goa: João de Endem.

D'Orta G (1567) *Aromatum, et simplicium aliquot medicamentorum apud Indos nascentium historia: Ant biennium quidem Lusitanica lingua per dialogos conscripta*. Antwerp: Plantin.

Driverius J (1532) *De missione sanguinis in pleuritide*. Louvain: B. Gravius.

Dryander J (1536) *Anatomia capitis humani*. Marburg: E. Cervicornus.

Dudith A (2002) *Epistulae. Pars VI: 1577–1580*. Budapest: Akadémiai Kiadó.

Du Fail N (1874) *Contes facétieuses*. Paris: P. Daffis.

Duso E (1582) *De tuenda valetudine*. Turin: Heirs of N. Bevilacqua.

Ellenbog U (1524) *Von den gifftigen Besen Tempffen vnd Reuchen der Metal*. Augsburg: Melchior Ramminger.

Elyot Sir T (1534) *The Castell of Health Gathered and Made. . . . Out of the Chiefe Authors of Physyke*. London: T. Berthelet.

Elyot Sir T (1541) *The Castell of Health. Corrected and Augmented*. London: T. Berthelet.

Eobanus Hessus H (1524) *Bonae valetudinis conseruandae praecepta*. Erfurt: E regione divi Servatii.

Erasmus D (1526) *Galeni medicorum principis Exhortatio ad bonas artes, praesertim medicinam, de optimo docendi genere, & qualem oporteat esse medicum*. Basle: J. Froben.

Erasmus D (1906–1947) *Opus epistolarum De. Erasmi Roterodami*. Oxford: Clarendon Press.

Erasmus D (1969) *Opera omnia. Ord. 1*, tomo 1. Amsterdam: North-Holland.

Erastus T (1571-3) *Disputationes de medicina nova Paracelsi, I-IV*. Basle: P. Perna.

Eustachi B (1563-4) *Opuscula anatomica*. Venice: V. Luchinus.

Eustachi B (1728) *Tabulae anatomicae*. Rome: R. Bernabò.

Falloppia G (1561) *Observationes anatomicae*. Venice: M. A. Ulmus.

Fernel J (1542) *De naturali parte medicinae*. Paris: A. Wechel.

Fernel J (1548) *De abditis rerum causis*. Paris: A. Wechel.

Fernel J (1554) *Medicina*. Paris: A. Wechel.

Fernel J (1567) *Universa medicina*. Paris: A. Wechel.

Fernel J (2003) *The Physiologia of Jean Fernel (1567)*, trans. and annotated. Forrester JM with an intro. Henry J and Forrester JM. Philadelphia: American Philosophical Society.

Fernel J (2005) *Jean Fernel's on the Hidden Causes of Things: Forms, Souls, and Occult Diseases in Renaissance Medicine, with an Edition and Translation of Fernel's De abditis rerum causis by John M. Forrester, Introduction and Annotations by John Henry and John M. Forrester*. Leiden and Boston: Brill.

Ferrand J (1610) *Traité de l'essence et guérison de l'amour ou mélancolie erotique*. Toulouse: Chez la veuve de J. Colomiez.

Ferrand J (1990) *A Treatise on Love Sickness*, trans. and ed. and with a critical introduction and notes. Beecher DA and Ciavolella M. Syracuse: Syracuse University Press.

Fioravanti L (1567) *Dello specchio di scientia universale*. Venice: Andrea Ravenoldo.

Fioravanti L (1582) *De chirugia*. Venice: Heirs of Melchior Sessa.

Foesius A (1588) *Oeconomia Hippocratis, alphabeti serie distincta: In qua dictionum apud Hippocratem omnium . . . usus explicatur . . . ita ut lexikon Hippocrateum merito dici possit*. Frankfurt: Heirs of A. Wechel, C. Marnius and J. Aubrius.

Forestus P (1591a) *De incerto, fallaci, urinarum iudicio, quo uromantes, ad perniciem multorum aegrotantium utuntur.* Leiden: F. Raphelengius.

Forestus P (1591b) *Observationum et curationum de febribus publice grassantibus . . . liber sextus: Accessit liber septimus.* . . . Leiden: Plantin for F. Raphelengius.

Forestus P (1597) *Observationum et curationum medicinalium liber XXVItus et XXVIImus: De penis, virgae, scroti et testiculorum affectionibus ac vitiis.* . . . Leiden: Plantin for F. Raphelengius.

Forestus P (1599) *Observationum et curationum medicinalium liber vigesimus octavus de mulierum morbis.* Leiden: Plantin for C. Raphelengius.

Forestus P (1610a) *Observationum et curationum chirurgicarum libri quinque.* Leiden: Ex officina Plantiniana Raphelengii.

Forestus P (1610b) *Observationum et curationum chirurgicarum libri quatuor posteriores.* Leiden: Ex officina Plantiniana Raphelengii.

Forestus P (1653) *Observationum et curationum medicinalium ac chirurgicarum opera omnia.* Rouen: J. and D. Berthelin.

Fracastoro G (1530) *Syphilis sive morbus Gallicus.* Verona: De Sabbio Brothers.

Fracastoro G (1546) *De sympathia et antipathia rerum: De contagione, contagiosis morbis et eorum curatione.* Venice: Heirs of Lucantonio Giunta.

Fracastoro G (1930) *De contagione, contagiosis morbis et eorum curatione*, trans. Wright WC. New York and London: G. P. Putnam's.

Fracastoro G (1984) *Fracastoro's Syphilis*, intro., text, trans. and notes. Eatough G. Liverpool: Francis Cairns.

Fracastoro G (2013) *Girolamo Fracastoro, Latin Poetry*, trans. Gardner J. Cambridge, MA and London: Harvard University Press.

Franco P (1895) *Chirurgie de Pierre Franco de Turriers en Provence composée en 1561, nouvelle edition.* . . Paris: Félix Alcan.

Fryer J (1567) *Hippocratis Aphorismi versibus scripti.* London: W. Seres.

Fuchs L (1531) *Compendiaria ac succincta admodum in artem medendi. . . . introductio.* Hagenau: J. Secerius.

Fuchs L (1541) *Methodus seu ratio compendiaria cognoscendi veram solidamque medicinam.* Lyons: S. Gryphius.

Fuchs L (1542) *De historia stirpium commentarii insignes.* Basle: J. Isingrin.

Galen (1490) *Opera omnia.* Venice: P. Pincius.

Galen (1502) *Opera omnia.* Venice: B. Benalius.

Galen (1517) *De sanitate tuenda*, trans. Linacre T. Paris: D. Mattheu for G. Hittorp.

Galen (1519) *Methodus medendi*, trans. Linacre T. Paris: D. Mattheu for G. Hittorp.

Galen (1525) *Opera omnia.* Venice: Heirs of Aldus.

Galen (1536) *Antidotarius liber. . . . translatus a Josepho Struthio . . . Galeni Astrologiae ad Aphrodiseum liber unus, Galeni De urinis liber unus.* Venice: J. A. Nicolini de Sabio.

Galen (1538) *Opera omnia, ad fidem complurium & perquam vetustorum exemplariorum ita emendata atque restituta, ut nunc primum nata, atque in lucem aedita, uideri possint.* Basle: Cratander.

Galen (1541–1542) *Opera quae extant omnia.* Venice: Giunta.

Galen (1541–1545) *Opera omnia.* Venice: G. Farri and Brothers.

Galen (1542) *Opera.* Basle: H. Frobenius and N. Episcopius.

Galen (1549) *Opera quae ad nos extant omnia.* H. Froben and N. Episcopius.

Galen (1565) *Opera quae extant omnia.* Venice: Giunta.

Galen (1956) *Galen On Anatomical Procedures: Translation of the Surviving Books by Charles Singer*. London, Oxford and New York: Oxford University Press.

Galen (1962) *Galen on Anatomical Procedures: The Later Books*, trans. Duckworth WHL, Lyons MC and Towers B. Cambridge: Cambridge University Press.

Galen (1968) *On the Usefulness of the Parts of the Human Body*, trans. May MT, vol. 2. Ithaca: Cornell University Press.

Gallus P (1950) *Bibliotheca medica, sive catalogus illorum qui ex professo Artem Medicam in hunc usque annum scriptis illustrarunt*. Basle: Conrad Waldkirch.

Gaurico L (1546) *Super diebus decretoriis . . . axiomata. . . . Isagogicus astrologiae tractatus medicis admodum opportunus*. Rome: V. & L. Doricus.

Geminus T (1545) *Compendiosa totius anatomiae delineatio aere exarata*. London: J. Herdford.

Geminus T (1955) *Compendiosa totius anatomie delineatio: A facsimile of the first English edition of 1553 in the version of Nicholas Udall*. London: Dawson's.

Gessner C (1545) *Bibliotheca Universalis*. Zurich: C. Froschover.

Gessner C (1554) *Thesaurus Euonymi Philiatri de remediis secretis, liber physicus, medicus, et partim etiam chymicus*. Zurich: A. Gesner.

Gessner C (1555a) *Appendix Bibliothecae Universalis*. Zurich: C. Froschover.

Gessner C (1555b) *De chirurgia scriptores optimi quique veteres et recentiores*. Zurich: A. and J. Gesner.

Gessner C (1559) *The Treasure of Euonymus, Conteyninge the Wonderfull Hid Secretes of Nature, Touchinge the Most Apte Formes to Prepare and Destyl Medicines, for the Conservation of Health*. London: John Daye.

Gessner C (1569) *Euonymus . . . de remediis secretis . . . Liber secundus nunc primum opera et studio Gaspari Wolfii in lucem editus*. Zurich: C. Froschover.

Gessner C (1576) *The New Jewell of Health*. London: H. Denham.

Gessner C (1577) *Epistolae medicinales*. Zurich: C. Froschover.

Gessner C (1581) *Enchiridion rei medicae triplicis*. Zurich: J. Gesner.

Gilino C (1497) *De morbo gallico*. Ferrara: L. de Rubeis.

Gilino GG (1937) *La relazione ai deputati dell'Ospedale Grande di Milano*, ed. Spinelli S. Milan: Tipografia Antonio Cordani.

Grisignano P (1543) *De pulsibus et urinis*. Salerno: Alifano Cilio.

Gross D and Steinmetzer J (2006) *Volcher Coiter (1534–1576) und die Konstituierung ärztlicher Autorität in der Vormoderne*. Aachen: Shaker Verlag.

Gryllus L (1566a) *De sapore*. Prague: G. Melantrich.

Gryllus L (1566b) *Oratio de peregrinatione studii medicinalis ergo suscepta*. Prague: G. Melantrich.

Guillemeau J (1609) *De l'heureux accouchement des femmes*. Paris: N. Buon.

Guinter J (1536) *Institutionum anatomicarum secundum Galeni sententiam ad candidatos medicinae libri quatuor*. Paris: S. de Colines.

Guinter J (1539) *Institutionum anatomicarum libri*. Basle: Robert Winter.

Guinter J (1571) *De medicina vetere et nova facienda commentarii*. Basle: P. Perna.

Guinter J and Vesalius A (1538) *Institutionum anatomicarum secundum Galeni sententiam . . . libri . . . Ab Andrea Wesalio Bruxellensi auctiores et emendatiores redditi*. Venice: D. Bernardino.

Guinter J and Vesalius A (2019) *Principles of Anatomy According to the Opinion of Galen*, trans. Nutton V. London and New York: Routledge.

Hart J (1623) *The Arraignement of Urines*. London: G. Ent for R. Mylbourne.

Harvey W (1628) *Exercitatio anatomica de motu cordis et sanguinis in animalibus.* Frankfurt: G. Fitzer.

Herberstein S (1871–2) *Notes upon Russia: Being a Translation of the Earliest Account of That Country, Entitled Rerum Moscoviticarum commentarii, by the Baron Sigismund von Herberstein,* ed. and trans. Major RH. London: The Hakluyt Society.

Hippocrates (1525) *Octaginta volumina . . . nunc tandem per Fabium Calvum Rhavennatem latinitate donata.* Rome: F. M. Calvus.

Hippocrates (1526) *Opera omnia.* Venice: Aldus and A. Asulanus.

Hippocrates (1588) *Opera quae extant, graece et latine . . . scholiis illustrata.* Venice: Giunta.

Hippocrates (1595) *Opera omnia quae extant: Nunc recens Latina interpretatione illustrata.* Frankfurt: Heirs of A. Wechel, C. Marnius and J. Aubrius.

Hrubetius P (1610) *Theses de peregrinatione.* Basle: J. J. Genath.

Huniadinus F (1586) *Ephemeron seu Itinerarium Bathoreum.* Cracow: Officina Lazari.

Ingrassia GF (1552) *De tumoribus praeter naturam.* Naples: M. Cancer.

Jasolino G (1576) *De aqua in pericardio.* Naples: O. Salvioni.

Jessen J (1595) *De domino Martino Biermanno . . . oratio.* Wittenberg: W. Meissner.

Jordanus T (1580) *Luis novae in Moravia exortae descriptio.* Frankfurt: A. Wechel.

Joubert L (1587) *La premiere et seconde partie des Erreurs populaires touchant la medecine* et le regime de santé. Paris: C. Micard.

Joubert L (1989) *Popular Errors,* trans. and annotated. de Rocher GD. Tuscaloosa and London: The University of Alabama Press.

Joubert L (1995) *The Second Part of the Popular Errors,* trans. and annotated. de Rocher GD. Tuscaloosa and London: The University of Alabama Press.

Junius H (1577) *Nomenclator omnium rerum.* Antwerp: C. Plantin.

Karlstadt von Bodenstein A (1557) *Wie sich meniglich dem Cyperlin podagra genennet waffnen solle. Unnd Bericht diser* Kreüter, so den himmelischen zeichen Zodiaci zugeachnet. Basle: B. Stähälin.

Karlstadt von Bodenstein A (1559) *Isagoge excellentissimi philosophi Arnoldi de Villa Nova, Rosarium, Chimicum.* Basle: G. Ringysen.

Kellwaye S (1593) *A Defensative Against the Plague.* London: J. Windet.

La Framboisière NA (1595a) *Canonum medicinalium libri tres.* Paris: M. Sonnius.

La Framboisière NA (1595b) *Les canons requis pour practiquer methodiquement la chirurgie.* Paris: M. Sonnius.

La Framboisière NA (1609) *L'estat des parties du corps humain, methodiquement dressé.* Paris: D. Langlois.

Laguna A (1536) *Anatomica methodus, seu de sectione humani corporis contemplatio.* Paris: J. Kerver.

Laguna A (1554) *Epitome omnium rerum et sententiarum, quae annotatu dignae in Commentariis Galeni in Hippocratem extant . . . Cui accessere nonnulla Galeni Enantiomata.* Lyons: G. Rouille.

Lange J (1589) *Epistolarum medicinalium volume tripartitum.* Frankfurt: A. Wechel.

Langton C (1547) *A Very Brefe Treatise Ordrely Declaring the Principal Partes of Physick, That Is to Say: – Thynges Naturall, Thynges Not Naturall, Thynges Against Nature.* London: Edward Whitchurch.

Langton C (undated) *An Introduction into Physicke, with an Universal Dyet.* London: E(dward) W(hitchurch).

Le Forestier T (1494?) *Tractatus contra pestilentiam, tenesmon et dysenteriam.* Rouen: G. Le Tailleur.

Leoniceno N (1492) *De Plinii et aliorum in medicina erroribus.* Ferrara: L. de Rubeis and A. de Grassis.

Leoniceno N (1497) *De epidemia quam morbum gallicum vocant.* Venice: Aldus Manutius.

Leoniceno N (1506) *De virtute formativa.* Venice: B. Locatellus.

Leoniceno N (1508) *In libros Galeni e greca in linguam latinam a se translatos prefatio communis. . . . De tribus doctrinis ordinatis secundum Galeni opus.* Venice: J. Pentius de Leucho.

Leoniceno N (1509) *De Plinii et plurium aliorum medicorum in medicina erroribus.* Ferrara: J. Macciochius.

Liébault J (1577) *Thesaurus sanitatis paratu facilis.* Paris: J. Du Puys.

Liébault J (1582a) *Trois livres de la santé, foecondité et maladies des femmes.* Paris: J. Du Puys.

Liébault J (1582b) *Trois livres de l'embellissement et ornement du corps humain.* Paris: J. Du Puys.

Lowe P (1597) *A Course of the Whole Art of Chyrurgerie Whereunto Is Annexed the Presages of Devyne Hyppocrates.* London: Thomas Purfoot.

Luisinus A (1566–7) *De morbo gallico omnia quae extant.* Venice: J. Zilettus.

Luther M (1967) Table Talk. In *Luther's Works,* ed. and tr. Tappert TG, vol. 54. Philadelphia: Westminster Press.

Lycosthenes C (1557a) *Prodigiorum ac ostentorum chronicon, quae praeter naturae ordinem, motum et operationem, et in superioribus et his inferioribus mundi regionibus ab exordio mundi usque ad haec nostra tempora, acciderunt.* Basle: H. Petri.

Lycosthenes C (1557b) *Wunderwerck oder Gottes unergründtliches Vorbilden, das er inn seinen gschöpffen allen, so geystlichen, so leyblichen in Fewr, Lufft, Wasser, Erden. . . . von Anbegin der Weldt, bisz zu unserer diser Zeit erscheynen, hören, brieven lassen.* Basle: H. Petri.

Lygaeus J (1555) *De humani corporis harmonia libri iiii.* Paris: J. Vascosanus.

Machiavelli N (1979) *Il principe e Discorsi.* Milan: Feltrinelli Economica.

Machiavelli N (2019) *Epistola della peste: Edizione critica secondo il ms, banco rari 29, a cura di Pasquale Stoppelli.* Rome: Edizioni di Storia e Letteratura.

Maggi B (1552) *De vulneribus sclopetorum.* In aa.vv. *Epistolae medicinales diversorum authorum.* Lyons: Heirs of Giacomo Giunta.

Manardi G (1556) *Epistolae medicinales.* Bologna: B. Bonardus.

Malingre M (1533) *Moralite de la maladie de chrestiente.* Paris: P. de Vingle.

Marcellus Virgilius A (1518) *Pedacii Dioscoridae Anazarbei De medica materia.* Florence: F. Giunta and Sons.

Marchant J (1598) *In Fr. Rosetti Apologiam, Declamatio.* Paris: Nicolaus Delouvain.

Marguerite de Navarre (1946) *Théâtre profane.* Geneva: Droz.

Martius H (1568) *Nonni medici clarissimi de omnium morborum curatione.* Strasbourg: J. Rihel.

Massa N (1536) *Anatomiae liber introductorius.* Venice: F. Bindoni and M. Pasini.

Massa N (1550) *Epistolae medicinales et philosophicae.* Venice: F. Bindoni and M. Pasini.

Mattioli PA (1544) *Libri cinque della historia et materia medica.* Venice: N. de Bascarini.

Mattioli PA (1550) *Il Dioscoride . . . con li suoi discorsi. . . . la seconda volta illustrati et diligentissime ampliati*. Venice: V. Valgrisi.

Mattioli PA (1554) *Commentarii in libros sex Pedacii Dioscoridis Anazarbei, de materia medica*. Venice: V. Valgrisi.

Mattioli PA (1561) *Epistularum medicinalium libri quinque*. Prague: G. Melantrich for V. Valgrisi.

Mattioli PA (1562) *Herbař: Ginak Bylínař*. Prague: G. Melantrich.

Mattioli PA (1573) *Il Dioscoride . . . con li suoi discorsi. . . . Hora di nuovo dal suo autore ricorretti, & in più di mille luoghi aumentati. . .* Venice: V. Valgrisi.

Mattioli PA (1583) *Commentarii in libros sex Pedacii Dioscoridis Anazarbei, de materia medica*. Venice: V. Valgrisi.

Melanchthon P (1540) *Commentarius de Anima*. Wittenberg: P. Seitz.

Melanchthon P (1977–) *Briefwechsel: Kritische und kommentierte Gesamtausgabe*. Stuttgart and Bad Cannstatt: Verlag Frommann-Holzboog.

Mercuriale G (1571) *Variarum lectionum libri quatuor*. Venice: G. Perchacinus for P. and A. Meietus.

Mercuriale G (1577) *De pestilentia*. Venice: P. Meietus.

Mercuriale G (1569) *Artis gymnasticae apud antiquos celeberrimae, nostris temporibus ignotae, libri sex*. Venice: Giunta.

Mercuriale G (1601) *De arte gymnastica*, ed. 5. Venice: Giunta.

Mercuriale G (2008) *De arte gymnastica*. Florence: Leo S. Olschki.

Mercuriale G and Crato von Krafftheim J (2016) *Une correspondance entre deux humanistes*, ed. Agasse JM and Pennuto C. Geneva: Droz.

Mercurio S (1601) *La commare o raccoglitrice*. Venice: G. B. Ciotti.

Milanesi G (ed) (1875) *Le lettere di Michelangelo Buonarotti*. Florence: Successori Le Monnier.

Mitchell WT (ed) (1980) *Epistolae academicae 1508–1596, Oxford Historical Society*, n.s. 26. Oxford: Clarendon Press.

Mizauld A (1551) *Planetologia, rebus astronomicis, medicis et philosophicis erudite referta*. Lyons: J. des Tournes.

Moffet T (1588) *Nosomantica Hippocratea, sive Hippocratis prognostica cuncta*. Frankfurt: Heirs of A. Wechel, C. Marnius and J. Aubrius.

Monacius JJ (1560) *Tres excellente & novelle description contre la peste & un remede tres singulier*. London: T. Purfoot.

Monardes N (1580) *Primera y segunda y tercera partes de la historia medicinal de las cosas que se traen de nuestras Indias Occidentales....* Seville: F. Diaz.

Mondino de' Liuzzi (1992) *Anothomia*, ed. Giorgi PP and Pasini GF. Bologna: Istituto per la Storia dell' Università di Bologna.

Montaigne M de (1955) *Journal de voyage en Italie par la Suisse et l'Allemagne en 1580 et 1581*, ed. Rat M. Paris: Classiques Garnier.

Montuus S (1537) *Dialexeis medicinales*. Lyons: J. Barbous.

Morel T (1528) *Tredecim orationes encomiasticae habitae Parisiis, Anno M.D. XXIII*. Paris: N. Savetier.

Moryson F (1903) *Itinerary*, ed. Hughes C. London: Sherratt and Hughes.

Mulcaster R (1581) *Positions Wherein Those Primitiue Circumstances Be Examined: Which Are Necessarie for the Training Up of Children Either for Their Skill in Their Booke or Health in Their Bodie*. London: T. Vautrollier for T. Chard.

Mulcaster R (1887) *Positions Wherein Those Primitiue Circumstances Be Examined: Which Are Necessarie for the Training up of Children Either for Their Skill in Their booke or Health in Their Bodie*. London: Harrison and Sons.

Orozco C (1540) *Annotationes in Interpretationes Aetii medici*. Basle: R. Winter.

Panizza L (1561) *De venaesectione in inflammationibus*. Venice: F. Camozzi.

Paracelsus von Hohenheim (1549) *Wundt und Leibarznei . . . Dabei von Auszziehung der fünften Wesenheit, Quinta Essentia, ausz bewerten Stucken der Arznei, zu wunderbarer Heylung leiblicher Gebrechen*. Frankfurt: C. Egenolff.

Paracelsus von Hohenheim (1560) *Libri quatuor de vita longa. Diligentia et opera Adami a Bodenstein recogniti*. Basle: n.p.

Paracelsus von Hohenheim T (1567) *Von der Bergsucht oder Bergkranckheiten*. Dillingen: S. Mayer.

Paracelsus von Hohenheim (1571) *De spiritibus planetarum sive metallorum. . . . Georg. Phedronis Rhodochaei pestis Epdemicae curatio*. Basle: P. Perna.

Paracelsus von Hohenheim (1575) *Operum latinorum redditorum tomus I (-II)*. Basle: P. Perna.

Paracelsus von Hohenheim T (1577a) *Von den Frantzosen*. Basle: P. Perna.

Paracelsus von Hohenheim T (1577b) *Aurora Thesaurusque philosophorum*. Basle: T. Guarinus.

Paracelsus von Hohenheim T (1603) *Erster (-zehender) Theil der Bücher und Schrifften*. Frankfurt: J. Wechel.

Paracelsus von Hohenheim T (1922–1933) *Theophrast von Hohenheim/Paracelsus: Sämtliche Werke I. Abteilung. Medizinische, naturwissentschaftliche und philosophische Schriften*, ed. Sudhoff K. Munich and Berlin: R. Oldenbourg.

Paracelsus von Hohenheim T (1941) *Four Treatises of Theophrastus von Hohenheim Called Paracelsus*, trans. Temkin CL, Rosen G, Zilboorg G and Sigerist HE. Baltimore and London: The Johns Hopkins University Press.

Paracelsus von Hohenheim T (1955–1986) *Theophrast von Hohenheim/Paracelsus: Sämtliche Werke II. Abteilung. Theologische und religionsphilosophische Schriften*, ed. K. Goldammer. Wiesbaden: Fritz Steiner Verlag.

Paracelsus von Hohenheim T (2008) *Paracelsus (Theophrastus Bombastus von Hohenheim 1493–1541) Essential Theoretical Writings*, ed. and trans. with a Commentary and intro. Weeks A. Leiden and Boston: Brill.

Paré A (1545) *La Maniere de traicter les playesn faictes tant par hacquebutes et aultres bastons a feu*. Paris: V. Gaultherot.

Paré A (1552) *La Maniere de traicter les playes faictes tant par hacquebutes que par fleches*. Paris: A. L'Angelie.

Paré A (1573) *Deux livres de chirurgie . . . II: Des monstres tant terrestres que marins avec leurs portraits*. Paris: A. Wechel.

Paré A (1585) *Oeuvres*. Paris G. Buon.

Paré A (1840–1) *Oeuvres complètes d'Ambroise Paré revues et collationnées . . . par J-F. Malgaigne*. Paris and London: Baillière.

Paré A (1968) *The Apologie and Treatise of Ambroise Paré Containing the Voyages Made unto Divers Places with Many of His Writings*. New York: Dover Publications Inc.

Paré A (1982) *Ambroise Paré, on Monsters and Marvels*, trans. Palliser JL. Chicago: The University of Chicago Press.

Peucer C (1554a) *Propositiones de causis liberarum actionum hominis ethicis et physicis*. Wittenberg: J. Crato.

Peucer C (1554b) *Propositiones de coctionibus et anni ratione.* Wittenberg: J. Crato.

Peucer C (1555) *Propositiones de origine et causis succini Prussiaci.* Wittenberg: J. Crato.

Peucer C (1557) *Propositiones de principiis rerum physicis.* Wittenberg: J. Crato.

Piccolomini A (1586) *Praelectiones anatomicae.* Rome: B. Bonfadinus.

Pictorius G (1550) *Dialogi...del modo di conservare la sanita.* Venice: V. Valgrisi.

Platter F (1583) *De corporis humani structura et usu.* Basle: A. Froben.

Platter F (1987) *Beschreibung der Stadt Basel 1610 und Pestbericht 1610/11, Basler Chroniken, Band 11.* Basle and Stuttgart: Schwabe & Co. AG Verlag.

Pratensis J (1527) *De pariente et partu.* Antwerp: n.p.

Previdelli G (1524) *Tractatus legalis de peste.* Bologna: J. B. Phaellus.

Purkircher G (1988) *Opera quae supersunt omnia,* ed. Okál M. Budapest: Akadémiai Kiadó.

Rabelais F (1532) *Hippocratis Aphorismi.* Paris: Gryphius.

Rabelais F (1944) *The Five Books of Gargantua and Pantagruel in the Modern Translation of Jacques Le Clerq.* New York: Random House.

Rabelais F (1964) *Le tiers livre.* Geneva: Librairie Droz.

Rauwolf L (1582) *Aigentliche Beschreibung der Raiss inn die Morgenländer.* Lauingen: Leonhard Reinmichel.

Ripa FJ de N (1538) *De peste.* Lyons: V. de Portonaris.

Rogano, L (1560) *De urinis libri III.* Tome: I. Salviani.

Rosario N (1572) *Contradictiones, dubia et paradoxa in libros Hippocratis, Celsi, Galeni, Aetii, Aeginetae, Avicennae: Cum eorundem conciliationibus.* Venice: F and G. Bindonus.

Roseler M (1554) *Aphorismi Hyppocrtatis carmine redditi.* Rostock: L. Ditius.

Rossi G (1572) *Historiarum Ravennatum libri decem.* Venice: Aldus Manutius the Younger.

Rousset F (1581) *Traitté nouveau de l'hystérotomotokie, ou enfantement Caesarien.* Paris: Denys du Val.

Sanches F (1581) *Quod nihil scitur.* Lyons: S. Gryphius.

Sanseverino F (1561) *Delle cento novelle scelte dai piu nobili scrittori.* Venice: F. Sansovino.

Sassonia E (1604) *De pulsibus tractatus absolutissimus, omnibus medicinae studiosis apprime necessarius & vtilis.* Frankfurt: Z. Palthenius.

Schiller J (1531) *De peste Britannica commentariolus vere aureus.* Basle: H. Petri.

Schmaus L (1518) *Lucubratiuncula de morbo Gallico et cura ejus noviter reperta cum ligno Indico.* Augsburg: S. Grimm and M. Wyrsung.

Scholz L (1610a) *Consiliorum medicinalium . . . liber.* Hanau: Heirs of J. Aubrius.

Scholz L (1610b) *Epistolarum philosophicarum: Medicinalium ac chymicarum a summis nostrae aetais philoophis ac medicis exaratarum volumen.* Hanau: Heirs of J. Aubrius.

Schrauf K (1899) *Acta facultatis medicae Universitatis Vindobonensis,* vol. II. Vienna: Auf Verlassung des medizinischen Doktorenkollegiums.

Schroeter J (1550) *De idea hippocraticae doctrinae.* Vienna: Egidius Aquila.

Servetus M (1553) *Christianismi Restitutio.* Lyons.

Severinus P (1571) *Idea medicinae philosophicae.* Basle: A. Henricpetri.

Severinus P (1979) *Petrus Severinus og hans Idea medicinae philosophicae,* trans. Skov H. Odense: Universitetsforlag.

Simoni S (1576) *Artificiosa curandae pestis methodus.* Leipzig: J. Steinmann.

Spach I (1591) *Nomenclator scriptorum medicorum, hoc est, elenchus qui artem medicam suis scriptis illustrarunt, secundum locos communes ipsius medicinae conscriptus*. Frankfurt: M. Lechler.

Spach I (1597) *Gynaeciorum sive de mulierum tum communibus, tum gravidarum, parientium, et puerperarum affectibus et morbis, libri Graecorum, Arabum, Latinorum veterum et recentium quotquot extant*. Strasbourg: L. Zetzner.

Stephanus C (1545) *De dissectione partium corporis humani*. Paris: S. de Colines.

Stephanus C (1546) *La dissection des parties du corps humain*. Paris: S. de Colines.

Struthius J (1555) *Sphygmicae artis iam mille ducentos annos perditae & desideratae*. Basle: J. Oporinus.

Sylvius J (1539) *Ordo et ordinis ratio in legendis Hippocratis et Galeni libris*. Paris: S. de Colines.

Sylvius J (1551) *Vaesani cujusdam calumniarum in Hippocratis Galenique anatomicam depulsio*. Paris: C. Barbé and the widow of I. Gazellus.

Sylvius J (1555) *In Hippocratis et Galeni physiologiae partem anatomicam Isagoge*. Paris: J. Hulpeau.

Tabernaemontanus JT (1564) *Gewisse unnd erfahren Practick, wie man, vor der Pestilentz hüten und bewaren*. Heidelberg: J. Mayer.

Tagliacozzi G (1597) *De curtorum chirurgia per insitionem*. Venice: G. Bindoni, jr.

Tarchagnota G (1549) *Galeno: A che guisa si possano, e conoscere, e curare le infirmità del'animo*. Venice: M. Tramezzino.

Thurneisser L (1574) *Quinta Essentia*. Munster: J. Ossenbruck,.

Tiraqueau A (1561) *Commentarii de nobilitate et jure primigeniorum*. Basle: Froben.

Trincavella V (1585) *Consiliorum medicinalium libri III: Epistolarum medicinalium libri III . . . Duae quaestiones*. Venice: C. Borgominerius.

Trincavella V (1586) *Omnia opera*. Lyons: Giunta and Guittius.

Trincavella V (1587) *Consilia medica . . . accessione CXXVIII consiliorum locupletata . . . Epistolae item philosophicis et medicis quaestiones insignitae expolitaeque*. Basle: C. Waldkirch.

Turinus A (1545) *Opera*. Rome: H. de Cartulariis.

Turner W (1551) *A New Herball*. London: S. Mierdman for J. Gybken.

Turner W (1562) *The Seconde Parte of William Turners Herball. . . . Here unto Is Joyned also a Book of the Bath of Baeth in England, and of the Vertues of the Same Wyth Diverse Other Bathes Most Holsum and Effectuall, Both in Almany and Englande*. Cologne: A. Birckman.

Valla G (1498) *Nicephori logica. . . . Rhazes de pestilentia, Galenus de inequali distemperantia, Galenus de bono corporis habitu, Galenus de confirmatione corporis humani, Galenus de praesagitura, Galenus de praesagio, Galeni introductorium, Galenus de succedaneis, Alexander Aphrodiseus de causis febrium, Psellus de victu humano*. Venice: S. Bevilaqua.

Valla G (1501) *De expetendis et fugiendis rebus*. Venice: Aldus Manutius.

Valles F (1556) *Controversiae medicae et philosophicae*. Alcalá: J. Brocar.

Valles F (1582) *Controversiae medicae et philosophicae, editio tertia ab eodem auctore denuo recognita et aucta*. Frankfurt: A. Wechel.

Valles F (1588) *De urinis, pulsibus ac febribus compendiariae tractationes*. Turin: Heirs of N. Bevilacqua.

Valleriola F (1573) *Observationes medicinales*. Lyons: A. Gryphius.

Valverde de Hamusco J (1556) *Historia de la composicion del cuerpo humano.* Rome: A. Salamanca and A. Lafreri.

Vasari G (1984) *Lives of the Artists.* Harmondsworth: Penguin.

Vernay P (1552) *Opuscules de divers autheurs médecins.* Lyons: J. de Tournes.

Vesalius A (1537) *Paraphrasis in nonum librum Rhazae medici Arabis clariss.* Louvain: R. Rescius.

Vesalius A (1538) *Tabulae Anatomicae Sex.* Venice: B. Vitalis.

Vesalius A (1539) *Epistola, docens venam axillarem dextri cubiti in dolore laterali secandam.* Basle: R. Winter.

Vesalius A (1544) *De humani corporis fabrica.* Basle: J. Oporinus.

Vesalius A (1546) *Epistola, rationem modumque propinandi radicis Chynae decocti . . . pertractans.* Basle: J. Oporinus.

Vesalius A (1551) *Anatomia deudsch, ein kurtzer Auszug der Beschreibung aller Glider menschlichs Leibs.* Nuremberg: J. P. Fabricius.

Vesalius A (1552) *De humani corporis fabrica.* Lyons: J. de Tournes.

Vesalius A (1555) *De humani corporis fabrica.* Basle: J. Oporinus.

Vesalius A (1564) *Anatomicarum Gabrielis Falloppii observationum examen.* Venice: Francesco di Franceschis.

Vesalius A (1568) *De humani corporis fabrica.* Venice: Francesco di Franceschis.

Vesalius A (1998–2009) *Vesalius, on the Fabric of the Human Body*, trans. Richardson WF and Carman JB. Novato, CA: Norman Publishing.

Vesalius A (2014) *Andreas Vesalius, the Fabric of the Human Body*, trans. Garrison DH and Hast MH. Basle: Karger.

Vesalius A (2015) *Vesalius: The China Root Epistle*, a new trans. and critical ed. Garrison DH. Cambridge: Cambridge University Press.

Veyras J, Guilhemet T and Joubert L (1581) *Traicte de chirurgie contenant la vraye methode de gverir playes d'arquebusade, selon Hippocrate, Galien & Paracelse.* Lyons: B. Barthélemy.

Vidius V (1544) *Chirurgia e graeco in latinum conversa.* Paris: P. Galterius.

Vigo G de (1514) *Practica in chirurgia, Practica in arte chirurgica copiosa.* Rome: S. Guilaneti and E. di Bologna.

Villamont J (1600) *Les voyages du Seigneur de Villamont.* Paris: C. de Montr'oeil and J. Richer.

Virdung JH (1532) *Nova medicinae methodus . . . ex mathematica ratione morbos curandi.* Ettlingen: V. Kobian.

Virdung JH (1584) *De cognoscendis et medendis morbis ex corporum coelestium positione Libri III. Cum argumentis et expositionibus Joannis Pauli Gallucii Soensis . . . Quibus accesserunt in eandem sententiam auctores alii.* Venice: D. Zenarius.

Vives JL (1555) *De anima.* Lyons: J. Frellon.

Von Gersdorff H (1517) *Feldtbuch der Wundartzney.* Strasbourg: Johannes Schott.

Von Hutten U (1519) *De guaiaci medicina et morbo gallico.* Mainz: J. Scheffer.

Von Hutten U (2015) *De guaiaci medicina et morbo gallico*, ed. Gauvin B. Paris: Les Belles Lettres.

Wecker JJ (1576) *Medicinae utriusque syntaxes ex Graecorum, Latinorum Arabumque thesauris . . . singulari fide, methodo ac industria collectae & concinnatae.* Basle: E. Episcopius and the Heirs of N. Episcopius.

Wecker JJ (1582) *De secretis libri XVII.* Basle: P. Perna.

Wecker JJ (1585) *A Compendious Chyrurgerie Gathered & Translated Especially Out of Wecker . . . with Certaine Annotations, Resolutions and Supplyes.* London: J. Winder for T. Man and W. Brome.

Weckerin A (1598) *Eine Köstlich New Kochbuch von allerhand Speisen . . . Nie allein vor Gesunde: Sondern auch und fürnehmlich vor Krancke in allerley Kranckheiten und Gebrästen: Auch Schwangere Weiber, Kindbetterinnen und alter schwache Leute.* Amberg: Michael Forster 1597.

Weyer J (1563) *De praestigiis daemonum et incantationibus ac veneficiis.* Basle: J. Oporinus.

Weyer J (1567) *Medicarum observationum rarum liber I.* Basle: J. Oporinus.

Weyer J (1583) *Arztney Buch: Von etlichen bisz anher unbekandten unnd unbeschrieben Kranckheiten.* Frankfurt: N. Bassee.

Weyer J (1991) *Witches, Devils and Doctors in the Renaissance, Johann Weyer, De praestigiis daemonum,* trans. Mora G. Binghamton, NY: Medieval & Renaissance Texts and Studies.

Zerbi G (1502) *Liber anathomiae corporis humani et singulorum membrorum illius.* Venice: B. Locatello.

Zum Trübel E (1528) *Ein vetterliche, gedruge gute zucht, lere und bericht christlich zu leben und sterben, an meine kynder und alle frumme Christen.* Strasbourg: n.p.

Zwinger T (1577) *Methodus apodemica.* Basle: E. Episcopius.

Zwinger T (1579) *Hippocratis Coi . . . viginti duo commentarii. . . . Sententiae insignes per locos communes methodice digestae.* Basle: E. Episcopius.

Zwinger T (1586–1587) *Theatrum humanae vitae.* Basle: E. Episcopius.

Zwinger T (1610) *Physiologia medica.* Basle: S. Henricpetri.

Secondary Literature

Abreu L (2020) Health Care and the Spread of Medical Knowledge in the Portuguese Empire, Particularly the Estado da India (Sixteenth to Eighteenth Centuries). In *Medical History* 64: 449–66.

Adelmann HM (1966) *Marcello Malpighi and the Evolution of Embryology.* Ithaca: Cornell University Press.

Agasse JM (2002–3) La bibliothèque d'un médecin humaniste: L'index librorum de Girolamo Mercuriale. In *Les Cahiers de l'humanisme* 3–4: 201–53.

Agasse JM (2006) *Girolamo Mercuriale, De arte gymnastica: L'art de la gymnastique.* Paris: Les Belles Lettres.

Agasse JM and Pennuto C (eds) (2016) *Girolamo Mercuriale, Johann Crato von Krafftheim: Une correspondance entre deux médecins humanistes.* Geneva: Droz.

Agrimi J and Crisciani C (1988) *Edocere medicos: Medicina scolastica nei secoli XIII–XV.* Naples: Guerini e Associati.

Agrimi J and Crisciani C (1994) *Les Consilia médicaux.* Turnhout: Brepols.

Allen P (1985) *The Concept of Woman: The Aristotelian Revolution 750 B.C-AD 1250.* Montreal: Eden.

Andreoni L and Fortuna S (2019) Nuovi contributi su Amato Lusitano e Ancona (1547–1555). In González Manjarrés MA (ed) *Amato Lusitano y la medicina de su tiempo.* Madrid: Escolar y Mayo: 101–21.

Andretta E (2011) *Roma medica: Anatomie d'un système médical au XVIᵉ siècle.* Rome: Ecole française de Rome.

Andretta E and Pardo-Tomás J (2019) Books, Plants, Herbaria: Diego Hurtado de Mendoza and His Circle in Italy (1539–1554). In *History of Science* 57: 1–25.

Ankarloo B, Clark S and Monter EW (2002) *Witchcraft and Magic in the Period of the Witch Trials: Athlone History of Witchcraft and Magic in Europe*, vol. 4. London: Bloomsbury.

Antonioli R (1976) *Rabelais et la médecine*. Geneva: Droz.

Arbenz E (ed) (1891) *Die Vadianische Briefsammlung der Stadtbibliothek St. Gallen, II, Mitteilungen zur vaterländische Geschichte 25.2*. St. Gallen.

Arber A (1986) *Herbals: Their Origin and Evolution. A Chapter in the History of Botany, 1470–1670*, ed. 3. Cambridge: Cambridge University Press.

Arcangeli A and Nutton V (eds) (2008) *Girolamo Mercuriale: Medicina e cultura nell'Europa del Cinquecento*. Florence: Leo S. Olschki editore.

Arikha N (2007) *Passions and Tempers: A History of the Humours*. New York: Ecco.

Arrizabalaga J (1998) The Death of a Medieval Text: The *Articella* and the Early Press. In French *et al.* (eds): 84–120.

Arrizabalaga J, Henderson J and French R (1997) *The Great Pox: The French Disease in Renaissance Europe*. New Haven and London: Yale University Press.

Ascheri M (1997) *I giuristi e le epidemie di peste (secolo XIV–XVI)*. Siena: Università di Siena.

Ashley-Montagu MF (1953) Vesalius and the Galenists. In Ashworth Underwood E (ed) *Science, Medicine, and History: Essays in Honour of Charles Singer*. Oxford: Oxford University Press: 374–85.

Assion P (1973) *Altdeutsche Fachliteratur*. Berlin: Erich Schmitt Verlag.

Assion P (1981) Der Hof Herzog Siegmunds von Tirol als Zentrum spätmittelalter Fachliteratur. In Keil (ed): 37–76.

Azzolini M (2010) The Political Uses of Astrology: Predicting the Illness and Death of Princes, Kings and Popes in the Italian Renaissance. In *Studies in History and Philosophy of Biological and Biomedical Sciences* 41: 135–45.

Badali R (2013) *Carmina medicalia. Studi e Testi 476*. Vatican: Biblioteca Apostolica Vaticana.

Bainton RH (1960) *Michael Servet, 1511–1553*. Gütersloh: Mohn.

Baker BJ, Crane-Kremer G, Dee MW, Gregoricka LA, Henneberg M, Lee C, Lukehart SA, Maber DC, Roberts CA, Stodder ALW, Stone AC and Winingear S (2020) Advancing the Study of Treponemal Disease in Past and Present. In *Yearbook of Physical Anthropology* 171 (Suppl. 70): 5–41. https://doi.org/10.1002/ajpa.23988.

Baker T (2016) Why All This Jelly? Jacopo Zabarella and Hieronymus Fabricius ab Aquapendente on the Usefulness of the Vitreous Humour. In Goldberg B, Ragland ER and Distelzweig P (eds) *Early Modern Medicine and Natural Philosophy*. Wiesbaden: Springer Verlag: 59–88.

Baldassari F and Zampieri F (2021) *Scientiae in the History of Medicine*. Rome and Bristol, CT: L'Erma di Bretschneider.

Baldo G (2014) *Realdo Colombo De re anatomica libri XV; Anatomia*. Paris: Les Belles Lettres.

Bamji A (2019) Health Passes, Print and Public Health in Early Modern Europe. In *Social History of Medicine* 32: 441–64.

Barbour R (2013) *Sir Thomas Browne: A Life*. Oxford: Oxford University Press.

Barcia Goyanes JJ (1994) *El mito de Vesalio.* Valencia: Universidad de Valencia.

Bastow SL (2007) *The Catholic Gentry of Yorkshire, Resistance and Accommodation.* Lewiston, Queenston and Lampeter: The Edwin Mellen Press.

Baur O, Bott B, Braunfels-Esche S, Keele KD, Ladendorf H and Putscher M (1984) *Leonardo da Vinci, Anatomie, Physiognomik, Proportion und Bewegung. Kölner medizinhistoriusche Beiträge* 1. Cologne: Institut für Geschichte der Medizin.

Beecher D (2015) Nicólas Monardes, John Frampton and the Medical Wonders of the New World. In Lopes Andrade *et al.*: 141–60.

Benedictow OJ (2004) *The Black Death, 1346–1353: The Complete History.* Woodbridge: The Boydell Press.

Benkert D (2020) *Ökonomien botanischen Wissens: Praktiken der Gelehrsamkeit in Basel um 1600.* Basle: Schwabe.

Benzenhöfer U and Triebs M (1992) Zu Theophrast von Hohenheims Auslegungen der *Aphorismen* des Hippokrates. In Telle J (ed) *Parerga Paracelsica; Paracelsus in Vergangenheit und Gegenwart.* Stuttgart: Steiner Verlag: 39–44.

Berriot-Salvadore E and Mironneau P (eds) (2003) *Ambroise Paré (1510–1590) Pratique et écriture de la science á la Renaissance: Actes du Colloque de Pau (6–7 Mai 1999).* Paris: Honoré Champion.

Beta S (2019) *Moi, un manuscrit: Autobiographie de l'Anthologie palatine.* Paris: Les Belles Lettres.

Bethencourt F and Egmond F (eds) (2007) *Correspondence and Cultural Exchange in Europe, 1400–1700.* Cambridge. Cambridge University Press.

Bigotti F (2019) *Physiology of the Soul: Mind, Body and Matter in the Galenic Tradition of the Late Renaissance (1550–1630).* Turnhout: Brepols.

Biow D (2002) *Doctors, Ambassadors, and Secretaries: Humanism and Professions in Renaissance Italy.* Chicago and London: The University of Chicago Press.

Biraben JN (1975–6) *Les hommes et la peste en France et dans les pays européens et méditerranéens.* Paris and The Hague: Mouton.

Birnbaum MB (1983) *Humanists in a Shattered World: Croatian and Hungarian Latinity in the Sixteenth Century.* Columbus, OH: Slavica Publishers, Inc.

Blair AM (2010) *Too Much to Know: Managing Scholarly Information Before the Modern Age.* New Haven and London: Yale University Press.

Blair AM (2017) The Dedication Strategies of Conrad Gessner. In Manning and Klestinec (eds): 169–210.

Blazina Tomic Z and Blazina V (2015) *Expelling the Plague: The Health Office and the Implementation of Quarantine in Dubrovnik 1377–1533.* Montreal and Kingston: McGill-Queen's University Press.

Bliquez LJ and Kazhdan A (1984) Four Testimonia to Human Dissection in Byzantine Times. In *Bulletin of the History of Medicine* 58: 554–7.

Bloch H (1986) *Monte Cassino in the Middle Ages.* Cambridge, MA: Harvard University Press.

Bloch M (1973) *The Royal Touch: Sacred Monarchy and Scrofula in England and France.* Montreal: McGill University Press.

Blumenfeld-Kosinski R (1990) *Not of Woman Born: Representation of Caesarean Birth in Medieval and Renaissance Culture.* Ithaca: Cornell University Press.

Blundell JWF (1864) *The Muscles and Their Story.* London: Chapman and Hall.

Blunt A (1938–9) The Tricilinium in Religious Art. In *Journal of the Warburg Institute* 2: 271–6.

Bonoli P (1826) *Storia di Forlì*, vol. VI. Forlì: Luigi Bordandini.

Bosman-Jelgersma HA (1989) Hoe Pieter van Foreest de geleerde Petrus Forestus Werd. In Houtzager (ed): 11–24.

Bosman-Jelgersma HA (ed) (1996a) *Pieter Van Foreest. De Hollandse Hippocrates.* Krommenie: Drukkerij Knijnenberg.

Bosman-Jelgersma HA (ed) (1996b) *Petrus Forestus medicus.* Duivendrecht: Drukkerij Stolwijk.

Boudon-Millot V (2014) *Galien de Pergame. Un médecin grec à Rome.* Paris: Les Belles Lettres.

Boudon-Millot V, Cobolet G and Jouanna J (eds) (2012) *René Chartier (1572–1654), éditeur et traducteur d'Hippocrate et Galien.* Paris: De Boccard.

Boudon-Millot V and Michaud F (eds) (2020) *La thériaque: Histoire d'un remède millénaire.* Paris: Les Belles Lettres.

Bouras-Vallianatos P and Zipser B (eds) (2019) *Brill's Companion to the Reception of Galen.* Leiden and New York: Brill.

Brady TA (2009) *German Histories in the Age of Reformations, 1400–1650.* Cambridge: Cambridge University Press.

Branca V (ed) (1981) *Giorgio Valla tra scienza e sapienza.* Florence: Leo S. Olschki.

Braudel F (1972) *The Mediterranean and the Mediterranean World in the Age of Philip II.* London: Collins.

Braudel F (1986) *L'Identité de la France: Les hommes et les choses.* Paris: Flammarion.

Bray RS (1996) *Armies of Pestilence: The Impact of Disease on History.* New York: Barnes and Noble.

Brendecke A (ed) (2015) *Praktiken der frühen Neuzeit: Akteure – Handlungen – Artefakte.* Cologne, Weimar and Vienna: Böhlau Verlag.

Brigden S (2012) *Thomas Wyatt: The Heart's Forest.* London: Faber and Faber.

Brinckhus G and Pachnicke C (eds) (2001) *Leonhart Fuchs 1501–1566: Mediziner und Botaniker.* Tübingen: Stadtmuseum.

Brockbank W (1956) The Man Who Was Vidius. In *Annals of the Royal College of Surgeons* 19: 269–95.

Brockliss L and Jones C (1997) *The Medical World of Early Modern France.* Oxford: Clarendon Press.

Bröer R (2002) Friedenspolitik durch Verketzerung: Johannes Crato (1519–1585) und die Denunziation der Paracelsisten als Arianer. In *Medizinhistorisches Journal* 37: 139–82.

Broomhall S (2004) *Women's Medical Work in Early Modern France.* Manchester and New York: Manchester University Press.

Burckhardt A (1917) *Geschichte der medizinischen Fakultät zu Basel 1460–1900.* Basle: Friedrich Reinhardt.

Burnett C (2011) Translations and Transmission of Greek and Islamic Science to Latin Christendom. In Lindberg DC and Shank MH (eds) *The Cambridge History of Science, Vol. II: Medieval Science.* Cambridge: Cambridge University Press: 341–64.

Burnett J (1982) The Giustiniani Medical Chest. In *Medical History* 26: 325–33.

Bylebyl JJ (1985) Disputation and Description in the Renaissance Pulse Controversy. In Wear, French and Lonie (eds): 223–45.

Bylebyl JJ (1990) Interpreting the *Fasciculo* Anatomy Scene. In *Journal of the History of Medicine and Allied Sciences* 45: 285–316.

Caccamo D (1970) *Eretici italiani in Moravia, Polonia, Transilvania.* Florence: Sansoni.

Cagle H (2018) *Assembling the Tropics: Science and Medicine in Portugal's Empire, 1450–1700.* Cambridge: Cambridge University Press.

Caiati MR, Fabbri MC, Van Hee R, Campanella B, Legnaioli S, Pagnotta S, Palleschi V and Poggialini F (2020) Vesalius' 'Philosopher', a Recently Found Drawing by Jan Steven van Calcar. In Van Hee (ed): 13–24.

Cairns F (1994) Fracastoro's *Syphilis, the Argonautic Tradition, and the Aetiology of Syphilis.* In *Humanistica Lovaniensia* 43: 246–61.

Canalis RF (2018a) Vesalius' Methods in the Production of the *Fabrica* with Emphasis on the Neuroanatomy Chapters. In Canalis and Ciavolella (eds): 131–70.

Canalis RF (2018b) Gabrielle Falloppia; Vesalius's Admirer and First Critic. In Canalis and Ciavolella (eds): 171–200.

Canalis RF and Ciavolella M (eds) (2018) *Andreas Vesalius and the "Fabrica" in the Age of Printing: Art, Anatomy, and Printing in the Italian Renaissance.* Turnhout: Brepols.

Canano GB (1925) *Musculorum humani corporis picturata dissectio (Ferrara 1541?). Facsimile Edition.* Florence: R. Lier & co.

Caplan J (2016) *Postal Culture in Europe 1500–1800.* Oxford: Voltaire Foundation.

Carey HM (1992) *Courting Disaster: Astrology at the English Court and University in the Later Middle Ages.* Basingstoke: Macmillan.

Carlino A (1999a) *Books of the Body: Anatomical Ritual and Renaissance Learning.* Chicago: Chicago University Press.

Carlino A (1999b) *Paper Bodies: A Catalogue of Anatomical Fugitive Sheets 1538–1687, Medical History Supplement 19.* London: The Wellcome Institute.

Carlino A (2012) Medical Humanism: Rhetoric and Anatomy at Padua, circa 1540. In Pender and Struever (eds): 111–28.

Carmichael AG (1986) *Plague and the Poor in Renaissance Florence.* Cambridge: Cambridge University Press.

Carmichael AG (1993a) Diseases of the Renaissance and Early Modern Europe. In Kiple KG (ed) *The Cambridge World History of Human Disease.* Cambridge: Cambridge University Press: 279–86.

Carmichael AG (1993b) Sweating Sickness. In Kiple KG (ed) *The Cambridge World History of Human Disease.* Cambridge: Cambridge University Press: 279–86.

Carmichael AG (2008) Universal and Particular: The Language of Plague, 1348–1500. In Nutton (2008a): 17–52.

Catani M and Sandrone S (2015) *Brain Research from Vesalius to Modern Neuroscience.* Oxford: Oxford University Press.

Cavallo S (2007) *Artisans of the Body.* Manchester: Manchester University Press.

Cavallo S and Storey T (2013) *Healthy Living in Renaissance Italy.* Oxford: Oxford University Press.

Cavallo S and Storey T (eds) (2017) *Conserving Health in Early Modern European Culture: Bodies and Environment in Italy and England.* London and Manchester: Manchester University Press.

Cavanagh GST (1983) A New View of the Vesalian Landscape. In *Medical History* 27: 77–9.

Cazes H and Carlino A (2003) Plaisir de l'anatomie, plaisir du livre: *La dissection des parties du corps humain* par Charles Estienne (Paris, 1546). In *Cahiers de l'Association Internationale des Études Françaises* 55: 251–69.

Cazort M, Kornell M and Roberts KB (1996) *The Ingenious Machine of Nature*. Ottawa: National Gallery of Canada.

Céard J, Fontaine MM and Margolin JC (eds) (1990) *Le Corps à la Renaissance*. Paris: Aux Amateurs de Livres.

Celati A (2014) Heresy, Medicine and Paracelsianism in Sixteenth-Century Italy: The Case of Girolamo Donzellini (1513–1587). In *Gesnerus* 71: 5–37.

Celati A (2015) Pigafetta, Antonio Francesco. In *DBI* 83. www.treccani.it/enciclopedia/antonio-francesco-pigafetta_(Dizionario-Biografico).

Celati A (2018a) Simoni, Pietro Simoni. In *DBI* 92: 765–7.

Celati A (2018b) *Contra medicos*: Physicians Facing the Inquisition in 16th-Century Venice. In *Early Science and Medicine* 23: 72–9.

Celati A (2018c) Heretical Physicians in Sixteenth-Century Italy: The Fortunes of Girolamo Massari, Guglielmo Grataroli, and Teofilo Panarelli. In *Society and Politics* 12: 11–31.

Celati A (2021) The Experience of the Physician Girolamo Donzellini in the 1575 Venetian Plague: Between Scientia and Heterodoxy. In Baldassari and Zampieri (eds): 189–216.

Cerasoli G (2004) L'inventario di palazzo Mercuriali a Forlì nel 1638. In *Studi Romagnoli* 55: 471–94.

Chambers DS (1990) A Mantuan in London in 1557: Further Research on Annibale Litolfi. In Chaney E and Mack P (eds) *England and the Continental Renaissance: Essays in Honour of J. B. Trapp*. Woodbridge: The Boydell Press: 73–108.

Chaney EP (1981) Philanthropy in Italy: English Observations on Italian Hospitals 1545–1789. In Riis T (ed) *Aspects of Poverty in Early Modern Europe*. Stuttgart: Klett-Cotta: 183–217.

Cipolla CM (1976) *Public Health and the Medical Profession in the Renaissance*. Cambridge: Cambridge University Press.

Cipolla CM (1979) *Faith, Reason and the Plague; a Tuscan Story of the Seventeenth Century*. Brighton: Harvester Press.

Cipolla CM (1981) *Fighting the Plague in Seventeenth Century Italy*. Madison: University of Wisconsin Press.

Clark Sir G (1964) *A History of the Royal College of Physicians*. Oxford: Clarendon Press, for the Royal College of Physicians.

Clayton M and Philo R (2012) *Leonardo da Vinci: Anatomist*. London: Royal Collection Enterprises Ltd.

Clemen O (1898) Andreas Frank von Kamenz. In *Neues Archiv für sächsische Geschichte* 19: 95–115; repr. in Clemen (1982–88): 13–23.

Clemen O (1903) Urtheile zweier Brauschweiger Stadtärtze über ihr Publikum im 16. Jahrhundert. In *Zeitschrift des historischen Vereins für Niedersächsen* 68: 536–7; repr. in Clemen (1982–88): 1,570–2.

Clemen O (1905) Der erste Stadtarzt vom Joachimsthal. In *Mitteilungen des Vereins für die Geschichte der Deutschen in Böhmen* 43: 120–1; repr. in Clemen (1982–88): 2,293–4.

Clemen O (1907a) Briefe von Georg Sturtz. In *Beiträge zur Geschichte der Stadt Buchholz* 6: 1–7; repr. in Clemen (1982–88): 3,51–8.

Clemen O (1907b) Klagelied des Stadtarztes von Schlaggenwald (Theodor Eccombertus) vom. Jahre. 1583. In *Mitteilungen des Vereins für die Geschichte der Deutschen in Böhmen* 45: 431–2; repr. in Clemen (1982–88): 3,137–8.

Clemen O (1909) Georg Pylander. In *Neues Archiv füt sächsische Geschichte* 30: 335–48; repr. in Clemen (1982–88): 261–75.

Clemen O (1911) *Alte Einblattdrücke*. Bonn: A. Marcus and E. Weber.

Clemen O (1912) Janus Cornarius. In *Neues Archiv für sächsische Geschichte* 33: 36–76; repr. in Clemen (1982–88): 4,16–56.

Clemen O (1923) Zur Literatur über die englischen Schweiß von 1529. In *Sudhoffs Archiv* 13: 1921: 85–97; repr. in Clemen 1982–88: 5,97–109.

Clemen O (1928) Ein unbekanntes Pestregiment, Dresden 1566. In *Archiv für Geschchte der Medizin* 20: 175–8; repr. in Clemen (1982–88): 5,339–42.

Clemen O (1929) Die Hamburger Handschrift Suypellex epistolica 1 fol. In *Archiv für Reformationsgeschichte* 26: 1–29; repr. in Clemen (1982–88): 5,383–412.

Clemen O (1943–4) Der fingierte (letzte) Briefwechsel zwischen der Kurfürstin Agnes und dem Kurfürst Moritz von Sachsen. In *Zeitschrift für Kirchengeschichte* 62: 1–28; repr. in Clemen (1982–88): 587–614.

Clemen O (1982–88) *Kleine Schriften zur Reformationsgeschichte*. Leipzig: Zentralantiquariat der Deuttschen Demokratischen Republik.

Clericuzio A and Ernst G (eds) (2008) *Il Rinascimento italiano e l'Europa: Volume quinto. Le scienze*. Rome: Fondazione Cassamarca.

Clouse ML (2011) *Government and Public Health in Philip II's Spain: Shared Interests, Competing Authorities*. Farnham: Ashgate.

Cohn SK Jr (2010) *Cultures of Plague: Medical Thinking at the End of the Renaissance*. Oxford: Oxford University Press.

Cohn SK Jr (2018) *Epidemics: Plague and Compassion from the Plague of Athens to AIDS*. Oxford: Oxford University Press.

Collinson P (1983) *Godly People*. London: Hambledon Press.

Colombi Ferretti A, Prati L and Tramonti U (2000) *Il complesso monumentale di San Mercuriale a Forlì. Restauri*. Forlì: La Greca.

Compier AH (2012) Rhazes in the Renaissance of Andreas Vesalius. In *Medical History* 56: 3–25.

Conforti M (2008) Chirurgi, mammane, ciarlatani: Pratica medica e controllo delle professioni. In Clericuzio and Ernst (eds): 323–40.

Connell SM (2016) *Aristotle on Female Animals: A Study of the Generation of Animals*. Cambridge: Cambridge University Press.

Copenhaver BP (1978) *Symphorien Champier and the Reception of the Occultist Tradition in France*. The Hague, Paris and New York: Mouton.

Cook ND (1998) *Born to Die: Disease and New World Conquest, 1492–1650*. Cambridge: Cambridge University Press.

Cooper A (2007) *Inventing the Indigenous: Local Knowledge and Natural History in Early Modern Europe*. Cambridge: Cambridge University Press.

Coste J (2007) *Représentations et comportements en temps d'épidémie dans la littérature imprimée de peste (1490–1725): Contribution á l'histoire culturelle de la peste en France à l'époque moderne*. Paris: Honoré Champion.

Crossgrove W (1994) *Die deutsche Sachliteratur des Mittelalters*. Bern: Peter Lang.

Cunningham A (1985) Fabricius and the 'Aristotle Project' in Anatomical Teaching and Research in Padua. In Wear *et al.* (eds): 195–222.

Cunningham A (1997) *The Anatomical Renaissance*. Aldershot: Scolar Press.

Cunningham A (2003) The Pen and the Sword: Recovering the Disciplinary Identity of Physiology and Anatomy Before 1800. II: Old Anatomy – the Sword. In *Studies in History and Philosophy of Science: Part C. Studies in History and Philosophy of Biological and Biomedical Sciences* 34: 51–76.

Cunningham A (2010) The Bartholins, the Platters, and Laurentius Gryllus: the peregrinatio medica in the 16th and 17th centuries. In *Grell, Cunningham and Arrizabalaga* (eds): 3–16.

Curry HA, Jardine N, Secord JA and Spary EC (eds) (2018) *Worlds of Natural History*. Cambridge: Cambridge University Press.

Cyrus C (2021) Five Strategies in Sixteenth-Century Tertiaries' Prayers Against Pestilence. *Academia Letters* Article 479. Accessed online on 8 August 2021. https://doi.org/10.20935/AL479.

DaCosta Kaufmann T (1995) *Court, Cloister, and City: The Art and Culture of Central Europe, 1450–1800*. Chicago: University of Chicago Press.

Dandrey P (2002) *Molière ou l'ésthétique du ridicule*, ed. 2. Paris: Klingsieck.

Danzi M (2016) Gessner balnéologue. In Leu and Ruoss (eds): 119–28.

Darwin J (2007) *After Tamerlane: The Global History of Empire Since 1405*. London: Allen Lane.

Daston L and Park K (1998) *Wonders and the Order of Nature, 1150–1750*. New York: Zone.

Davies J (2009) *Culture and Power: Tuscany and Its Universities 1537–1609*. Leiden and Boston: Brill.

Davis NZ (1975) *Society and Culture in Early Modern France*. London: Duckworth.

Dawbarn F (2003) New Light on Dr. Thomas Moffet; the Triple Roles of an Early Modern Physician, Client, and Patronage-Broker. In *Medical History* 47: 3–22.

Dean-Jones LA (1994) *Women's Bodies in Classical Greek Science*. Oxford: Clarendon Press.

De Blasi N (1966) Bentivoglio, Ercole. In *DBI* 8: 614–16.

Deer Richardson L (1985) The Generation of Disease: Occult Causes and Diseases of the Total Substance. In Wear *et al.* (eds): 175–94.

Debus AG (1965) *The English Paracelsians*. London: Oldbourne.

Debus AG (1987) *Chemistry, Alchemy and the New Philosophy, 1550–1700*. London: Variorum.

Debus AG (1991) *The French Paracelsians: The Chemical Challenge to Medical and Scientific Tradition in Early Modern France*. Cambridge: Cambridge University Press.

Decamp E (2016) *Civic and Medical Worlds in Early Modern England: Performing Barbery and Surgery*. Basingstoke: Palgrave Macmillan.

De Ferrari A (1978) Casseri, Giulio Cesare. In *DBI* 21: 433–7.

De Ferrari A (1983) Corti, Matteo. In *DBI* 29: 795–7.

Dekoster K (2021) Dissecting Violence. Autopsy, Medical Expertise and Criminal Justice in Early Modern Flanders. In *Social History of Medicine* 34: 285–304.

Delisle C (2004) The Letter: Private Text or Public Place? The Mattioli-Gesner Controversy About the Aconitum Primum. In *Gesnerus* 61: 164–76.

Delisle C (2006) Une correspondence scientifique à la Renaissance: Les *Lettres médicinales* de Conrad Gesner. In Beaurepaire PY, Häseler J and McKenna A (eds) *Réseaux de correspondance à l'âge classique*. St. Etienne: Publications de l'Université de St. Etienne: 33–43.

Delisle C (2008) *Establishing the Facts: Conrad Gessner's Epistolae Morales Between the Particular and the General*. PhD Diss. University of London, London.

Demaitre L (2013) *Medieval Medicine: The Art of Healing, from Head to Toe.* Santa Barbara, Denver and Oxford: Praeger.

De Moulin D (1998) *A History of Surgery with Emphasis on the Netherlands.* Dordrecht, Boston and Lancaster: Martinus Nijhoff Publishers.

De Ridder-Symoens H (ed) (1996) *A History of the University in Europe. Volume II: Universities in Early Modern Europe (1500–1800).* Cambridge: Cambridge University Press.

De Ridder-Symoens H (2010) The Mobility of Medical Students from the Fifteenth to the Eighteenth Century: The Institutional Context. In Grell *et al.* (eds): 47–89.

De Vecchi B (1932) I libri di un medico umanista fiorentino del sec. XV. In *La Bibliofilia* 34: 293–301.

De Waardt H (1996) Chasing Demons and Curing Mortals: The Medical Practice of Clerics in the Netherlands. In Marland and Pelling (eds): 179–204.

Dickens AG (1947) Robert Parkyn's Narrative of the Reformation. In *English Historical Review* 59: 58–83.

Dietz Moss J (2012) The Promotion of the Bath Waters by Physicians in the Renaissance. In Pender and Struever (eds): 60–82.

Dirix T (2014) *In Search of Andreas Vesalius: The Quest for the Lost Grave.* Tielt: Lannoo Campus.

Dobson J and Walker RM (1979) *Barbers and Barber-surgeons of London: A History of the Barbers' and Barber-surgeons' Companies.* Oxford: Blackwell Scientific Publications.

Donaldson IML (2010) Two States of Some Plates in the *Compendiosa* of Thomas Geminus (1545). In *The Library* 11 (1): 89–104.

Donaldson IML (2015) Ambroise Paré's Accounts of New Methods for Treating Gunshot Wounds and Burns. In *Journal of the Royal College of Medicine* 108: 457–61.

Donato MP (ed.) (2019) *Medicine and the Inquisition in the Early Modern World.* Leiden: Brill.

Dross F (2010) Vom zuverlässigen Urteile: Äutorität, reichsstädtische Ordnung und der Verlust "armer Glieder Christi" in der Nürnberger Sondersiechenschau. In *Medizin, Gesellschaft und Geschichte* 29: 9–46.

Dross F (2020a) Vergesellschaftung unter Ansteckenden – für eine Körpergeschichte der Seuche. In *NTM* 28: 195–202.

Dross F (2020b) *De officiis:* Doctors' Oaths and Appointments in Early Modern Nuremberg. In Mendelsohn *et al.* (eds): 110–32.

Du Broc de Segange L and Morel LF (1887) *Les Saints patrons des corporations et protecteurs spécialement invoqués dans les maladies et dans les circonstances critiques de la vie*, vol. 2. Paris: Librairie Bloud et Barral.

Duffy E (1992) *The Stripping of the Altars: Traditional Religion in England 1400–1580.* New Haven and London: Yale University Press.

Dumaître P (1986) *Ambroise Paré: Chirurgien de 4 rois de France.* Paris: Perrin.

Durling RJ (1961) A Chronological Census of Renaissance Editions and Translations of Galen. In *Journal of the Warburg and Courtauld Institutes* 24: 230–305.

Durling RJ (1990) Girolamo Mercuriale's *De modo studendi.* In *Osiris*, ser. 2.6: 181–95.

Dyer A (1997) The English Sweating Sickness of 1551: An Epidemic Anatomized. In *Medical History* 41: 562–84.

Eamon W (1994) *Science and the Secrets of Nature: Books of Secrets in Medieval and Early Modern Culture*. Princeton: Princeton University Press.

Eamon W (2005) The Charlatan's Trial an Italian Surgeon in the Court of King Philip II. In *Cronos* 8: 3–30.

Eccles A (1982) *Obstetrics and Gynaecology in Tudor and Stuart England*. London: Croom Helm.

Eckart EA (1996) *The Structures of Plague in Early Modern Europe: Central Europe, 1560–1640*. Basle: Karger.

Egmond MF (2018a) On Northern Shores: Sixteenth-Century Observations of Fish and Seabirds (North Sea and North Atlantic). In MacGregor A (ed) *Naturalists in the Field: Collecting, Recording and Preserving the Natural World from the Fifteenth to the Twenty-First Century*. Leiden and Boston: Brill: 129–48.

Egmond MF (2018b) *Conrad Gessners Thierbuch: Die Originalzeichnungen*. Darmstadt: WBG.

Egmond MF (2018c) European Exchanges and Communities. In Curry *et al.* (eds): 78–93.

Egmond MF (2021) Sixteenth-Century University Gardens in a Medical and Botanical Context. In Baldassari and Zampieri (eds): 89–120.

Eikermann D and Kaiser G (2012) *Die Pest in Berlin, 1576: Eine wiederentdeckte Pestschrift von Leonhart Thurneisser zum Thurn (1531–1596)*. Rangsdorf: Basilisken-Presse.

Eisenstein E (1979) *The Printing Press as an Agent of Change*. Cambridge: Cambridge University Press.

Elaut L (1974) De derde en de vierde druk van Vesalius' Fabrica: 1568, 1604. In *Scientiarum Historia* 6: 124–34.

Elton GR (1953) An Early Tudor Poor Law. In *Economic History Review* 6: 55–67.

Emmart EW (1940) *The Badianus Manuscript (Codex Barberini, Latin 241) Vatican Library: An Aztec Herbal of 1552*. Baltimore: Johns Hopkins University Press.

Endo H (2020) *Surgeons Chests from the Mary Rose*. Accessed online on 21 May 2021. https://www.matteringpress.org/books/boxes/read/boxes-figs-56.xhtml.

Enenkel KL and De Jong JL (eds) (2019) *Artes Apodemicae and Early Modern Travel Culture, 1550–1700*. Leiden: Brill.

Eriksson R (1959) *Andreas Vesalius' First Public Anatomy at Bologna 1540: An Eye-Witness Report by Baldasar Heseler medicinae scolaris Together with His Notes on Matthaeus Curtius' Lectures on Anatomia Mundini*. Uppsala and Stockholm: Almqvist and Wiksell.

Esposito A (2013) Alla corte dei Papi: Archiatri pontifici ebrei tra'400 e'500. In Andretta E and Nicoud M (eds) *Être médecin à la cour (Italie, France, Espagne, xiiie–xviiie siècle)*. Florence: Sismel-Edizioni del Galluzzo: 17–33.

Evans RJW (1984a) *Rudolf II and His World: A Study in Intellectual History 1576–1612*. Oxford: Clarendon Press.

Evans RJW (1984b) *The Making of the Habsburg Monarchy, 1550–1700: An Interpretation*. Oxford: Clarendon Press.

Fausti D (ed) (2004) *La complessa scienza dei semplici. Atti delle Celebrazioni per il V Centenario della Nascita di Pietro Andrea Mattioli, Atti dell' Accademia delle Scienze di Siena detta De' Fisiocritici, serie XV, Supplement 200, tom 20*. Siena: Tipografia Senese.

Favaretti Camposampiero M and Scribano E (eds) (forthcoming) *Galen and the Early Moderns*. Cham: Springer.

Fay I (2015) *Health and the City: Disease, Environment and Government in Norwich, 1200–1575.* Woodbridge: Boydell and Brewer.

Ferrari G (1987) Public Anatomy Lessons and the Carnival; the Anatomy Theatre of Bologna. In *Past and Present* 117: 50–106.

Ferrari G (1996) *L'esperienza del passato: Alessandro Benedetti, filologo e medico umanista.* Florence: L. S. Olschki.

Ferrari G (ed) (1998) *Alessandro Benedetti, Historia corporis sive Anatomice.* Florence: Giunti.

Ferrari G (2008) Tra medicina e chirurgia: La rinascita dell'anatomia e la dissezione come *spettacolo.* In Clericuzio and Ernst (eds): 341–68.

Ferretto S (2012) *Maestri per il metodo di trattar le cose: Bassiano Lando, Giovan Battista da Monte e la scienza della medicina nel xvi secolo.* Padua: CLEUP.

Ferri S (ed) (1997) *Pietro Andrea Mattioli, Siena 1501-Trento 1578: La vita, le opera.* Perugia: Quattroemme.

Fichtner PS (2001) *Emperor Maximilian II.* New Haven and London: Yale University Press.

Fierz M (1983) *Girolamo Cardano, 1501–1576.* Boston: Birkhäuser.

Findlen P (1996) *Possessing Nature: Museums, Collecting and Scientific Culture in Early Modern Italy.* Berkeley, Los Angeles and London: University of California Press.

Findlen P (1999) The Formation of a Scientific Community: Natural History in Sixteenth-Century Italy. In Grafton and Siraisi (eds): 369–400.

Findlen P (2017) The Death of a Naturalist: Knowledge and Community in Late Renaissance Italy. In Manning and Klestinec (eds): 127–68.

Finger H (1990) *Gisbert Longolius, ein niederrheinischer Humanist.* Düsseldorf: Droste,

Finger H and Benger A (1987) *Der Kölner Professor Gisbert Longolius – Leibarzt Erzbischof Hermanns von Wied – und die Reste seiner Bibliothek in der Universitätsbibliothek Düsseldorf.* Düsseldorf: Universität Düsseldorf.

Firpo L (1971) Borgarucci, familia. In *DBI* 12: 565–8.

Firpo M (1984) 'Gli spirituali'. L'accademia di Mantova e il formulario di fede del 1542: Controllo del dissenso religioso e Nicodemismo. In *Rivista di storia e letteratura religiosa* 20: 40–111.

Fisch MH, Schullian DM and Rodenwald LJ (1947) *Nicolaus Pol, Doctor, 1494: With a Critical Edition of His Guaiac Tract.* New York: Reisner.

Fischer-Homberger E (1983) *Medizin vor Gericht. Gerichtsmedizin von der Renaissance bis zur Aufklärung.* Bern, Stuttgart and Vienna: Verlag Hans Huber.

Flemming R (2000) *Medicine and the Making of Roman Women: Gender, Nature, and Authority from Celsus to Galen.* Oxford: Oxford University Press.

Flood JL (2003) 'Safer on the Battlefield Than in the City': England, the 'Sweating Wickness', and the Continent. In *Renaissance Studies* 17: 147–76.

Flood JL and Shaw D (1997) *Johannes Sinapius (1505–1560): Hellenist and Physician in Germany and Italy.* Geneva: Droz.

Florescu R and McNally RT (1973) *Dracula, a Biography of Vlad the Impaler, 1431–1476.* London: E. P. Dutton.

Flügge S (1998) *Hebammen und heilkundige Frauen: Recht und Rechtswirklichkeit im 15. und 16. Jahrhundert.* Frankfurt and Basle: Stroemfeld Verlag.

Fontaine MM (1984) Quaresprenant: L'image littéraire et la contestation de l'analogie médicale. In Coleman JA and Scollen-Jimack CM (eds) *Rabelais in Glasgow.* Glasgow: University of Glasgow: 87–112.

Forster LW (1967) *Janus Gruter's English Years*. Oxford: Oxford University Press.

Fortuna S (2019a) Editions and Translations of Galen from 1490 to 1540. In Bouras-Vallianatos and Zipser (eds): 437–52.

Fortuna C (2019b) L'insegnamento di Nicolò Leoniceno e la sua incidenza nella storia della medicina italiana ed europea. In Lonigo (ed): 81–96.

Fortuna S (2020) Pseudo-Galenic Texts in the Editions of Galen (1490–1689). In *Medicina dei Secoli* 32: 117–38.

Foscati A (2019) 'Nonnatus dictus quod casa defunctae matris prodiit': Postmortem Caesarean Section in the Late Middle Ages and Early Modern Period. In *Social History of Medicine* 32: 465–80.

Fossel V (1913) Die *Epistolae medicinales* des Humanisten Andreas Dudith 1533–1589. In *Sudhoffs Archiv* 6: 34–51.

Foust CM (1992) *Rhubarb, the Wondrous Drug*. Princeton: Princeton University Press.

Frank R (2003) Fracastoro: Poetry vs. Prose. In *International Journal of the Classical Tradition* 9: 524–34.

Frasca-Spada M and Jardine N (eds) (2000) *Books and the Sciences in History*. Cambridge: Cambridge University Press.

French RK (1979) *De Juvamentis Membrorum* and the Reception of Galenic Physiological *Anatomy*. In *Isis* 70: 96–109.

French RK (1985) Berengario da Carpi and the Use of Commentary in Anatomical Teaching. In Wear *et al.* (eds): 42–74.

French RK (1994) *William Harvey's Natural Philosophy*. Cambridge: Cambridge University Press.

French RK (1999) *Dissection and Vivisection in the European Renaissance*. Aldershot and Brookfield, VT: Ashgate.

French RK, Arrizabalaga J, Cunningham A and García Ballester L (eds) (1998) *Medicine from the Black Death to the French Disease*. Aldershot and Brookfield, VT: Ashgate.

Friedenwald H (1939) Immortality through Writ of Error: Dionysius: a Portuguese Jewish Court Physician with Notes on Brudus Lusitanus, His Son, and on Pierre Brissot. In *Bulletin of the History of Medicine* 7: 249–56.

Funk H (2021) Thomas Penny and the Preservation of Conrad Gessner's Botanical Legacy. In *Journal of the History of Collections* 33: 1–9.

Furdell EL (2001) *The Royal Doctors 1485–1714: Medical Personnel at the Tudor and Stuart Courts*. Rochester, NY: University of Rochester Press.

Gadebusch-Bondio MC (ed) (2014) *Medical Ethics: Premodern Negotiations Between Medicine and Philosophy. Aurora. Schriften der Villa Vigoni, Band 2*. Stuttgart: Franz Steiner Verlag.

Gairdner J (ed) (1891) *Letters and Papers of the Reign of Henry VIII*, vol. XIII.2. London: Stationery Office.

Gambaccini P (2004) *Mountebanks and Medicasters, a History of Italian Charlatans from the Middle Ages to the Present*. Jefferson, NC and London: McFarland & Company, Inc.

García Ballester L (1984) *Los Moriscos y la medicina: Un capitulo de la medicina y la ciencia marginadas en la España del siglo XVI*. Barcelona: Editorial Labor S.A.

García Ballester L (1985) Academicism Versus Empiricism in Practical Medicine in Sixteenth-Century Spain with Regard to Morisco Practitioners. In Wear *et al.* (eds): 246–70, 338–42; repr. as Ch. VIII in García Ballester (2001).

García Ballester L (1993) The Inquisition and Minority Medical Practitioners in Counter-Reformation Spain. In Grell and Cunningham (eds): 156–91; repr. as Ch. IX in Garcia Ballester (2001).

García Ballester L (2001) *Medicine in a Multicultural Society*. Aldershot and Burlington, VT: Ashgate.

Garofalo I (2004) Agostino Gadaldino (1515–1575) et le Galien latin. In Boudon-Millot V and Cobolet G (eds) *Lire les médecins grecs à la Renaissance: Aux origines de l'édition médicale: Actes du colloque international de Paris, 19–20 septembre 2003*. Paris: Bibliothèque interuniversitaire de médecine: 283–322.

Geltner G (2019) *Roads to Health: Infrastructure and Urban Wellbeing in Later Medieval Italy*. Philadelphia: University of Pennsylvania Press.

Gentilcore D (1994) 'All That Pertains to Medicine': *Protomedici* and *protomedicati* in Early Modern Italy. In *Medical History* 58: 121–42.

Gentilcore D (1995) 'Charlatans, Mountebanks and Other Similar People': The Regulation and Role of Itinerant Practitioners in Early Modern Italy. In *Social History* 20: 297–314.

Gentilcore D (1998) *Healers and Healing in Early Modern Italy*. Manchester: Manchester University Press.

Gentilcore D (2006) *Medical Charlatanism in Early Modern Italy*. Oxford: Oxford University Press.

Geyer-Kordesch J and MacDonald F (1999) *Physicians and Surgeons in Glasgow: The History of the Royal College of Physicians and Surgeons of Glasgow 1599–1858*. London and Rio Grande: The Hambledon Press.

Giacomelli C (2021) Medica Patavina. Codici di medicina a Padova, tra Bessarione, Niccolò Leonico Tomeo e Marco Antonio della Torre (?). In *Revue d'histoire des textes* 16: 75–113.

Gielen E and Goyens M (eds) 2018) *Towards the Authority of Vesalius: Studies on Medicine and the Human Body from Antiquity to the Renaissance and Beyond*. Turnhout: Brepols.

Giese E and Von Hagen B (1958) *Geschichte der medizinischen Fakultät der Friedrich-Schiller-Universität Jena*. Jena: Fischer.

Gigliotti GL (1990) The Alexandrian Fracastoro: Form and Meaning in the Myth of Syphilus. In *Renaissance and Reformation* 14: 261–70.

Gillet JFA (1860–61) *Crato von Crafftheim und seine Freunde: Ein Beitrag zur Kirchengeschichte*. Frankfurt: H.L. Brönner.

Gilly C (1977) Zwischen Erfahrung und Spekulation: Theodor Zwinger und die religiöse und kulturelle Krise seiner Zeit. In *Basler Zeitschrift für Geschichte und Altertumskunde* 67: 57–137.

Gilly C (1991) Das Sprichwort 'Die Gelehrten Die Verkehrten' oder der Verrat der Intellektuellen im Zeitalter der Glaubenspaltung. In Rotondò A (ed) *Forme e destinazione del Messaggio religioso: Aspetti della propaganda religiosa nel Cinquecento*. Florence: Leo S. Olschki editore: 229–375.

Gilly C (1998) 'Theophrastia sancta' – Paracelsianism as Religion in Conflict with the Established Churches. In Telle J (ed): 151–85.

Ginzburg C (1970) *Il nicodemismo: Simulazione e dissimulazione religiosa nell'Europa del '500*. Turin: Einaudi.

Gleason MW (2009) Shock and Awe: The Performance Dimension of Galen's Anatomical Demonstrations. In Gill C, Whitmarsh T, and Wilkins J (eds) *Galen and the World of Knowledge*. Cambridge: Cambridge University Press: 85–114.

Gliozzi G (1972) Brasavola, Antonio. In *DBI* 14: 51–2.

Gliozzi G (1974) Canano, Giovanni Battista, il Giovane. In *DBI* 17: 714–16.

Gnudi MT and Webster JP (1950) *The Life and Times of Gaspare Tagliacozzi*. New York: H. Reichner.

Godman P (1998) *From Poliziano to Machiavelli. Florentine Humanism in the High Renaissance*, Princeton: Princeton University Press.

Goodwin G and Bevan M (2004) Robert Jacob. In *ODNB* 46: 942–3.

Gowland A (2006) *The Worlds of Renaissance Melancholy: Robert Burton in Context*. Cambridge: Cambridge University Press.

Grafton A (1980) The Importance of Being Printed. In *The Journal of Interdisciplinary History* 11: 265–86.

Grafton A (1992) *New Worlds, Ancient Texts: The Power of Tradition and the Shock of Discovery*. Cambridge, MA and London: The Belknap Press of Harvard University Press.

Grafton A (2001) *Bring Out Your Dead: The Past as Revelation*. Cambridge, MA and London: Harvard University Press.

Grafton A (2012) *What Was History?* Cambridge: Cambridge University Press.

Grafton A (2017) A Medical Man Among Ecclesiastical Historians: John Caius, Matthew Parker and the History of Cambridge University. In Manning and Klestinec (eds): 85–100.

Grafton A and Siraisi NG (eds) (1999) *Natural Particulars: Nature and the Disciplines in Renaissance Europe*. Cambridge, MA: The MIT Press.

Grafton A and Siraisi NG (2001) Between the Election and My Hopes: Girolamo Cardano and Medical Astrology. In Newman and Grafton (eds): 69–131.

Granjel LS (1980) *La medicina española renacentista*. Salamanca: Universidad de Salamanca.

Gray L (2001) *The Self-Perception of Chronic Physical Incapacity Among the Labouring Poor. Pauper Narratives and Territorial Hospitals in Early Modern Rural Germany*. PhD Diss. University College London, London.

Gray L (2002) The Experience of Old Age in the Narratives of the Rural Poor in Early Modern Germany. In Ottaway RS, Botelho LA and Kittredge K (eds) *Power and Poverty: Old Age in the Pre-Industrial Past*. Westport and London: Greenwood Press: 107–24.

Gray L (2007) Hospitals and the Lives of the Chronically Sick: Self-experience and Coping with Illness in the Narratives of the Rural Poor in Early Modern Germany. In Henderson *et al.* (eds): 297–316.

Green D (2003) *The Double Life of Doctor Lopez: Spies, Shakespeare and the Plot to Poison Elizabeth I*. London: Century.

Green MH (2008) *Making Women's Medicine Masculine: the Rise of Male Authority in Pre-modern Gynaecology*. Oxford: Oxford University Press.

Green MH (ed) (2014) Pandemic Disease in the Medieval World: Rethinking the Black Death. In *The Medieval Globe* I: 1–326.

Green MH (2019) *Gloriosissimus Galienus*: Galen and Galenic Writings in the Eleventh and Twelfth-Century Latin West. In Bouras-Vallianatos and Zipser (eds): 319–42.

Grell OP (ed) (1998) *Paracelsus: The Man and His Reputation, His Ideas and Their Transformation*. Leiden: Brill.

Grell OP and Cunningham A (eds) (1993) *Medicine and the Reformation*. London and New York: Routledge.

Grell OP, Cunningham A and Arrizabalaga J (eds) (2010) *Centres of Medical Excellence?: Medical Travel and Education in Europe, 1500–1789*. Farnham: Ashgate.

Grendler PF (2002) *The Universities in the Italian Renaissance*. London and Baltimore: Johns Hopkins University Press.

Grierson P (1978) John Caius' Library. In Prichard MJ and Skemp JB (eds) *The Biographical History of Gonville and Caius College, VII.1*. Cambridge: Cambridge University Press: 509–25.

Griffin C (2020) Disentangling Commodity Histories: *Pauame* and Sassafras in the Early Modern Global World. In *Journal of Early Modern Global History* 15: 1–18.

Grmek MD (1978) Contribution à la bibliographie de Vidius. In *Revue d'histoire des Sciences* 31: 289–99.

Grunberg B (2006) Les apothicaires de la Péninsule ibérique aux Indes espagnoles (XVIᵉ siècle). In Collard F and Samama E (eds) *Pharmacopoles et apothicaires: Les <pharmaciens> de l'Antiquité au Grand Siècle*. Paris: L'Harmattan: 151–66.

Guest CEL (2014) Art, Antiquarianism and Early Anatomy. In *Medical Humanities* 40: 97–104.

Guilday P (1914) The English Catholic Refugees at Louvain, 1559–1575 (Vatican Library, MS. Regina. 2020. F. 445–446. In aa.vv. *Mélanges d'histoire offerts à Charles Moeller*. Louvain: Bureau du Receuil; Paris: A Picard et Fils: Vl. 2: 175–89.

Gundert B (2006) Zu den Quellen der Basler Galen-Ausgabe (1538). In Müller *et al.* (eds): 81–100.

Gunnoe CD and Shackelford J (2009) Johannes Crato von Krafftheim (1519–1585): Imperial Physician, Irenicist, and Anti-Paracelsian. In Plummer ME and Barnes R (eds) *Ideas and Cultural Margins in Early Modern Germany: Essays in Honor of H. C. Erik Midelfort*. Farnham and Aldershot: Ashgate: 201–16.

Gutwirth E (2004) Amatus Lusitanus and the Location of Sixteenth Century Cultures. In Ruderman DB and Veltri G (eds) *Cultural Intermediaries: Jewish Intellectuals in Early Modern Europe*. Philadelphia: University of Pennsylvania Press: 216–38.

Guy JA (1988) *Tudor England*. Oxford and New York: Oxford University Press.

Győry T (1901) *Morbus hungaricus: Eine medico-historische Quellenstudie, zugleich ein Beitrag zur Geschichte der Türkenherrschaft in Ungarn*. Jena: Gustav Fischer.

Győry T (1912) *Die morbus Brunogallicus (1577): Ein Beitrag zur Geschichte der Syphilisepidemien*. Giessen: A. Töpelmann.

Hadass O (2018) *Medicine, Religion and Magic in Early Stuart England: Richard Napier's Medical Practice*. University Park, PA: The Pennsylvania State University Press.

Hagenmeyer C (1981) Die Entstehung des 'Zwölfbändigen Buches der Medizin' zu Heidelberg. In Keil (ed): 538–45.

Hale J (1994) *The Civilization of Europe in the Renaissance*. London: Fontana Press.

Hall TS (1975) *History of General Physiology 600 B.C. to A,D. 1900. Volume One, from Pre-Socratic Times to the Enlightenment*. Chicago and London: The University of Chicago Press.

Hammond EA (1975) Doctor Augustine, Physician to Cardinal Wolsey and Henry VIII. In *Medical History* 19: 215–49.

Harding V (2019) Plague in Early Modern London: Chronologies, Localities, and Environments. In Engelmann L, Henderson J and Lynteris C (eds) *Plague and the City*. London: Routledge: 39–68.

Hardingham GJ (2005) *The Regimen in Late Medieval England*. PhD Diss. Cambridge University, Cambridge.

Harig G (1974) *Bestimmung der Intensität im medizinischen System Galens*. Berlin: Akademie Verlag.

Harkness DE (2007) *The Jewel House: Elizabethan London and the Scientific Revolution*. New Haven and London: Yale University Press.

Harley D (1990) A Sword in a Madman's Hand: Professional Opposition to Popular Consumption in the Waters Literature of Southern England and the Midlands, 1570–1870. In Porter (ed): 48–55.

Harley D (2000) Rychard Bostok of Tandridge, Surrey (c. 1530–1605), Paracelsian Propagandist and Friend of John Dee. In *Ambix* 47: 29–36.

Harper-Bill C (2004) Robert Sherborn. In *ODNB* 50: 283–4.

Haye T (2019) Lorenz Gryll (d. 1560): A Traveller in Search of Medical Training. In Enenkel and De Jong (eds): 75–91.

Heesakkers CL (1996) Petrus Forestus in gedichten en brieven: Een overzicht van het material en een editie van zijn correspondentie met Johannes Heurnius. In Bosman-Jelgersma (ed): (1996b) 119–244.

Helm J (2001) Religion and Medicine: Anatomical Education at Wittenberg and Ingoldstadt. In Helm J and Winkelmann A (eds) *Confessions and the Sciences in the Sixteenth Century*. Leiden: Brill: 51–68.

Henderson J (1994) *Piety and Charity in Late Medieval Florence*. Oxford: Clarendon Press.

Henderson J (2006) *The Renaissance Hospital: Healing the Body and Healing the Soul*. New Haven and London: Yale University Press.

Henderson J (2019) *Florence Under Siege: Surviving Plague in an Early Modern City*. New Haven and London: Yale University Press.

Henderson J, Horden P and Pastore A (eds) (2007) *The Impact of Hospitals in Europe 1000–2002*. Amsterdam: Rodopi.

Henderson J, Jacobs F and Nelson J (eds) (2021) *Representing Infirmities: Diseased Bodies in Renaissance Italy*. London and New York: Routledge.

Heyd U (1964) An Unknown Turkish Treatise by a Jewish Physician Under Suleyman the Magnificent. In *Eretz Israel: Archaeological, Historical and Geographical Studies* 1: 48–53.

Heyman P, Cochez C and Hukić M (2018) The English Sweating Sickness: Out of Sight, Out of Mind? In *Acta Medica Academica* 47: 102–16.

Hieronymus F (1991) 'Habent sua fata libelli': Ein Widmungsgedicht Johannes Cratos und ein Lutherbild in der Bibliothek eines Jesuiten. In *Gutenberg Jahrbuch* 66: 230–43.

Hieronymus F (2005) *Theophrast und Galen – Celsus und Paracelsus. Medizin, Naturphilosophie und Kirchenreform im Basler Buchdruck bis zum dreissigjährigen Krieg*. Basle: Universitätsbibliothek.

Hillman D and Mazzio C (eds) (1997) *The Body in Parts. Fantasies of Corporeality in Early Modern Europe*. London: Routledge.

Hirai H (2007) Semence, vertu formatrice et intellect agent chez Nicolò Leoniceno entre la tradition arabo-latine et la renaissance des commentaires grecs. In *Early Science and Medicine* 12: 134–65.

Hirai H (2011) *Medical Humanism and Natural Philosophy: Renaissance Debates on Matter, Life, and the Soul*. Leiden and Boston: Brill.

Hobart B (2020) *La Peste à la Renaissance: L'imaginaire d'un fléau dans la littérature au XVIᵉ siècle*. Paris: Garnier.

Hobson A (1975) The *iter italicum* of Jean Matal. In Hunt RW (ed) *Studies in the Book Trade in Honour of Graham Pollard*. Oxford: Oxford Bibliographical Society: 33–61.

Hobson A (1999) *Renaissance Book Collecting: Jean Grolier and Diego Hurtado de Mendoza, Their Books and Bindings*. Cambridge: Cambridge University Press.

Horne PR (1958) Reformation and Counter-Reformation at Ferrara: Antonio Musa Brasavola and Giambattiusta Cinthio Giraldi. In *Italian Studies* 13: 62–82.

Houtzager HL (ed) (1989) *Pieter van Foreest. Een Hollands medicus in de zestiende eeuw*. Amsterdam: Rodopi.

Houchon M (2003) Définition et Description: Ambroise Paré chirurgien méthodique et rationale. In Berriot-Salvadore and Mironneau (eds): 201–28.

Huguet-Termes T (2001) New World Materia Medica in Spanish Renaissance Medicine: From Scholarly Reception to Practical Impact. In *Medical History* 45: 359–76.

Huguet-Termes T (2009) Medical Hospitals and Welfare in the Context of the Hapsburg Empire. In Huguet-Termes T *et al.* (eds): 64–85.

Huguet-Termes T, Arrizabalaga J and Cook HJ (eds) (2009) *Health and Medicine in Hapsburg Spain: Agents, Practices, Representations: Medical History, Supplement 29*. London: The Wellcome Trust Centre for the History of Medicine at UCL.

Huisman F (1996) Civic Roles and Academic Definitions: The Changing Relationship Between Surgeons and Urban Government in Groningen, 1550–1800. In Marland and Pelling (eds): 69–100.

Hurd Mcad KC (1938) *A History of Women in Medicine: From the Earliest Times to the Beginning of the Nineteenth Century*. Haddam, CT: The Haddam Press.

Hurren ET (2011) *Dying for Victorian Medicine: English Anatomy and Its Trade in the Dead Poor, 1832 to 1929*. London: Palgrave Macmillan.

Ieraci-Bio AM (2017) Giorgio Valla e la medicina: Disegni anatomici e nomenclatura delle parti del corpo umano nel Mutin. α. W.5.5. (gr. 165). In *Galenos* 11: 227–45.

Jacobs F (2002) (Dis)assembling: Marsyas, Michelangelo, and the Accademia del Disegno. In *The Art Bulletin* 84: 426–48.

Jacquart D (1980) Le regard d'un médecin sur son temps: Jacques Despars (1380?–1458). In *Bibliothèque de l'École des Chartes* 138: 35–86.

Jacquart D (1998) Medical Scholasticism. In Grmek MD (ed) *Western Medical Thought from Antiquity to the Middle Ages*. Cambridge, MA and London: Harvard University Press: 273–90.

Janssen FA (2005) The Rise of the Typographical Paragraph. In Enenkel KAE and Neuber W (eds) *Cognition and the Book: Typologies and Formal Organisation of Knowledge in the Printed Book of the Early Modern Period*. Leiden and Boston: Brill: 9–32.

Joffe SN (2014) *Andreas Vesalius, the Making, the Madman and the Myth*. Bloomington: Author House.

Johns A (1998) *The Nature of the Book: Print and Knowledge in the Making*. Chicago: Chicago University Press.

Jones PM (1984) *Medieval Medical Miniatures*. London: The British Library.

Jones PM (1988) Thomas Lorkyn's Dissections, 1564/5 and 1566/7. In *Transactions of the Cambridge Bibliographical Society* 9 (3): 209–29.

Jones PM (1995) Reading Medicine in Tudor Cambridge. In Nutton and Porter (eds): 153–83.

Jones PM (1996) Book Ownership and the Lay Culture of Medicine in Tudor Cambridge. In Marland and Pelling (eds): 49–68.

Jones WRD (1988) *William Turner, Tudor Naturalist, Physician and Divine*. London and New York: Routledge.

Jones WRD (2004) Turner, William. In *ODNB* 55: 674–7.

Jouanna J (2008) Mercuriale, commentateur et éditeur d'Hippocrate. In Arcangeli and Nutton (eds): 269–300.

Jütte R (1988) 'Wo kein Weib ist, da seufzet der Kranke': Familie und Krankheit im 16. Jahrhundert. In *Jahrbuch des Instituts für Geschichte der Medizin der Robert Bosch Stiftung* 8: 7–24.

Jütte R (1991) *Ärzte, Heiler und Patienten: Medizinische Alltag im frühen Neuzeit*. Munich and Zurich: Artemis & Winkler.

Jütte R (1993) Valentin Rösswurm: Zur Sozialgeschichte des Paracelsismus im 16. Jht. In Dilg P and Rudolph H (eds) *Resultate und Desiderate der Paracelsus-Forschung. Sudhoffs Archiv, Beiheft 31*. Stuttgart: Steiner: 97–112.

Jurina K (1985) *Vom Quacksalber zum Doctor Medicinae*. Cologne: Bohlau Verlag.

Kahn D (2007) *Alchimie et paracelsisme en France à la fin de la Renaissance, 1567–1625*. Geneva: Droz.

Kahn D and Hirai H (eds) (2019) Pseudo-Paracelsus: Forgery and Early Modern Alchemy, Medicine and Natural Philosophy. In *Early Science and Medicine* 24: 415–572.

Kalff S (2018) Torinese Plague and Roman Fever: Court Physicians and Their Impact on Health Policy in Late Sixteenth Century Italy: Francesco Alessandri (1529–1587) and Marsilio Cagnati (1543–1612). In *Medizinhistorisches Journal* 53: 241–62.

Karant-Nunn SC (1987) *Zwickau in Transition, 1500–1547: The Reformation as an Agent of Change*. Columbus: Ohio State University Press.

Karant-Nunn SC (1997) *The Reformation of Ritual: An Interpretation of Early Modern Germany*. London and New York: Routledge.

Kassell L (2005) *Medicine and Magic in Elizabethan England: Simon Forman, Astrologer, Alchemist and Physician*. Oxford: Clarendon Press.

Katz DS (1994) *Jews in the History of England*. Oxford: Clarendon Press.

Kaufman D (1893) Jacob Mantino: Une page d'histoire de la Renaissance. In *Revue des Études juives* 28: 30–60, 207–38.

Kavvadia M (2015) *Making Medicine in Post-Tridentine Rome: Girolamo Mercuriale's De arte gymnastica. A Different Reading of the Book*. PhD Diss. European University Institute, Florence.

Kavvadia M (2021) Sources and Resources of Court Medicine in Mid-Sixteenth Rome: Erudition as an Epistemological and Ethical Claim. In Baldassari and Zampieri (eds): 171–88.

Keele KD and Pedretti C (1978–80) *The Drawings of Leonardo da Vinci in the Collection of Her Majesty the Queen at Windsor Castle*. New York: Harcourt Jovanovitch.

Keil G (ed) (1982) *Fachprosa-Studien: Beiträge zur mittelalterlichen Wissenschafts- und Geistesgeschichte*. Berlin: Erich Schmitt Verlag.

Keil G (ed) (1993) *"Ein teutsch puech machen": Untersuchungen zur landessprachlichen Vermittlung medizinischen Wissens. Ortolf-Studien 1*. Wiesbaden: Dr. Ludwig Reichert Verlag.

Keil G (1995) Mittelalterliche Konzepte in der Medizin des Paracelsus. In Zimmermann (ed): 173–94.

Kellett CE (1961) Sylvius and the Reform of Anatomy. In *Medical History* 5: 101–16.

Kemp M (2006) *Leonardo: Experience, Experiment and Design*. London: V & A.

Kerwin W (2005) *Beyond the Body: The Boundaries of Medicine and English Renaissance Drama*. Amherst and Boston: The University of Massachusetts Press.

Keynes, Sir G (1962) *Dr. Timothie Bright (1550–1615): A Survey of His Life with a Bibliography of His Writings*. London: The Wellcome Historical Medical Library.

King H (1998) *Hippocrates' Woman: Reading the Female Body in Ancient Greece*. London: Routledge.

King H (2004) *The Disease of Virgins: Green Sickness, Chlorosis and the Problems of Puberty*. London: Routledge.

King H (2007) *Midwifery, Obstetrics and the Rise of Gynaecology: The Uses of a Sixteenth-Century Compendium*. Aldershot: Ashgate.

King H (2013) *The One-Sex Body on Trial: The Classical and Early Modern Evidence*. Farnham and Burlington, VT: Ashgate.

Kinzelbach A (2014a) 'Erudite and Honoured Artisans'? Performers of Body Care and Surgery in Early Modern German Towns. In *Social History of Medicine* 27: 668–88.

Kinzelbach A (2014b) Women and Healthcare in Early Modern German Towns. In *Renaissance Studies* 28: 619–38.

Kinzelbach A (2020a) Negotiating on Paper: Councilors, Medical Officers and Patients in an Early Modern City. In Mendelsohn *et al.* (eds): 162–81.

Kinzelbach A (2020b) Leprosaria: The Simultaneity of Segregation and Integration in Early Modern South German Towns. In Stevens Crawshaw *et al.* (eds): 46–66.

Kirkup J (2006) *The Evolution of Surgical Instruments: An Illustrated History from Ancient Times to the Twentieth Century*. Novato: Historyofscience.com.

Klebs AC (1938) Incunabula scientifica et medica. In *Osiris* 4: 1–359.

Klestinec C (2010) Medical Education in Padua: Students, Faculty and Facilities. In Grell *et al.* (eds): 193–211.

Klestinec C (2011) *Theaters of Anatomy: Students, Teachers and Traditions of Dissection in Renaissance Italy*. Baltimore: Johns Hopkins University Press.

Kilbansky R, Panofsky E and Saxl F (1964) *Saturn and Melancholy*. London: Nelson.

Kocher PH (1947) The Physician as Atheist in Elizabethan England. In *Huntington Library Quarterly* 10: 229–49.

Koelbing HM (1967) *Renaissance der Augenheilkunde 1540–1630*. Bern: Huber.

König KG (1961) *Der Nürnberger Stadtarzt Dr Georg Palma (1543–1591)*. Stuttgart: Fischer.

Kornell MN (1989) Rosso Fiorentino and the Anatomical Text. In *The Burlington Magazine* 131 (1041): 842–7.

Kornell MN (1993) *Artists and the Study of Anatomy in Sixteenth-Century Italy*. PhD Diss. University of London, London.

Kornell MN (1998) Drawings for Bartolomeo Passarotti's Book on Anatomy. In Currie S (ed) *Drawing 1400–1600: Invention and Innovation*. London: Ashgate: 172–88.

Kornell MN (2000) Vesalius' Method of Articulating the Skeleton and a Drawing in the Collection of the Wellcome Library. In *Medical History* 44: 97–110.

Kornell MN (2018) Jan Steven van Calcar (c. 1515 – c. 1546), Vesalius's Illustrator. In Canalis and Ciavolella (eds): 99–130.

Kornell MN (2022) *Flesh and Bones: The Art of Anatomy*. Los Angeles: Getty Research Institute.

Kosmin JF (2018) Midwifery Anatomized: Vesalius. Dissection and Reproductive Authority in Early Modern Italy. In *The Journal of Medieval and Early Modern Studies* 48: 79–104.

Krause C (1879) *Helius Eobanus Hessus, sein Leben und Seine Werke: Ein Beitrag zur Cultur- und Gelehrtengeschichte des 16. Jahrhunderts*. Gotha: Perthes.

Kunstmann H (1963) *Die Nürnberger Universität Altdorf und Böhmen*. Cologne and Graz: Böhlau Verlag.

Kusukawa S (1993) *Aspectio divinorum operum:* Melanchthon and Astrology for Lutheran Medics. In Grell and Cunningham (eds): 33–56.

Kusukawa S (2012) *Picturing the Book of Nature: Image, Text and Argument in Sixteenth-Century Human Anatomy and Medical Biology*. Chicago: Chicago University Press.

Labowsky L (1961) Manuscripts from Bessarion's Library Found in Milan. In *Medieval and Renaissance Studies* 5: 108–31.

Labowsky L (1979) *Bessarion's Library and the Biblioteca Marciana. Sussidi eruditi 31*. Rome: Edizioni di storia e letteratura.

Lambrecht K (2002) Stadt und Geschichtskultur: Breslau und Krakau im 16. Jahrhundert. In Bahlcke J and Strohmeyer A (eds) *Die Konstruktion der Vergangenheit: Geschichtsdenken, Traditionsbildung und Selbstdarstellung im frühneuzeitlichen Ostmitteleuropa*. Berlin: Duncker & Humblot: 245–64.

Lammel HU (2018) Hofmedizin als interdisziplinäre Forschungsaufgabe – eine Bilanz/Court Medicine as Interdisciplinary Challenge – a Review. In *Medizinhistorisches Journal* 53: 197–216.

Landucci Ruffo P (1981) Le fonti della medicina nell'enciclopedia di Giorgio Valla. In Branca V (ed) *Giorgio Valla tra scienza e sapienza*. Florence: Olschki: 55–68.

Lanning JT (1985) *The Royal Protomedicato: The Regulation of the Medical Professions in the Spanish Empire*. Durham, NC: Duke University Press.

Latham S (2010) *"Lady Alcumy": Elizabethan Gentlewomen and the Practice of Chymistry*. PhD Diss. Victoria University of Wellington, Wellington.

Laurenza D (2003) *La ricerca dell'armonia: Rappresentazioni anatomiche nel Rinascimento*. Florence: L. S. Olscki.

Laurenza D (2011) In Search of a Phantom; Marcantonio della Torre and Leonardo's Late Anatomical Studies. In Nova A and Laurenza D (eds) *Leonardo's Anatomical World: Language, Context and "Disegno"*. Venice: Marsilio.

Laurenza D (2012a) Art and Anatomy in Renaissance Italy: Images from a Scientific Revolution. In *Metropolitan Museum of Art Bulletin* 69 (3): 1–48.

Laurenza D (2012b) Contenuto, canoni visive e techniche nella illustrazioni anatomiche del Rinascimento: Riflessioni in margine ad una tavola di Berengario da Carpi. In Olmi and Pancino (eds): 27–44.

Laven M (2016) Recording Miracles in Renaissance Italy. In *Past and Present* 230 (Suppl. 11): 191–212.

Lee S and Wallis P (2004) Chambre, John. In *ODNB* 42: 198–9.

Legrand E (1885) *Bibliographie Hellénique*. Paris: Ernest Leroux.

Lehoux F (1976) *Le cadre de vie des médecins parisiens aux XVIe et XVIIe siècles*. Paris: Picard.

Lenz R (ed) (1984) *Leichenpredigten als Quelle historischer Wissenschaften*. Marburg: Böhlau Verlag.

Leong E (2018) *Recipes and Everyday Knowledge: Medicine, Science, and the Household in Early Modern England*. Chicago: University of Chicago Press.

Leu UB (2014) Die Bedeutung Basels als Druckort im 16. Jahrhundert. In Christ-von Wedel C, Grosse S and Hamm B (eds) *Basel als Zentrum des geistigen Austauschs in der frühen Reformation*. Tübingen: Mohr Siebeck.

Leu UB (2016a) *Conrad Gessner (1516–1565): Universalgelehrter und Naturforscher der Renaissance*. Zürich: Verlag Neue Züricher Zeitung.

Leu UB (2016b) Conrad Gessners Netzwerk. In Leu and Ruoss (eds): 61–74.

Leu UB and Ruoss M (eds) (2016) *Facetten eines Universums: Conrad Gessner 1516–1565*. Zürich: Verlag Neue Züricher Zeitung.

Lewis GM (1986) The Faculty of Medicine. In McConica J (ed) *The History of the University of Oxford. Vol. III: The Collegiate University*. Oxford: Clarendon Press: 213–56.

Lind LR (1959) *Berengario da Carpi, a Short Introduction to Anatomy*. Chicago: University of Chicago Press.

Lind LR (1975) *Studies in Pre-Vesalian Anatomy; Biography, Translations, Documents*. Philadelphia: American Philosophical Society.

Lindemann M (2010) *Medicine and Society in Early Modern Europe*, ed. 2. Cambridge: Cambridge University Press.

Lincs D (1922) <u>*The Dynamics of Learning in Early Modern Italy: Arts and Medicine at the University of Bologna*</u>. Cambridge, MA and London: Harvard University Press.

Livi Bacci M (2008) *Conquest: The Destruction of the American Indios*. Cambridge and Malden, MA: Polity Press.

Lo M (2018) Cut, Copy and English Anatomy: Thomas Geminus and the Reordering of Vesalius's Canonical Body. In Canalis and Ciavolella (eds): 225–53.

Long PO (2011) *Artisan/Practitioners and the Rise of the New Sciences: 1400–1600*. Corvallis: Oregon State University Press.

Lonie IM (1985) The 'Paris Hippocratics': Teaching and Research in Paris in the Second Half of the Sixteenth Century. In Wear *et al.* (eds): 155–74.

Lonigo A (2019) *Nicolò Leoniceno 1428–1524 Un umanista veneto nella storia della Medicina: Atti del Convegno in Lonigo per il 590 anniversario della nascita*. Contro: Riccardo editore.

Lopes Andrade AM (2018) Conrad Gessner Edits Brudus Lusitanus: The Trials and Tribulations of Publishing a Sixteenth Century Treatise on Dietetics. In Stuckzynski CB and Feitler B (eds) *Portuguese Jews, New Christians and 'New Jews': A Tribute to Roberto Bachmann*. Leiden and Boston: Brill: 189–205.

Lopes Andrade AM, De Miguel C and Nunes Torrao JM (eds) (2015) *Humanismo e Ciencia: Antiguedad e Renascimento*. Aveiro, Coimbra and So Paolo: UA Editora.

López Piñero JM and Pardo Tomás J (1996) *La influencia de Francisco Hernandez (1515–1587) en la constitución de la botánica y la materia médica modernas*. Valencia: Universitat de Valencia, CSIC.

López Terrada ML (2007) The Control of Medical Practice Under the Spanish Monarchy During the Sixteenth and Seventeenth Centuries. In Navarro Brotóns V and Eamon W (eds) *Beyond the Black Legend: Spain and the Scientific Revolution*. Valencia: Publicacions de la Universitat de Valencia: 283–94.

López Terrada ML (2009) Medical Pluralism in the Iberian Kingdoms: The Control of Extra-Academic Practitioners in Valencia. In Huguet-Termes *et al.* (eds): 7–25.

Lorenz B (1983) Notizen zu Privatbibliotheken deutscher Ärzte des 15.–17. Jahrhunderts. In *Sudhoffs Archiv* 67: 190–8.

Louthan H (1994) *Johannis Crato and the Austrian Habsburgs: Reforming a Counter-Reform Court*. Princeton, NJ: Princeton Theological Seminary.

Louthan H (1997) *The Quest for Compromise: Peacemakers in Counter-Reformation Vienna*. Cambridge: Cambridge University Press.

Loviconi L (2020) *Le diagnostic différentiel au Moyen Âge: Distinguer les maladies d'apparence voisine*. Paris: Classiques Garnier.

Lowry MJC (1974–5) Two Great Venetian Libraries. In *Bulletin of the John Rylands Library* 57: 128–66.

Ludwig F (1909) Dr Simon Simonius in Leipzig. In *Neues Archiv für sächsische Geschichte und Altertumskunde* 30: 209–90.

Ludwig W (1999) *Vater und Sohn im 16. Jahrhundert: Der Briefwechsel des Wolfgang Reichart . . . mit seinem Sohn Zeno (1520–1543)*. Hildesheim: Weidmann.

Lundin M (2012) *Paper Memory: A Sixteenth-Century Townsman Writes His World*. Cambridge, MA and London: Harvard University Press.

MacCulloch D (2003) *Reformation: Europe's House Divided 1490–1700*. London: Penguin.

MacCulloch D (2018) Thomas Cromwell. *A Revlolutionary Life*. New York: Viking.

MacDonald M (1981) *Mystical Bedlam: Madness, Anxiety, and Healing in Seventeenth-Century England*. Cambridge: Cambridge University Press.

Maclean I (1980) *The Renaissance Notion of Woman: A Study in the Fortunes of Scholasticism and Medical Science in European Intellectual Life*. Cambridge: Cambridge University Press.

Maclean I (2000) The Diffusion of Learned Medicine in the Sixteenth Century Through the Printed Book. In Bracke W and Deumens H (eds) *Medical Latin from the Late Middle Ages to the Eighteenth Century*. Brussels: Koninklijke Academie voor Geneeskunde van Belgie: 93–114.

Maclean I (2002) *Logic, Signs and Nature in the Renaissance*. Cambridge: Cambridge University Press.

Maclean I (2004) *De libris propriis: The Editions of 1544, 1550, 1557, 1562 with Supplementary Material*. Milan: FrancoAngeli.

Maclean I (2008) The Medical Republic of Letters Before the Thirty Years War. In *Intellectual History Review* 18: 15–30.

Maclean I (2009) *Learning and the Market Place: Essays in the History of the Early Modern Book*. Leiden and Boston: Brill.

Maclean I (2017) A Medical Collection Anatomized: The *Catalogus Bibliothecae Hieremiae Martii* (1572). In Manning and Klestinec (eds): 101–23.

Maddison F, Pelling M and Webster C (eds) (1977) *Essays on the Life and Work of Thomas Linacre c.1460–1524*. Oxford: Clarendon Press.

Madonia C (1980) Simone Simoni da Lucca. In *Rinascimento* 20: 161–97.

Maloney G and Savoie R (1985) *Cinq Cent Ans de Bibliographie Hippocratique 1473–1982*. St-Jean-Chrystostome: Les Éditions du Sphinx.

Manfron A (ed) (1998) *La biblioteca di un medico del quattrocento: I codici di Giovanni di Marco da Rimini nella Biblioteca Malatestiana*. Turin: Umberto Allemandi.

Mann S (2020) 'A Double Cure': Prayer as Therapy in Early Modern England. In *Social History of Medicine* 33: 1055–76.

Manning G and Klestinec C (eds) (2017) *Professors, Physicians and Practices in the History of Medicine: Essays in Honor of Nancy Siraisi.* Cham: Springer.

Marchesi S (1678) *Supplemento istorico dell'antica città di Forli.* Forlì: Gioseffe Selua.

Marcus H (2020) *Forbidden Knowledge: Medicine, Science and Censorship in Early Modern Italy.* Chicago: University of Chicago Press.

Margócsy D, Somos M and Joffe SN (2018) *The* Fabrica *of Andreas Vesalius: A Worldwide Descriptive Census, Ownership and Annotations of the 1543 and 1555 Editions.* Leiden and Boston: Brill.

Marland H (ed) (1993) *The Art of Midwifery: Early Modern Midwives in Europe.* London and New York: Routledge.

Marland H and Pelling M (eds) (1996) *The Task of Healing: Medicine, Religion and Gender in England and the Netherlands, 1450–1800.* Rotterdam: Erasmus Publishing.

Martin R (1989) *Witchcraft and the Inquisition in Venice, 1550–1650.* Oxford: Basil Blackwell.

Martinez Millan J (2000) *La Corte de Carlos V, tercera parte, Los Servidores de las Casas Reales*, vol. V. Madrid: Sociedad Estatal para la Conmemoración de los Centenarios de Felipe II y Carlos V.

Martínez Navarro MdelR (2018) Cristóbal de Castillejo y el *milagro americano*: El palo santo de Indias y el *mal de bubas* en clave bufonesca, política y anticortesana. In *Temas Americanistas* 40: 92–118.

Marx F (1915) *A. Cornelius Celsus, De medicina. Corpus medicorum latinorum I.* Leipzig: Teubner.

Mattern SP (2020) Galen, Lykos of Macedon, and Rivalry for the Legacy of Quintus. In Pietrobelli A (ed) *Contre Galien: Critques d'une autorité médicale de l'Antiquité à l'âge moderne.* Paris: Honoré Champion: 31–44.

Matthews LG (1962) *History of Pharmacy in Britain.* Edinburgh and London: E & S Livingstone Ltd.

Maurette P (2018) The Organ of Organs: Vesalius and the Wonders of the Human Hand. In *The Journal of Medieval and Early Modern Studies* 48: 79–104.

McClive C and King H (2007) When Is a Foetus Not a Foetus? Diagnosing False Conceptions in Early Modern France. In Dasen V (ed) *L'embryon humain à travers l'histoire.* Gollion: Infolio: 223–38.

McDonald G (2013) Thomas More, John Clement and the Palatine Anthology. In *Bibliothèque d'Humanisme et Renaissance* 75 (2): 259–70.

McVaugh MD (1998) Therapeutic Strategies: Surgery. In Grmek MD (ed) *Western Medical Thought from Antiquity to the Middle Ages.* Cambridge, MA and London: Harvard University Press: 273–90.

Mendelsohn JA, Kinzelbach A and Schilling R (eds) (2020) *Civic Medicine, Physician, Polity and Pen in Early Modern Europe.* London and New York: Routledge.

Merisalo O, Kuha M and Niiranen S (eds) (2019) *Transmission of Knowledge in the Late Middle Ages and the Renaissance.* Bibliologia, Elementa ad librorum studia pertinentia 53. Turnhout: Brepols.

Michel SH (2015) Die ältesten Statuten der medizinischen Fakultät der Universität Rostock. In *Medizinhistorisches Journal* 50: 295–306.

Midelfort HCE (1980) Protestant Monastery? A Reformation Hospital in Hesse. In Brooks PN (ed) *Reformation Principle and Practice: Essays in Honour of Arthur Geoffrey Dickens*. London: Routledge: 71–93.

Midelfort HCE (1999) *A History of Madness in Sixteenth-Century Germany*. Stanford: Stanford University Press.

Mikkeli H (1999) *Hygiene in the Early Modern Medical Tradition*. Helsinki: The Finnish Academy of Science and Letters.

Militzer K (1975) *Das Markgröninger Heilig-Geist-Spital im Mittelalter: Ein Beitrag zur Wirtschaftsgeschite des 15. Jahrhunderts*. Sigmaringen: Jan Thorbecke Verlag.

Milt B (1959) *Vadian als Arzt*. St. Gallen: Verlag der Fehr'schen Buchhandlung.

Mitchell WT (ed) (1980) *Epistolae academicae 1508–1596*. Oxford Historical Society, n.s. 26. Oxford: Clarendon Press.

Mocarelli L (2008) Guilds Reappraised: Italy in the Early Modern Period. In *International Review of Social History* 53 (Suppl.): 159–78.

Mocarelli L (2018) Il Sistema delle arti. In Ago R (ed) *Storia del lavoro in Italia. Vol. III: L'età moderna: Trasformazioni e risorse del lavoro tra associazioni di mestiere e pratiche individuali*. Rome: Castelvecchi: 19–50.

Moëll H (1984) *Ulrich von Hutten, Guajak och Franska Sjukan: Sydsvenska Medicinhistoriska Sällskapets Årsskrift, Supplement 3*. https://www.antikvariat.net/en/rod50695-ulrich-von-hutten-guajak-och-franska-sjukan-moell-hans-antikvariat-roda-rummet-ab.

Monahan E (2016) *The Merchants of Siberia: Trade in Early Modern Eurasia*. Ithaca and London: Cornell University Press.

Monahan E (2021) Locating Rhubarb: Early Modernity's Relevant Obscurity. In Findlen P (ed) *Early Modern Things: Objects and Their Histories, 1500–1800*, ed. 2. London: Routledge: 297–322.

Mondrain B (1997) Éditer et traduire les médecins grecs au XVIe siècle: L'exemple de Janus Cornarius. In Jacquart D (ed) *Les voies de la science grecque: Études sur la transmission des textes de l'Antiquité au dix-neuvième siècle*. Paris: De Boccard: 391–417.

Montagne V (2017) *Médecine et rhétorique à la Renaissance: Le cas du traité de peste en langue vernaculaire*. Paris: Classiques Garnier.

Montfort ML (2018) *Janus Cornarius et la redécouverte d'Hippocrate à la Renaissance*. Turnhout: Brepols.

Moore N and Bakewell S (2004) Chambre, John. In *ODNB* 10: 1009–10.

Moote AL and Moote DG (2004) *The Great Plague: The Story of London's Most Deadly Year*. Baltimore: The Johns Hopkins University Press.

Moran BT (1991) *The Alchemical World of the German Courts: Occult Philosophy and Chemical Medicine in the Circle of Moritz of Hessen, 1572–1632*. Stuttgart: Franz Steiner Verlag.

Moran BT (2019) *Paracelsus: An Alchemical Life*. London: Reaktion Books.

Morys P (1982) *Medizin und Pharmazie in der Kosmologie Leonhard Thurneissers zum Thurn (1531–1596)*. Husum: Matthiesen Verlag.

Mudry A (2013) Disputes Surrounding the Discovery of the Stapes in the Mid-16th Century. In *Otology & Neurotology* 34 (3): 588–92.

Müller CW, Brockmann C and Brunschön CW (eds) (2006) *Ärzte und ihre Interpreten: Medizinische Fachtexte der Antike als Forschungsgegenstand der Klassischen Philologie. Fachconferenz zu Ehren von Diethard Nickel*. Munich and Leipzig: K. G. Saur.

Müller I (1970) Die Entwicklung der Schiffspharmazie. In *Deutsche Apotheker Zeitung* 110: 1241–9.

Müller-Jahncke WD (1983) Agrippa von Nettesheim in Antwerpen: Ein Beitrag zur Geschichte des 'Englischen Schweiß'. In Dilg P (ed) *Perspective der Pharmaziegeschichte: Festschrift für Rudolf Schmitz zum 65. Geburtstag.* Graz: Akademische Druck- u. Verlagsanstalt: 243–68.

Mugnai Carrara D (1979) Profilo di Nicolò Leoniceno. In *Interpres* 2: 169–212.

Mugnai Carrara D (1983) Una polemica umanistica-scolastica circa l'interpretazione delle tre dottrine ordinate di Galeno. In *Annali dell'Istituto e Museo di storia della scienza di Firenze* 8: 31–57.

Mugnai Carrara D (1989) La polemica "De cane rabida" di Nicolò Leoniceno, Nicolò Zocca e Scipione Carteromaco: Un episodio di filologia medico-umanista. In *Interpres* 9: 196–236.

Mugnai Carrara D (1991) *La biblioteca di Nicolò Leoniceno tra Aristotele e Galeno; cultura e libri di un medico umanista.* Florence: L.S. Olschki.

Mugnai Carrara D and Conforti M (2008) L'insegnamento della medicina delle università. In Clericuzio and Ernst (eds): 455–78.

Mungert RS (1949) Guiacum, the Holy Wood from the New World. In *Journal of the History of Medicine and Allied Sciences* 4: 196–229.

Munkhoff R (2014) Poor Women and Parish Public Health in Sixteenth-Century London. In *Renaissance Studies* 28: 579–96.

Muratori G (1969) Academic Career and Anatomical Teaching of G. B. Cananus at St. Dominic and the Anatomical Theatres of the University of Arts and Medicine of Ferrara. In *Acta Anatomica* (Suppl. 56): 308–24.

Muratori G and Menini C (1947) Contributi allo studio della storia dell' anatomia e della medicina nell'Ateneo ferrarese nel 1500. In *Annali dell'Università di Ferrara* 5: 19–103.

Murphy H (2019) *A New Order of Medicine: The Rise of Physicians in Reformation Nuremberg.* Pittsburgh: University of Pittsburgh Press.

Murphy H (2020) Skin and Disease in Early Modern Medicine: Jan Jessen's *De cute et cutaneis affectibus* (1601). In *Bulletin of the History of Medicine* 94: 197–214.

Nance B (2001) *Turquet de Mayerne as Baroque Physician.* Amsterdam and New York: Rodopi.

Nance B (2005) Wondrous Experience as Text: Valleriola and the *Observationes Medicinales*. In Furdell EL (ed) *Textual Healing: Essays in Medieval and Early Modern Medicine.* Leiden: Brill: 101–18.

Nauck ET (1956) Der Ingolstädter medizinische Lehrplan aus der Mittte des 16. Jahrhunderts. In *Sudhoffs Archiv* 40: 1–14.

Nauert CG (1979) Humanists, Scientists, and Pliny: Changing Approaches to a Classical Author. In *The American Historical Review* 84: 72–85.

Nauert CG (1980) Caius Plinius Secundus. In Cranz FE (ed) *Catalogus Translationum et Commentariorum*, vol. 4. Washington, DC: Catholic University of America Press: 297–422.

Nayar SJ (2019) *Renaissance Responses to Technological Change.* Cham: Springer Nature.

Newman WR and Grafton AT (eds) (2001) *Secrets of Nature: Astrology and Alchemy in Early Modern Europe.* Cambridge, MA: MIT Press.

Newton H (2018) *Misery to Mirth: Recovery from Illness in Early Modern England.* Oxford: Oxford University Press.

Nicholl C (2004) *Leonardo da Vinci: The Flight of the Mind*. London: Penguin.

Nobre de Carvalho T (2015) Estratégias, patronos e favores em *Colóquios dos Simples* de Garcia de Orta. In Lopes Andrade *et al.* (eds): 63–94.

Nolte C (2020) Domestic Care in the Sixteenth Century: Expectations, Experiences, and Practices from a Gendered Perspective. In Ritchey S and Strocchia S (eds) *Gender, Health and Healing, 1250–1550*. Amsterdam: Amsterdam University Press: 215–43.

Nutton V (1974) Niccolò Moranghelli, a libellous physician. In *Medicalo History* 17: 83–8.

Nutton V (1981) Continuity or Rediscovery? The City Physician in Classical Antiquity and Mediaeval Italy. In Russell (ed): 9–46.

Nutton V (1983) The Seeds of Disease: An Explanation of Contagion and Infection from the Greeks to the Renaissance. In *Medical History* 27: 1–34.

Nutton V (1985a) Harvey, Goulston and Galen. In *Koroth* 8: 112–22.

Nutton V (1985b) Humanist Surgery. In Wear *et al.* (eds): 75–99.

Nutton V (1985c) Murders and Miracles: Lay Attitudes Towards Medicine in Classical Antiquity. In Porter (ed): 23–54.

Nutton V (1987a) *John Caius and the Manuscripts of Galen: Proceedings of the Cambridge Philological Society, Supplementary 13*. Cambridge: The Cambridge Philological Society.

Nutton V (1987b) 'Qui magni Galeni doctrinam in re medica primus revocavit' Matteo Corti und der Galenismus im medizinischen Unterricht der Renaissance. In Keil G, Moeller B and Trusen W (eds) *Der Humanismus und die oberen Fakultäten, Mitteilungen XIV der Kommission fur Humanismusforschung*. Weinheim: VDA: 173–84.

Nutton V (1988a) *Prisci dissectionum professores*: Greek Texts and Renaissance Anatomists. In Dionisotti AC, Grafton A and Kraye J (eds) *The Uses of Greek and Latin, Historical Essays*. London: The Warburg Institute: 111–26.

Nutton V (1988b) Rabelais's Copy of Galen. In *Etudes Rabelaisiennes* 22: 181–7.

Nutton V (1989) Pieter van Foreest and the Plagues of Europe; Some Observations on the *Observationes*. In Houtzager (ed): 25–39.

Nutton V (ed) (1990a) *Medicine at the Courts of Europe 1500–1837*. London: Croom Helm.

Nutton V (1990b) The Anatomy of the Soul in Early Renaissance Medicine. In Dunstan GR (ed) *The Human Embryo: Aristotle and the Arabic and European Traditions*. Exeter: University of Exeter Press: 136–57.

Nutton V (1990c) Medicine, Diplomacy and Finance: The Prefaces to a Hippocratic Commentary of 1541. In Henry J and Hutton S (eds) *New Perspectives on Renaissance Thought: Essays in the History of Science, Education and Philosophy in Memory of Charles B. Schmitt*. London: Duckworth: 230–44.

Nutton V (1990d) The Reception of Fracastoro's Theory of Contagion: The Seed that Fell Among Thorns? In *Osiris*, ser. 2, 6: 196–234.

Nutton V (1993) Wittenberg Anatomy. In Grell and Cunningham (eds): 11–32.

Nutton V (1995) Der Luther der Medizin: Ein paracelsisches Paradoxon. In Zimmermann (ed): 105–12.

Nutton V (1996) "Idle Old Trots, Coblers and Costardmongers"; Pieter van Foreest on Quackery. In Bosman-Jelgersma (ed): 243–56.

Nutton V (1997a) Hellenism Postponed: Some Aspects of Renaissance Medicine, 1490–1530. In *Sudhoffs Archiv* 81: 158–70.

Nutton V (1997b) The Rise of Medical Humanism: Ferrara, 1464–1555. In *Renaissance Studies* 11: 2–19.

Nutton V (1998) An Early Reader of Vesalius' *Fabrica*. In *Vesalius* 3: 73–4.

Nutton V (1999) "A Diet for Barbarians": Introducing Renaissance Medicine to Tudor England. In Grafton and Siraisi (eds): 275–94.

Nutton V (2003) André Vésale et l'anatomie parisienne. In *Cahiers de l'Association Internationale des Études Françaises* 55: 239–49.

Nutton V (2005) Books, Printing and Medicine in the Renaissance. In *Medicina nei Secoli* 17: 421–42.

Nutton V (2006) Medicine and Philology in Renaissance Paris. In Müller *et al.* (eds): 49–59.

Nutton V (ed) (2008a) *Pestilential Complexities: Understanding Medieval Plague: Medical History, Supplement 27.* London: The Wellcome Trust Centre for the History of Medicine at UCL.

Nutton V (2008b) "It's the Patient's Fault": Simone Simoni and the Plague of Leipzig, 1575. In *Intellectual History Review* 18: 5–13.

Nutton V (2008c) The Pleasures of Erudition: Mercuriale's *Variae lectiones*. In Arcangeli and Nutton (eds): 191–202.

Nutton V (2008d) Greek Medical Astrology and the Boundaries of Medicine. In Akasoy A, Burnett C and Yoeli-Tlalim R (eds) *Astro-Medicine: Astrology and Medicine, East and West.* Florence: Sismel – Edizioni del Galluzzo: 17–31.

Nutton V (2009) Biographical Accounts of Galen, 1340–1660. In Rütten T (ed) *Geschichte der Medizingeschichtsschreibung: Historiographie unter dem Diktat literarischer Gattungen von der Antike bis zur Aufklärung.* Remscheid: Gardez! Verlag: 201–32.

Nutton V (2011) Understanding Contagious Diseases: Baillou's Notes on Julien Le Paulmier's *De morbis contagiosis*. In *Medicina & Storia* 11: 141–51.

Nutton V (2012a) Vesalius Revised: His Annotations to the 1555 *Fabrica*. In *Medical History* 56: 415–43.

Nutton V (2012b) *Physiologia*: From Antiquity to Jacob Bording. In Horstmanshoff M, King H and Zittel C (eds) *Blood, Sweat and Tears – the Changing Concepts of Physiology from Antiquity into Early Modern Europe.* Leiden and Boston: Brill: 27–40.

Nutton V (2013) *Ancient Medicine*, ed. 2. London and New York: Routledge.

Nutton V (2014) The Doctor and the Magistrate: A Lawyer's View of Medical Ethics. In Gadebusch-Bondio (ed): 211–20.

Nutton V (2015) Books, Printing and Medicine in the Renaissance. In *Medicina nei Secoli* 17: 421–42.

Nutton V (2017a) *Johann Guinter and Andreas Vesalius, Principles of Anatomy According to the Opinion of Galen.* London and New York: Routledge.

Nutton V (2017b) John Caius, Historian. In Manning and Klestinec (eds): 69–84.

Nutton V (2017c) Pieter Van Foreest: The Physician as Writer on Surgery. *Journal of the History of Medicine and Allied Sciences* 72: 87–97.

Nutton V (2018a) *An Autobibliography by John Caius.* London and New York: Routledge.

Nutton V (2018b) 1538, a Year of Vesalian Innovation. In *Journal of Medieval and Early Modern Studies* 48: 42–60.

Nutton V (2019) The Transmission of Medical Knowledge Between Script and Print. In Merisalo *et al.* (eds): 73–83.

Nutton V (2020a) *Galen: A Thinking Doctor in Imperial Rome.* London and New York: Routledge.

Nutton V (2020b) Vesalius in England, 1544–1547. In Van Hee (ed): 93–100.

Nutton V (2020c) *Abiit . . . noster Celsus ad excelsos*: Some Lost Editions of Celsus. In *Medicina nei Secoli* 32: 247–62.

Nutton V (2022) *Galen and the Latin De Voce: A New Edition and English Translation.*

Nutton V and Bos G (2011) *Galen, on Problematical Movements.* Cambridge: Cambridge University Press.

Nutton V and D'Alessio S (2021) *Santorio Santori and the Emergence of Quantified Medicine, 1614–1790*, ed. Barry J and Bigotti F. Cham: Springer Verlag.

Nutton V and Nutton C (2003) The Archer of Meudon: A Curious Absence of Continuity in the History of Medicine. *Journal of the History of Medicine and Allied Sciences* 58: 401–27.

Nutton V and Porter R (eds) (1995) *The History of Medical Education in Britain.* Amsterdam and Atlanta: Rodopi.

Offner R (2018) Neue Daten zur Biographie des Klausenburger Arztes Thomas Jordanus (1540–1586) Epidemiologe, Balneologe und Protomedicus von Mähren. In *Sudhoffs Archiv* 102: 89–112.

Ogilvie BW (2006) *The Science of Describing: Botany in Renaissance Europe.* Chicago: Chicago University Press.

Ogilvie BW (2011) How to Write a Letter: Humanist Correspondence Manuals and the Late Renaissance Community of Naturalists. In *Jahrbuch für Europäische Wissenschaftskultur* 6: 13–38.

Olmi G and Pancino A (eds) (2012) *Anatome: Sezione, scomposizione, raffigurazione del corpo nell'età moderna.* Bologna: Bononia University Press.

O'Malley CD (1964) *Andreas Vesalius of Brussels (1514–1564).* Berkeley and London: University of California Press.

O'Malley CD (ed) (1970) *The History of Medical Education.* Los Angeles: University of California Press.

Ongaro G (1971) La scoperta della circolazione pulmonare e la diffusione della *Christianismi Restitutio* di Michele Serveto nel XVI secolo in Italia e nel Veneto. In *Episteme* 5: 3–44.

Ongaro G (1981) La medicina nello Studio di Padova e nel Veneto. In Folena G (ed) *Storia della cultura veneta. Vol. III.: Dal primo Quattrocento al concilio di Trento.* Vicenza: Neri Pozza Editore, part 3: 75–134.

Ongaro G (1994) L'insegnamento clinico di Giovan Battista da Monte (1489–1551): Una revisione critica. In *Physis: Rivista internazionale di storia della scienza* 31: 358–69.

Ongaro G, Rippa Bonati M and Thiene G (eds) (2006) *Harvey e Padova.* Padua: Antilia.

Orme N and Webster M (1995) *The English Hospital 1070–1570.* New Haven and London: Yale University Press.

O'Rourke Boyle M (1996) *Divine Domesticity: Augustine of Thagaste to Teresa of Avila.* Leiden: Brill.

Ortiz T (1993) From Hegemony to Subordination: Midwives in Early Modern Spain. In Marland (ed): 95–114.

Overwien O (2019) *Medizinische Lehrewerke aus dem spätantiken Alexandrien: Die Tabulae Vindobonenses und Summaria alexandrinorum zu Galens De Sectis. Scientia Graeco-Arabica 24.* Berlin and Boston: W. de Gruyter.

Pagel W (1982) *Paracelsus: An Introduction to Philosophical Medicine in the Era of the Renaissance*, ed. 2. Basle: Karger.

Pagel W (1984) *The Smiling Spleen: Paracelsianism in Storm and Stress.* Basle: Karger.

Palmer RJ (1978) *The Control of Plague in Venice and Northern Italy, 1348–1600.* PhD Diss. University of Kent, Canterbury.

Palmer RJ (1981a) Physicians and the State in Post-Medieval Italy. In Russell (ed): 47–62.

Palmer RJ (1981b) Nicolò Massa, His Family and His Fortune. In *Medical History* 25: 385–410.

Palmer RJ (1983) *The Studio of Venice and Its Graduates in the Sixteenth Century.* Padua: Lint.

Palmer RJ (1985) Medical Botany in Northern Italy in the Renaissance. In *Journal of the Royal Society of Medicine* 77: 149–57.

Palmer RJ (1990a) Medicine at the Papal Court in the Sixteenth Century. In Nutton (ed): 49–78.

Palmer RJ (1990b) "In This Our Lightye and Learned Tyme": Italian Baths in the Era of the Renaissance. In Porter (ed): 14–22.

Palmer RJ (1993) Physicians and the Inquisition in Sixteenth-Century Venice. In Grell and Cunningham (eds): 118–33.

Palmer RJ (2008) Girolamo Mercuriale and the Plague of Venice. In Arcangeli and Nutton (eds): 51–66.

Palumbo M (2007) Manardi, Giovanni. In *DBI* 68: 420–2.

Panse M (2012) *Hans von Gersdorff 'Feldbuch der Wundearznei': Produktion, Präsentation und Rezeption von Wissen.* Wiesbaden: Reichert Verlag.

Pardo Tomás J (2012) Opening Bodies in the New World: Anatomical Practices in Sixteenth-Century New Spain. In Olmi and Pancino (eds): 185–202.

Park K (1985) *Doctors and Medicine in Early Renaissance Florence.* Princeton: Princeton University Press.

Park K (1992) Medicine and Society in Medieval Europe, 500–1500. In Wear A (ed) *Medicine in Society: Historical Essays.* Cambridge: Cambridge University Press.

Park K (1994) The Criminal and the Saintly Body: Autopsy and Dissection in Renaissance Italy. In *Renaissance Quarterly* 47: 1–33.

Park K (2006) *Secrets of Women: Gender, Generation and the Origins of Human Dissection.* London: Zone Books.

Park K and Henderson G (1991) "The First Hospital Among Christians": The Ospedale di Santa Maria Nuova in Early Sixteenth-Century Florence. In *Medical History* 35: 164–88.

Pastore A (2006) L'organizzazione sanitaria nella Repubblica di Venezia all'epoca di William Harvey. In Ongaro *et al.* (eds): 201–20.

Pastore A (2007) *Le regole dei corpi, Medicina e disciplina nell'Italia moderna.* Bologna: il Mulino.

Paulus J (1994) Alchemie und Paracelsismus um 1600: Siebzig Porträts. In Telle J (ed) *Analecta Paracelsica, Studien zum Nachleben Theophrast von Hohenheims im deutschen Kulturgebiet der frühen Neuzeit.* Stuttgart: Franz Steiner Verlag: 335–405.

Pelling M (1985) Healing the Sick Poor: Social Policy and Disability in Norwich 1550–1640. In *Medical History* 29: 115–37.

Pelling M (1996) Compromised by Gender: The Role of the Male Medical Practitioner in Early Modern England. In Marland and Pelling (eds): 101–34.

Pelling M (2003) *Medical Conflicts in Early Modern London: Patronage, Physicians and Irregular Practitioners 1550–1640*. Oxford: Oxford University Press.

Pelling M and Webster C (1979) Medical Practitioners. In Webster (ed): 165–236.

Pender S and Struever NS (eds) (2012) *Rhetoric and Medicine in Early Modern Europe*. Farnham and Burlington, VT: Ashgate.

Pennuto C (2008) *Simpatia, fantasia e contagio: Il pensiero medico e il pensiero filosofico di Girolamo Fracastoro*. Rome: Edizioni di Storia e Letteratura.

Perilli L (2012) A Risky Enterprise: The Aldine Edition of Galen, the Failures of the Editors, and the Shadow of Erasmus of Rotterdam. In *Early Science and Medicine* 17: 446–66.

Perini L (2002) *La vita e i tempi di Pietro Perna*. Rome: Edizioni di Storia e Letteratura.

Perkins W (1996) *Midwifery and Medicine in Early Modern France: Louise Bourgeois*. Exeter: University of Exeter Press.

Petit C, Swain S and Fischer KD (2021) *Pseudo-Galenica: The Formation of the Galenic Corpus from Antiquity to the Renaissance*. Warburg Institute Colloquia 34. London: The Warburg Institute.

Pettigrew THJ (2007) *Shakespeare and the Practice of Physic: Medical Narratives on the Early Modern English Stage*. Newark: University of Delaware Press.

Pielmeyer K (1981) *Statuten der deutschen medizinischen Fakultäten im Mittelalter*. MD Diss. University of Bonn, Bonn.

Pietrobelli A (2008) *Histoire du texte, edition critique et traduction annotée du livre I du commentaire de Galien au Régime des maladies aigües d'Hippocrate*. Thesis. Université Paris-IV Sorbonne, Paris.

Pietrobelli A (Forthcoming) Peut-on retrouver des manuscrits perdus? Les marginalia de Caius et de Scaliger dans les éditions imprimées de Galien. In Ieraci-Bio AM, Raiola T and Roselli A (eds) *Actes du VIIe Colloque international sur l'ecdotique des textes médicaux greca (Procida, 11–13 June 2013)*. Paris: Actes du VIe Colloque International.

Pigozzi M (2012) Bologna: Dall'anatomia agli esemplari del corpo. In Olmi and Pancino (eds): 87–116.

Platt FJ (2004) James, John. In *ODNB* 26: 714–15.

Pollack L (1993) *With Faith and Physic: The Life of a Tudor Gentlewoman Lady Grace Mildmay (1552–1620)*. London: Collins and Brown.

Pomata G (1998) *Contracting a Cure: Patients, Healers, and the Law in Early Modern Bologna*. Baltimore: The Johns Hopkins University Press.

Pomata G (2010) Sharing Cases: The *Observationes* in Early Modern Medicine. In *Early Science and Medicine* 15: 193–236.

Pomata G and Siraisi NG (eds) (2005) *Historia, Empiricism and Erudition in Early Modern Medicine*. Cambridge, MA: Harvard University Press.

Pormann PE and Savage-Smith E (2007) *Medieval Islamic Medicine*. Edinburgh: Edinburgh University Press.

Porter RS (ed) (1985) *Patients and Practitioners: Lay Perceptions of Medicine in Pre-Industrial Society*. Cambridge: Cambridge University Press.

Porter RS (ed) (1990) *The Medical History of Waters and Spas: Medical History, Supplement 10*. London: Wellcome Institute for the History of Medicine.

Porterfield A (2005) *Healing in the History of Christianity*. Oxford: Oxford University Press.

Portmann M (2018) The *Paragone* on Anatomical Treatises During the Sixteenth Century. In *Paragone Past and Present* 1: 65–77.

Preti C (2009) Pietro Andrea Mattioli. In *DBI* 72: 308–12.

Preto P (1978) *Peste e Società a Venezia nel 1576*. Vicenza: Neri Pozza.

Preto P (ed) (1979) *Venezia e la peste*. Venice: Marsilio.

Pugliano V (2018) Natural History in the Apothecary's Shop. In Curry *et al.* (eds): 44–60.

Pugliano V (2020) Accountability, Autobiography and Belonging: The Working Journal of a Sixteenth-Century Diplomatic Physician between Venice and Damascus. In Mendelsohn *et al.* (eds): 183–209.

Pullan B (1971) *Rich and Poor in Renaissance Venice*. Oxford: Basil Blackwell.

Quaranta C (2018) Francesco Severi, da Argenta. In *DBI* 92: 354–7.

Rädle F (1982) Carmina Heidelbergensia inedita (saec. XVI ex.). In Green DH, Johnson LP and Wuttke D (eds) *From Wolfram and Petrarch to Goethe and Grass: Studies in Literature in Honour of Leonard Forster*. Baden Baden: Valentin Koerner: 323–79.

Raffaelli R (1983) Notizie intorno a Francesco Severi, il medico di Argenta. In *Studi Urbinati B* 3 (56): 91–136.

Raffaelli R (1984) Francesco Severi e i suoi amici. In Salmons J and Moretti W (eds) *The Renaissance in Ferrara and its European Horizons*. Cardiff: University of Wales Press: 245–62.

Ramenovsky AF (1987) *Vectors of Death: The Archaeology of European Contact*. Albuquerque: University of New Mexico Press.

Rankin AM (2008) Becoming an Expert Practitioner: Court Experimentalism and the Medical Skills of Anna of Saxony (1532–1585). In *Isis* 98: 23–53.

Rankin AM (2013) *Panaceia's Daughters: Noblewomen as Healers in Early Modern Germany*. Chicago: University of Chicago Press.

Raschieri AA (2012) Giorgio Valla, Editor and Translator of Ancient Scientific Texts. In Olmos P (ed) *Greek Science in the Long Run. Essays on the Greek Scientific Tradition (4th c. BCE–16th c. CE)*. Newcastle: Cambridge Scholars Publishing: 127–49.

Raven CE (1947) *The English Naturalists*. Cambridge: Cambridge University Press.

Rawcliffe C (1984) The Hospitals of Later Medieval London. In *Medical History* 28: 1–21.

Rawcliffe C (1999) *Medicine for the Soul: The Life, Death and Resurrection of an English Medieval Hospital*. Stroud: Sutton Publishing.

Rawles S and Screech MA (1987) *A New Rabelais Bibliography, Editions of Rabelais Before 1626*. Geneva: Droz.

Reed AW (1925–26) John Clement and His Books. In *The Library*, ser. 4 (6): 329–39.

Reeds KM (1991) *Botany in Medieval and Renaissance Universities*. New York and London: Garland.

Reeve MD (1983) Celsus. In Reynolds LD (ed) *Texts and Transmission: A Survey of the Latin Classics*. Oxford: Clarendon Press.

Reff DT (2005) *Plagues, Priests, Demons: Sacred Narratives and the Rise of Christianity in the Old World and the New*. Cambridge: Cambridge University Press.

Rex R (1990–1991) Thomas Vavasour. In *Recusant History* 20: 175–90.

Rice EK (1980) Paulus Aegineta. In Cranz FE and Kristeller PO (eds) *Catalogus translationum et commentariorum*, vol. 4. Washington, DC: Catholic University of America Press: 145–91.

Richards J (2012) Useful Books: Reading Vernacular Regimens in Sixteenth-Century England. In *Journal of the History of Ideas* 73: 247–71.

Riddle JM (1980) Dioscorides. In Cranz FE and Kristeller PO (eds) *Catalogus Translationum et Commentariorum*, vol. 4. Washington, DC: Catholic University of America Press: 1–143.

Rinaldi M (2006) *"Compendia vel potius dispendia"*: Girolamo Mercuriale e gli strumenti della formazione medica. In *Medicina e Storia* 11: 45–62.

Roberts ES (ed) (1912) *The Works of John Caius, M.D., Second Founder of Gonville and Caius College and Master of the College 1559–1573*. Cambridge: Cambridge University Press.

Roberts J (1990) An Introduction to Leonardo's Anatomical Drawings In Ames-Lewis F and Bednarek A (eds) *Nine Lectures on Leonardo da Vinci*. London: Birkbeck College: 53–62.

Roberts KB and Tomlinson JDW (1992) *The Fabric of the Body: European Traditions of Anatomical Illustration*. Oxford: Oxford University Press.

Roberts RS (1962) The Personnel and Practice of Medicine in Tudor and Stuart England, Part I: The Provinces. In *Medical History* 6: 363–82.

Roberts RS (1965) The Early History of the Import of Drugs into Britain. In Poynter RS (ed) *The Evolution of Pharmacy in Britain*. London: Pitman Medical Publishing: 165–86.

Robinson H (ed.) (1846–7) *Original Letters Relative to the English Reformation*, 2 Vols. Cambridge: Cambridge University Press.

Rocca J (2003) *Galen on the Brain: Anatomical Knowledge and Physiological Speculation in the Second Century AD*. Leiden: Brill.

Rocca J (2008) Anatomy. In Hankinson RJ (ed) *The Cambridge Companion to Galen*. Cambridge: Cambridge University Press: 242–62.

Roger E (2020) 'To Be Shut Up': New Evidence for the Development of Quarantine Regulations in Early Tudor England. In *Social History of Medicine* 33: 1077–96.

Ross SG (2016) *Everyday Renaissances: The Quest for Cultural Legitimacy in Venice*. Cambridge, MA and London: Harvard University Press.

Rossetti L (2006) La Laurea di Harvey a Padova. In Ongaro *et al.* (eds): 195–200.

Roth M (1892) *Andreas Vesalius Bruxellensis*. Berlin: Georg Reimer.

Roth M (1895) Vesaliana. In *Virchows Archiv* 141: 462–78.

Rotondò A (1974) *Studi e richerche di storia ereticale italiana del Cinquecento*. Turin: Giappichelli.

Rotondò A (1991) *Forme e destinazione del messaggio religioso*. Florence: L. S. Olschki.

Rowe K (1997) "God's Handy Worke": Divine Complicity and the Anatomist's Touch. In Hillmann and Mazzio (eds): 285–309.

Rowse AL (1953) *The England of Elizabeth*. London: The Reprint Society.

Rubin Pinault J (1992) *Hippocratic Lives and Legends*. Leiden, New York and Cologne: E. J. Brill.

Ruderman DB (1988) *Kabbalah, Magic and Science: The Cultural Universe of a Sixteenth Century Jewish Physician*. Cambridge, MA and London: Harvard University Press.

Ruisinger MM (2020) Die Pestarztmaske im Deutschen Medizinhistorischen Museum Ingolstadt. In *NTM* 28: 235–52.

Rumberg P (2011) '*Oculata fide*': Learning, Looking and the Anatomical Theatre. In Harris J, Nethersole S and Rumberg P (eds) '*una insalata di più erbe*': *A Festschrift for Patricia Lee Rubin*. London: The Courtauld Institute of Art: 83–7.

Russell AW (ed) (1981) *The Town and State Physician in Europe from the Middle Ages to the Enlightenment: Wolfenbütteler Forschungen, Band 12*. Wolfenbüttel: Herzog August Bibliothek.

Rütten T (2008) Traduzioni e commenti del corpus ippocratico e galenico. In Clericuzio and Ernst (eds): 479–96.

Sacchi MP (2020) Valenziano, Luca. In *DBI* 97. www.treccani.it/enciclopedia/luca-valenziano_(Dizionario-Biografico).

Salas LA (2020) *Cutting Words: Polemical Dimensions of Galen's Anatomical Experiments*. Leiden and Boston: Brill.

Salmon JHM (1979) *Society in Crisis: France in the Sixteenth Century*. London: Methuen.

Samuel E (2004) Lopes [Lopes], Rodrigo [Ruy, Roger] (c.1517–1594). In *ODNB* 34: 429–31.

Santing K (2010) Pieter van Foreest and the Acquisition and Travelling of Medical Knowledge in the Sixteenth Century. In Grell *et al*. (eds): 49–70.

Saunders JB de CM and O'Malley CD (1982) *The Anatomical Drawings of Andreas Vesalius*. New York: Bonanza Books.

Savage-Smith E (1995) Attitudes towards Dissection in Medieval Islam. In *Journal of the History of Medicine and Allied Sciences* 50: 67–110.

Savino C (2019) 'Galenic' Forgeries of the Renaissance: An Overview on Commentaries Falsely Attributed to Galen. In Bouras-Vallianatos and Zipser (eds): 453–71.

Savino C (2020) *Il medico di Utopia. Giovanni Battista Rasario (1517–1578) traduttore e falsario di testi medici greci*. Udine: Forum.

Sawday J (1995) *The Body Emblazoned: Dissection and the Body in Renaissance Culture*. London: Routledge.

Schefer HW (1990) *Das Berufsethos des Arztes Paracelsus, Gesnerus, Supplement 42*. Aarau, Frankfurt and Salzburg: Verlag Sauerländer.

Schen CS (2002) *Charity and Lay Piety in Reformation London. 1500–1620*. Farnham and Burlington VT: Ashgate.

Schlegelmilch S (2020) Promoting a Good Physician: Letters of Application to German Civic Authorities, 1500–1700. In Mendelsohn *et al*. (eds): 88–109.

Schlegelmilch U (2021) Ärzte als Informanten, Fürstenerzieher und Kanzleibeamte: Medizinerkarrieren am anhaltischen Hof im 16. Jahrhundert. In Hilber M and Taddei E (eds) *In fürstlicher Nähe – Ärzte bei Hof (1450–1800), Innsbrucker Historische Studien* 33: 127–47.

Schleiner W (2014) Early Modern Medical Ethics and Medical Humor. In Gadebusch-Bondio (ed): 175–84.

Schmitt CB (1974) The University of Pisa in the Renaissance. In *History of Universities* 3: 3–17.

Schmitt CB (1977) The Correspondence of Jacques Daléchamps (1513–1588). In *Viator* 8: 399–434.

Schmitt CB (1989) *Reappraisals in Renaissance Thought*. London: Variorum Reprints.

Schmitt CB and Bono JJ (1979) An Unknown Letter of Jacques Daléchamps to Jean Fernel: Local Autonomy Versus Centralized Government. In *Bulletin of the History of Medicine* 53: 100–27.

Schmitz R (2005) *Geschichte der Pharmazie: Band 2: Von der Frühen Neuzeit bis zur Gegenwart*, with the assistance of Friedrich C and Müller-Jahncke WD. Eschborn: Govi.

Schoenfeldt M (1999) *Bodies and Selves in Early Modern England: Physiology and Inwardness in Spenser, Shakespeare, Herbert and Milton*. Cambridge: Cambridge University Press.

Schullian DM and Belloni L (1954) *Giovanni Tortelli, on Medicine and Physicians; Gian Giacomo Bartolotti, On the Antiquity of Medicine. Two Histories of Medicine of the XVth Century*. Milan: Starchi.

Schultz B (1985) *Art and Anatomy in Renaissance Italy*. Ann Arbor, MI: UMI Research Press.

Schultz B (1986) A Fifteenth-Century Papal Brief on Human Dissection. In *Medical Heritage*, January: 50–6.

Scott T (2002) *Society and Economy in Germany, 1300–1600*. Basingstoke and New York: Palgrave.

Screech MA (1958) *The Rabelaisian Marriage: Aspects of Rabelais's Religion, Ethics & Comic Philosophy*. London: Edward Arnold.

Screech MA (1976) The Earliest Reference to a Gargantua and Pantagruel (*Gargantua rex, Pantagruel filius eius*); Petrus Baptista Cremonensis' *Epistolae tres*. In *Études Rabelaisiennes* 13: 69–78.

Semenzato C (1995) *The Anatomy Theatre: History and Restoration*. Padua: Università degli Studi.

Serrai A (1990) *Conrad Gesner*. Rome: Bulzoni.

Shackelford J (2004) *A Philosophical Path for Paracelsian Medicine: The Ideas, Intellectual Context, and Influence of Petrus Severinus (1540–1602)*. Copenhagen: Museum Tusculanum Press.

Sharples RW and Van der Eijk PJ (2008) *Nemesius, on the Nature of Man*. Liverpool: Liverpool University Press.

Shaw J and Welch E (2011) *Making and Marketing Medicine in Renaissance Florence*. Amsterdam and New York: Rodopi.

Sheridan B (2010) Whither Childbearing? Gender, Status, and the Professionalization of Medicine in Early Modern France. In Long KP (ed) *Gender and Scientific Discourse in Early Modern Culture*. Farnham and Burlington, VT: Ashgate: 239–58.

Sicherl M (1976) *Handschriftliche Vorlagen der Editio princeps des Aristoteles*. Mainz: Akademie der Wissenschaften und der Literatur.

Simons P and Kornell MN (2008) Annibal Caro's After-Dinner Speech (1536) and the Question of Titian as Vesalius's Illustrator. In *Renaissance Quarterly* 41: 1069–97.

Singer C and Rabin C (1946) *A Prelude to Modern Science*. Cambridge: Cambridge University Press.

Siraisi NG (1987) *Avicenna in Renaissance Italy: The Canon and Medical Teaching in Italian Universities After 1500*. Princeton: Princeton University Press.

Siraisi NG (1990) *Medieval and Early Modern Medicine: An Introduction to Knowledge and Practice*. Chicago: University of Chicago Press.

Siraisi NG (1997) *The Clock and the Mirror: Girolamo Cardano and Renaissance Medicine*. Princeton: Princeton University Press.

Siraisi NG (2001) *Medicine and the Italian Universities, 1250–1600*. Leiden: Brill.

Siraisi NG (2007) *History, Medicine, and the Traditions of Renaissance Learning.* Ann Arbor: University of Michigan Press.

Siraisi NG (2008) Mercuriale's Letters to Zwinger and Humanist Medicine. In Arcangeli and Nutton (eds): 77–96.

Siraisi NG (2013) *Communities of Learned Experience: Epistolary Medicine in the Renaissance.* Baltimore: Johns Hopkins University Press.

Siraisi NG (2016) Baudouin Ronsse as Writer of Medical Letters. In Blair A and Goeing AS (eds) *For the Sake of Learning: Essays in Honor of Tony Grafton.* Leiden and Boston: Brill: 123–39.

Skaarup BO (2015a) *Anatomy and Anatomists in Early Modern Spain.* Farnham and Burlington, VT: Ashgate.

Skaarup B (2015b) The Unexpected Success of a Spanish Anatomy Book: Juan Valverde de Amusco's *Historia de la composicion del cuerpo humano* (Rome, 1556), and Its Many Later Editions. In Kirwan R and Mullins S (eds) *Specialist Markets in the Early Modern Book World.* Leiden: Brill: 123–41.

Slack P (1979) Mirrors of Health and Treasures of Poor Men: The Uses of the Vernacular Medical Literature of Tudor England. In Webster (ed): 235–52.

Slack P (1990) *The Impact of Plague in Tudor and Stuart England.* Oxford: Clarendon Press.

Slater J, López Terrado ML and Pardo-Tomás J (eds) (2014) *Medical Cultures of the Early Spanish Empire.* Farnham and Burlington: Ashgate.

Smith WD (1979) *The Hippocratic Tradition.* Ithaca: Cornell University Press.

Sonderkamp JAM (1987) *Untersuchungen zur Überlieferung der Schriften des Theophanes Chrysobalantes (sog. Theophanes Nonnos).* Bonn: Dr. Rudolf Habelt GMBH.

Soulier D (2020a) The Start of Andreas Vesalius' Career at the Imperial Court According to His Letters to Benedetto Varchi. In Van Hee (ed): 37–52.

Soulier D (2020b) *Vésale anatomisé: Réception et diffusion du De humani corporis fabrica en Europe (1543–1628).* PhD Diss. Université Côte d'Azur, Nice.

Soulier D (2021) The Anatomy Theatre in Renaissance Italy: A Space of Justice? In Malland L (ed) *The Spaces of Renaissance Anatomy Theatre.* Wilmington: Vernon Press.

Stauber R (1908) *Die Schedelsche Bibliothek. Studien und Darstellungen aus dem Gebiete der Geschichte 6.* Freiburg im Breisgau: Herdersche Verlagshandlung.

Steeno M, Biesbrouck M and Godderis T (2020) Six Previously Unknown Letters from Andreas Vesalius to Octavius Landus concerning the Accident of the Spanish Prince Don Carlos in 1562. In Van Hee (ed): 53–92.

Stefanizzi S (2011) *Il De Balneis di Tomasso Giunta (1553).* Florence: Leo S. Olschki.

Stein C (2003) *Die Behandlung der Franzosenkrankheit in der Frühen Neuzeit am Beispiel Augsburgs, Medizin, Gesellschaft und Geschichte, Beiheft 19.* Stuttgart: Institut für Geschichte der Medizin Stuttgart.

Stein C (2009) *Negotiating the French Pox in Early Modern Germany.* Farnham and Burlington: Ashgate.

Stein C (2014) 'Getting' the Pox: Reflections by an Historian on How to Write the History of Early Modern Disease. In *Nordic Journal of Science and Technology Studies* 2: 53–9.

Steinmann M (1967) *Johannes Oporinus, ein Basler Buchdrucker um die Mitte des 16. Jahrhunderts.* Basle and Stuttgart: Helbing & Lichtenhahn.

Stephens W (1979) *Giants in those Days.* Lincoln: University of Nebraska Press.

Stevens Crawshaw J (2012) *Plague Hospitals: Public Health for the City in Early Modern Venice.* Farnham: Ashgate.

Stevens Crawshaw J (2014) Families, Medical Secrets and Public Health in Early Modern Venice. In *Renaissance Studies* 597–616.

Stevens Crawshaw J (forthcoming) A Sense of Time: Experiencing Plague and Quarantine in Early Modern Italy. In *I Tatti Studies in the Italian Renaissance*.

Stevens Crawshaw J, Benyovsky Latin I and Vongsathorn K (eds) (2020) *Tracing Hospital Boundaries Integration and Segregation in South Eastern Europe and Beyond, 1050–1970.* Leiden and Boston: Brill, Rodopi.

Stevenson LG (1965) 'New Diseases' in the Seventeenth Century. In *Bulletin of the History of Medicine* 39: 1–21.

Sticker G (1927) Die Entwicklung der medizinischen Fakultät an der Universität Würzburg. In Frisch F and Flury F (eds) *Festschrift zum 46. Deutschen Ärztetag in Würzburg vom 6 bis 10. September 1927.* Würzburg: H. Stürz A.G: 1–168.

Stilwell MB (1970) *The Awakening Interest in Science During the First Century of Printing, 1450–1550: An Annotated Checklist of First Editions Viewed from the Angle of Their Subject Content – Astronomy – Mathematics – Medicine – Natural Science – Physics – Technology.* New York: Bibliographical Society of America.

Stolberg M (2003) A Woman Down to Her Bones: The Anatomy of Sexual Difference in Early Modern Europe. In *Isis* 94: 273–99.

Stolberg M (2014) Bed-side teaching and the Acquisition of Practical Skills in Mid sixteenth-century Padua. In *Journal of the History of Medicine and Allied Sciences* 69: 633–664.

Stolberg M (2015) *Uroscopy in Early Modern Europe.* Farnham and Burlington, VT: Ashgate.

Stolberg M (2018a) Teaching Anatomy in Post-Vesalian Padua: An Analysis of Student Notes. In *The Journal of Medieval and Early Modern Studies* 48 (1): 61–7.

Stolberg M (2018b) Learning Anatomy in Late-Sixteenth Century Padua. In *History of Science* 56: 381–402.

Stolberg M (2019) A Sixteenth-Century Physician and His Patients: The Practice Journal of Hiob Finzel, 1565–1589. In *Social History of Medicine* 32: 221–40.

Stolberg M (2020) The Many Uses of Writing: A Humanist Physician in Sixteenth-Century Prague. In Mendelsohn *et al.* (eds): 67–87.

Stolberg M (2021a) *Gelehrte Medizin und ärztlicher Alltag in der Renaissance.* Berlin: De Gruyter Oldernbourg.

Stolberg M (2021b) The Doctor-Patient Relationship in the Renaissance. In *European Journal for the History of Medicine and Health* 1: 1–29.

Stolberg, M. (2022). *Learned Physicians and Everyday Medical Practice in the Renaissance.* Berlin: De Gruyter.

Stone G (2004) Ridley, Mark. In *ODNB* 46: 942–3.

Stout FJ (2015) *Exploring Russia in the Elizabethan Commonwealth: The Muscovy Company and Giles Fletcher the Elder (1546–1611).* Manchester: Manchester University Press.

Strauss G (1959) *Sixteenth Century Germany: Its Topography and Topographers.* Madison: University of Wisconsin Press.

Strocchia ST (2019) *Forgotten Healers: Women and the Pursuit of Health in Late Renaissance Italy*. Cambridge, MA: Harvard University Press.

Sudhoff K (1894–99) *Bibliographia Paracelsica*. Berlin: W. Reimer.

Sugg R (2012) The Anatomical Web: Literary Dissection from Castiglione to Cromwell. In Pender and Struever (eds): 83–103.

Sumillera RG (2020) *Political Medicine in Early Modern Spain, or how Physicians Counsel the King*. In *The Sixteenth Century Journal* 51: 419–44.

Taccari E (1971) Botallo, Leonardo. In *DBI* 13: 350–2.

Tait R (2020) The Editions of Gabriele Zerbi's *De cautelis medicorum* and Their Influence. In *Journal of the Warburg and Courtauld Institutes* 83: 327–36.

Talvacchia B (1999) *Taking Positions: On the Erotic in Renaissance Culture*. Princeton: Princeton University Press.

Taviner M, Thwaites G and Gant V (1998) The English Sweating Sickness, 1485–1551: A Viral Pulmonary Disease? In *Medical History* 42: 96–8.

Telle J (ed) (1998) *Transformation of Paracelsism 1500–1800: Alchemy, Chemistry and Medicine (Glasgow-Symposium 15–19 September 1993)*. Leiden: Brill.

Telle J (2008) Bodenstein, Adam of. In Koertge N (ed) *New Dictionary of Scientific Biography*. Detroit, York and London: Thomson Gale: I, 308–9.

Temkin O (1977) *The Double Face of Janus and Other Essays in the History of Medicine*. Baltimore: The Johns Hopkins University Press.

Thiery M (2014) *Female Genital Organs in Vesalius' Iconography*. In Van Hee (ed.): 161–80.

Thomas D (2006) Thomas Vicary and His *Anatomie of Man's Body*. In *Medical History* 50: 235–46.

Thomas K (1973) *Religion and the Decline of Magic*. Harmondsworth: Penguin.

Tongiorgi Tomasi L (1989) Gherardo Cibo: Visions of Landscape and the Botanical Sciences in a Sixteenth-Century Artist. In *Journal of Garden History* 9 (4): 99–216.

Traister BH (2001) *The Notorious Astrological Physician of London: Works and Days of Simon Forman*. Chicago and London: The University of Chicago Press.

Trevor-Roper HR (1985) The Paracelsian Movement. In *Renaissance Essays*. London: Secker and Warburg: 149–99.

Trevor-Roper HR (1990) The Court Physicians and Paracelsianism. In Nutton (ed): 79–94.

Trevor-Roper HR (2006) *Europe's Physician: The Various Lives of Sir Theodore de Mayerne*. New Haven and London: Yale University Press.

Triebs M (1995) *Die medizinische Fakultät der Universität Helmstedt (1576–1810)*. Wiesbaden: Harrassowitz Verlag.

Tröhler U (ed) (1991) *Felix Platter (1536–1614) in seiner Zeit*. Basle: Schwabe & Co.

Uhlig P (1938) Arzt und Apotheker in Altzwickau. In *Sudhoffs Archiv* 30: 301–5.

Urbansky S (2020) *Beyond the Steppe Frontier: A History of the Sino-Russian Border*. Princeton: Princeton University Press.

Vagenheim G (2008) Una collaborazione tra antiquario ed erudito: I disegni e le epigrafi di Pirro Ligorio nel *De arte gymnastica di Girolamo Mercuriale*. In Arcangeli and Nutton (eds): 127–58.

Van Glabbeek F and Biesbrouck M (2020) Giovanni Baptista Canani (1515–1579) and Andreas Vesalius (1514–1564). In Van Hee (ed): 101–48.

Van Hee R (ed) (2014) *Art of Vesalius*. Antwerp and Apeldoorn: Garant.

Van Hee R (ed) (2020) *In the Shadow of Vesalius*. Antwerp and Apeldoorn: Garant.

Van Hee R and Biesbrouck M (eds) (2018) *Tijdgenotem uit de leefwereld van Andreas Vesalius*. Antwerp and Apeldoorn: Garant.

Van Leersum EC and Martin W (1910) *Miniaturen das lateinischen Galenos-Handschrift der kgl. Oeffentl. Bibliothek in Dresden Db 92–93 in phototypischer Reproduktion*. Leiden: A. W. Sijthoff.

Van Lieburg MJ (1989) Pieter van Foreest en de tol de stadsmedicus in de Noord-Nederlandse steden van de 16e eeuw. In Houtzager (ed): 41–72.

Ventura I (2009–10) Theory and Practice in Amatus' Lusitanus *Curationum medicinalium centuriae; The Case of Fevers*. In *Koroth* 20: 139–79.

Ventura I (2019) Galenic Pharmacology in the Middle Ages: The Reception of Galen's *On the Capacities of Simple Drugs* and Its Reception Between the Sixth and the Fourteenth Century. In Bouras-Vallianatos and Zipser (eds): 393–433.

Verdigi M (1997) *Simone Simoni filosofo e medico nel'500*. Lucca: Maria Pacino Fazzi Editore.

Vollmuth R (2001) *Traumatologie und Feldchirurgie an der Wende vom Mittelalter zur Neuzeit, exemplarisch dargestellt anhand der "Grossen Chirurgie" des Walter Hermann Ryff*. Stuttgart: Franz Steiner Verlag.

Vons J (ed) (2016) *La Fabrique de Vésale: La mémoire d'un livre*. Paris: Bibliothèque interuniversitaire de Santé.

Vons J (2014) Jacques Grévin (1538–1570) et la nomenclature anatomique française. In Giacomotto-Charra V and Silvi C (eds) *Lire, choisir, écrire. La vulgarisation des savoirs du Moyen Âge à la Renaissance*. Paris: Etudes et rencontres de l'École des Chartes 43: 133–47.

Vons J and Velut S (2008) *André Vésale. Résumé de ses livres sur la Fabrique du corps humain*. Paris: Les Belles Lettres.

Waddell MA (2021) *Magic, Science and Religion in Early Modern Europe*. Cambridge: Cambridge University Press.

Walker DP (1972) *The Ancient Theology*. London: Duckworth.

Wallis F (2018) Pre-Modern Surgery: Wounds, Words and the Paradox of 'Tradition'. In Schlich T (ed) *The Palgrave Handbook of the History of Surgery*. London: Palgrave Macmillan: 49–70.

Walloe L (2008) Medieval and Modern Bubonic Plague: Some Clinical Continuities. In Nutton (ed): 59–73.

Walter T (2020) Ärztebriefe (16. und 17. Jahrhundert). In Becker EM (ed) *Handbuch Brief: Von der Frühen Neuzeit bis zur Gegenwart*, vol. 2. Berlin and Boston: De Gruyter, Oldenbourg 2020: 705–15.

Walter T (forthcoming) Stadt – Hof – Universität. Akademische Ärzte in den Städten und Residenzen des Alten Reich. In Fouquet G, Meinhardt M and Schwinges RC (eds) *Personen, Wissen, Karrieren: Bildung und Professionalisierung in Residenzstädten (1470–1540)*. Ostfildern: Thorbecke.

Walter T, Ghorbani A and Van Andel T (2021) The Emperor's Herbarium: The German Physician Leonhard Rauwolf (1535? – 96) and His Botanical Field Studies in the Middle East. In *History of Science* 59: 1–22.

Walton MT (1981) Stinking Air, Corrupt Water, and the English Sweat: A Footnote to the Quality of Life in Fifteenth-Century London. In *Journal of the History of Medicine and Allied Sciences* 36: 67–8.

Walton MT (1982) Thomas Forestier and the 'False Lechys' of London. In *Journal of the History of Medicine and Allied Sciences* 37: 71–3.

Wangensteen OH and Wangensteen SD (1978) *The Rise of Surgery: From Empiric Craft to Scientific Discipline*. London: Dawson's.

Wear AG (1985) Puritan Perceptions of Illness in Seventeenth Century England. In Porter (ed): 55–99.

Wear AG (1995) Early Modern Europe, 1500–1700. In Conrad LI, Neve M, Nutton V, Porter R and Wear A (eds) *The Western Medical Tradition 800 BC to AD 1800*. Cambridge: Cambridge University Press.

Wear AG (1996) Religious Beliefs and Medicine in Early Modern England. In Marland and Pelling (eds): 145–70.

Wear AG (2000) *Knowledge and Practice in English Medicine, 1550–1580*. Cambridge: Cambridge University Press.

Wear A, French R and Lonie IM (eds) (1985) *The Medical Renaissance of the Sixteenth Century*. Cambridge: Cambridge University Press.

Webster C (1977) Thomas Linacre and the Foundation of the College of Physicians. In Maddison *et al.* (eds): 198–222.

Webster C (ed) (1979) *Health, Medicine and Mortality in the Sixteenth Century*. Cambridge: Cambridge University Press.

Webster C (1993) Paracelsus: Medicine as Popular Protest. In Grell and Cunningham (eds): 57–77.

Webster C (2008) *Paracelsus: Medicine, Magic and Mission at the End of Time*. New Haven and London: Yale University Press.

Welker L (1988) *Das "Iatromathematische Corpus". Untersuchungen zu einem alemannischen astrologisch-medizinischen Kompendium des Spätmittelalters mit Textausgabe und einem Anhang: Michael Puffs von Schrick 'Von den ausgebrannten Wässern' in der handschriftlichen Fassung des Codex Zürich, Zentralbibliothek, C 102 b*. Zurich: Juris Druck +Verlag.

Wells FC (2013) *The Heart of Leonardo*. Stuttgart: Springer.

Wenkebach E (1925) *John Clement, ein englischer Humanist und Arzt des sechzehnten Jahrhunderts. Ein Lebensbild in Umrissen. Studien zur Geschichte der Medizine 18*. Leipzig: J. A. Barth.

Whiteley R (2019) Figuring Pictures and Picturing Figures. Images of the Pregnant Body and the Unborn Child in England, 1540–c. 1680. In *Social History of Medicine* 33: 241–66.

Whittet TD (1964) The Apothecary in Provincial Guilds. In *Medical History* 8: 245–73.

Wiesner ME (1993) The Midwives of South Germany and the Public/Private Dichotomy. In Marland (ed): 77–94.

Wilson NG (1992) *From Byzantium to Italy: Greek Studies in the Italian Renaissance*. London: Duckworth.

Wiswe H (1970) *Kulturgeschichte der Kochkunst*. Munich: Heinz Moos Verlag.

Wolf ER (1997) *Europe and the People Without History*, ed. 2. Berkeley, Los Angeles and London: University of California Press.

Woolfson J (1998) *Padua and the Tudors: English Students in Italy 1485–1603*. Cambridge: James Clarke & Co. Ltd.

Woolfson J (ed) (2005) *Palgrave Advances in Renaissance Historiography*. London: Palgrave Macmillan.

Wootton D (2006) *Bad Medicine: Doctors Doing Harm Since Hippocrates*. Oxford: Oxford University Press.

Wykes A (1969) *Doctor Cardano, Physician Extraordinary*. London: Friedrich Muller.

Wylie JAH and Collier LH (1981) The English Sweating Sickness (*sudor anglicus*): A Reappraisal. In *Journal of the History of Medicine and Allied Sciences* 36: 425–45.

Wyman AL (1984) The Surgeoness: The Female Practitioner of Surgery 1400–1800. In *Medical History* 28: 22–41.

Yates FA (1992) *The Art of Memory*. London: Pimlico.

Zahn P (2009/2010) Nürnberger Ärzte des 15.-17. Jahrhunderts in ihren humanistischen Gedenkschriften. In *Pirckheimer Jahrbuch* 24: 145–95.

Zambelli P (1965). Giovanni Mainardi e la polemica sull'astrologia. In *aa.vv. L'opera e il pensiero di Giovanni Pico della Mirandola nella storia dell'Umanesimo*. Florence: Istituto Nazionale di Studi sul Rinascimento: 228–35.

Zampieri F (2021) The University of Padua Medical School from the Origins to the Early Modern Time: A Historical Overview. In Baldassari and Zampieri (eds): 23–67.

Zemla M (2016) Adam Huber of Riesenpach (1545–1613) and His Translation of the Book on Regimen Within the Context of the Prague Medical Milieu. In *Ancient Medicine and Science* 21: 531–46.

Zimmermann V (1986) *Rezeption und Rolle der Heilkunde in landessprachigen handschriftlichen Kompendien des Spätmittelalters*. Wiesbaden: Franz Steiner Verlag.

Zimmermann V (ed) (1995) *Paracelsus. Das Werk – Die Rezeption, Beiträge zum 500. Geburtstag von Theophrastus Bombastus von Hohenheim, genannt Paracelsus (1493–1541) an der Universität Basel am 3. und 4. Dezember 1993*. Wiesbaden: Fritz Steiner Verlag.

Zinner E (1964) *Geschichte und Bibliographie der astronomischen Literatur in Deutschland zur Zeit der Renaissance*, ed. 2. Stuttgart: Anton Hiersemann.

Index

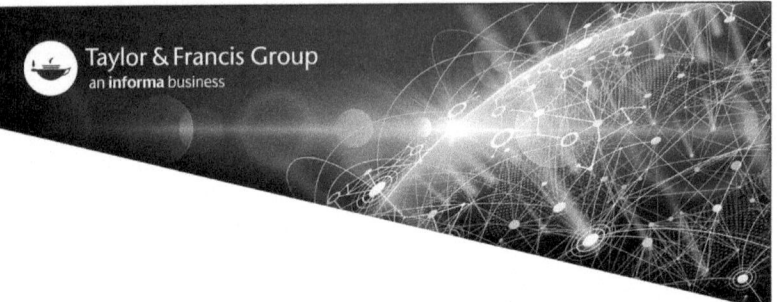
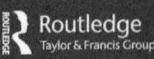
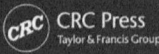